Review of
RADIOLOGY

Review of RADIOLOGY

Sixth Edition

Rajat Jain
MD (MAMC) DNB FICR FRCR (UK) MNAMS

Fellow, Body Imaging
University of Ottawa, Canada
Consultant and Head, Department of Radiology
Shree Aggarsain International Hospital
Ex Faculty, Maulana Azad Medical College
New Delhi, India

Virendra Jain
MBBS (UCMS) MD (MAMC) FRCR (UK)

Consultant Radiologist
University Hospitals of Derby and Burton
NHS Foundation Trust, UK

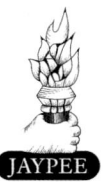

JAYPEE BROTHERS MEDICAL PUBLISHERS
The Health Sciences Publisher
New Delhi | London

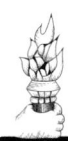

Jaypee Brothers Medical Publishers (P) Ltd

Headquarters
Jaypee Brothers Medical Publishers (P) Ltd
EMCA House, 23/23-B
Ansari Road, Daryaganj
New Delhi 110 002, India
Landline: +91-11-23272143, +91-11-23272703
+91-11-23282021, +91-11-23245672
Email: jaypee@jaypeebrothers.com

Corporate Office
Jaypee Brothers Medical Publishers (P) Ltd
4838/24, Ansari Road, Daryaganj
New Delhi 110 002, India
Phone: +91-11-43574357
Fax: +91-11-43574314
Email: jaypee@jaypeebrothers.com

Overseas Office
J.P. Medical Ltd
83 Victoria Street, London
SW1H 0HW (UK)
Phone: +44 20 3170 8910
Fax: +44 (0)20 3008 6180
Email: info@jpmedpub.com

Website: www.jaypeebrothers.com
Website: www.jaypeedigital.com

© 2021, Jaypee Brothers Medical Publishers

The views and opinions expressed in this book are solely those of the original contributor(s)/author(s) and do not necessarily represent those of editor(s) of the book.

All rights reserved. No part of this publication may be reproduced, stored or transmitted in any form or by any means, electronic, mechanical, photocopying, recording or otherwise, without the prior permission in writing of the publishers.

All brand names and product names used in this book are trade names, service marks, trademarks or registered trademarks of their respective owners. The publisher is not associated with any product or vendor mentioned in this book.

Medical knowledge and practice change constantly. This book is designed to provide accurate, authoritative information about the subject matter in question. However, readers are advised to check the most current information available on procedures included and check information from the manufacturer of each product to be administered, to verify the recommended dose, formula, method and duration of administration, adverse effects and contraindications. It is the responsibility of the practitioner to take all appropriate safety precautions. Neither the publisher nor the author(s)/editor(s) assume any liability for any injury and/or damage to persons or property arising from or related to use of material in this book.

This book is sold on the understanding that the publisher is not engaged in providing professional medical services. If such advice or services are required, the services of a competent medical professional should be sought.

Every effort has been made where necessary to contact holders of copyright to obtain permission to reproduce copyright material. If any have been inadvertently overlooked, the publisher will be pleased to make the necessary arrangements at the first opportunity. The **CD/DVD-ROM** (if any) provided in the sealed envelope with this book is complimentary and free of cost. **Not meant for sale.**

Inquiries for bulk sales may be solicited at: jaypee@jaypeebrothers.com

Review of Radiology

First Edition: 2016
Second Edition: 2017
Third Edition: 2018
Fourth Edition: 2019
Fifth Edition: 2020

Sixth Edition: 2021, **Reprint:** 2024, **2025**

ISBN: 978-93-5465-369-8

Printed at: Samrat Offset Pvt. Ltd.

Preface

Review of Radiology, the book is intended to help students in understanding the basic concepts of the subject with the help of images, who are preparing for the postgraduate medical entrance examination (PGMEE). It is a concise review of key radiology principles to help students not just in understanding radiology which they might have missed during their clinics in MBBS but also to help them in applications of imaging modalities for various clinical conditions like in medicine and surgery. Considering the changing pattern of exam and introduction of NEET at Pan India level, we feel that application-based questions are future of entrance exams at postgraduate level. We would like to state that, this book is not a substitute for comprehensive textbooks of radiology at any level, however, we have tried to cover all the commonly asked topics in entrance exams in a concise format so that students can finish the reading of this book in two days. Some facts are presented in the boxes on the side so that they can be easily revised in the end. We feel that after reading this book, a student preparing for postgraduate entrance examination will not feel the need to refer any other radiology books or courses.

This book is a concise and considerably shorter, still complete version than the full-length, standard radiology textbook. Most of this book evolved from the latest editions of **Grainger and Sutton's Textbooks of Radiology**, CT and MRI imaging—Haaga and AIIMS- MAMC-PGI CME series. All the facts in the book are checked multiple number of times to give an accurate and up-to-date content to the students.

The material is organized into 4 sections and seven chapters. Section–A includes General Radiology (Chapter 1), Section–B includes, Neuroradiology (Chapter 2), Cardio-thoracic Radiology (Chapter 3), Gastrointestinal and Genitourinary System (Chapter 4) and Musculoskeletal Radiology (Chapter 5). Section–C includes Radiotherapy and Chemotherapy (Chapter 6), and Nuclear Scans (Chapter 7). Image based questions and AIIMS new pattern questions with answer are included at the end of the book.

Difficult concepts are explained stepwise and in form of flowcharts with special high yield points in separate boxes adjacent to text wherever relevant. More than 150 images and more than 50 flow diagrams and tables will help the students not just to understand the text but also to memorize the material quickly in a way to aid in long-term retention.

Each chapter begins with a concise theory of each topic, followed by multiple-choice questions (MCQs) and their clear, concise, proper explanations with references of the standard textbooks and/or, research papers wherever required to avoid repetition of the text. Various states PG, AIIMS and JIPMER examination questions had been separated from PGI questions, so that the students can easily concentrate different examinations according to their choice.

Each chapter has high yield points in the boxes which are predicted and highly expected new questions for future examination, based on current examination pattern.

The IBQ section would definitely help the students in preparing for the different types of questions based in images expected to be asked in the examination. The online pool of questions is going to be a backbone for the preparation of IBQs in any examination not just for radiology but for other subjects too.

Finally the Section-D has a collection of important factual information of radiology including the investigations of choices, important systemic signs and important principles of radiology which might be helpful to solve questions from any clinical subject if understood rightly.

How to Read this Book

The best way to read this book is to read the theory given at the beginning of the chapter first and then solve the MCQs. The MCQs of a particular system are arranged randomly without mentioning the years. Absolute care has been taken to avoid repetition of the MCQs as lot of time is wasted in solving the same MCQ again and again. We want to stress on this fact that nowadays in the exams, same questions are not repeated but same topics are repeated and hence students are advised to focus more on the theoretical concepts rather than just MCQs. It is this reason that, deliberately years of the questions and superscript on important lines have not been put as we believe that each line written is a potential MCQ. We suggest that section A, C and D should be read together where section C should be read in associating with other clinical subjects like medicine, surgery, orthopedics, pediatrics, gynecology-obstetrics as they are interlinked.

We wish that our students will go through this book thoroughly and will do excellent in their examinations.

Best wishes for your postgraduate medical entrance examination. Your queries and feedback will always be welcomed. You are free to contact at email: reviewofradiology@gmail.com

Rajat Jain
Virendra Jain

Tips for Winners

- Confidence is the key to success. Believe in yourself because if you won't nobody else will.
- Do not be daunted by the efforts others put in because everybody is a different person and you only can find a pace and method to prepare that is conducive to exclusively yourself and thus maximizes your potential.
- Never believe a person who says that you can not do something. People will tell you certain things can't be done when they can't do them themselves.
- Studying smarter than others is much more important than studying harder when it comes to competitive exams.
- It is a level playing field... so forget your past performances whether good or bad because in the end everybody is preparing for the same one day game. Hence, it is important to take your best shot on that very day.
- It is never too late to start, seriously. There are a large number of success stories of people who started out late. However, the sooner the better still holds good even for those people especially in a rank based system.
- Never doubt yourself and your capabilities. Even the brightest of minds have their episodes of insecurity and uncertainty. In such times try this technique. Close your eyes and recall a past episode during which you were under stress and you handled it well, exceeding your own expectations. The feeling of being in control will return your confidence in no time and the doubt will vanish.
- BEG/BORROW/STEAL/KILL/ROB OR LOOT... but always lay your hands on the question papers of the previous few years because even if none of the questions are repeated (of which there is a slim chance of happening), you'll at least be familiar with the pattern and the type of questions asked in that exam.
- Weeks before the exam, have an honest conversation with yourself, reassure yourself about your preparation and come to terms with the lacunae. A day before the exam, reassess the state and decide how much you expect from the exam..
- Get adequate rest, starting a week before exam... large multicentric studies have proven that it is common sense to.
- While taking the exam, take your time while marking each answer because it is marked in ink. And one wrong question takes away more than even leaving one at the end. So take your time while answering. This is where the importance of practice tests lie.
- Guessing is a tricky game. Exclude all the choices you are SURE cannot be the answer then mark your favorite letter!! In cases of all choices being new, go for the first one you think is the answer. Apart from saving time most often changing your mind leads to a wrong answer.
- Personally I don't believe in leaving any question unmarked, but it is a personal decision and should heavily depend on the state of rest of the paper and number of unmarked answers.
- After the exam, celebrate!!!! No matter what ...and hope for the best.

Cool Quotes (to be Read when on a Break)
- Motivation will almost always beat mere talent.
- A mind troubled by doubt cannot focus on the course to victory.
- Do what you can, with what you have, where you are.
- Many of life's failures are people who did not realize how close they were to success when they gave up.
- The art of being wise is knowing what to overlook.
- Obstacles are those frightful things you see when you take your eyes off your goal.
- Too many people overvalue what they are not and undervalue what they are.
- Though no one can go back and make a brand new start, anyone can start from now and make a brand new ending.
- The real contest is always between what you've done and what you're capable of doing. You measure yourself against yourself and nobody else.
- The difference between a successful person and others is not a lack of strength, not a lack of knowledge, but rather a lack of will.
- According to aerodynamic laws, the bumblebee cannot fly. Its body weight is not the right proportion to its wingspan. Ignoring these laws, the bee flies anyway.
- The mind is like a parachute—it works only when it is open.
- Yesterday is a cancelled check; Tomorrow is a promissory note; Today is the only cash you have, so spend it wisely.
- Never mistake knowledge for wisdom. One helps you make a living, the other helps you make a life.
- The more I want to get something done, the less I call it work.
- The secret of success is to do the common things uncommonly well.
- Hard work beats talent when talent doesn't work hard.
- Successful and unsuccessful people do not vary greatly in their abilities. They vary in their desires to reach their potential.
- You must do the very thing you think you cannot do.
- Your goal should be out of reach but not out of sight.

Acknowledgments

We would like to thank our family members for their constant and unconditional support at every step in our life including but not limited to preparing the manuscript and editing is even time.

We are also very thankful to our friends for providing critical feedback at every time when it is required with special mention of Dr Nishith Kumar (Associate Professor of Radiology, VMMC, New Delhi), Dr. Swati Gupta (Associate Professor of Radiology, MAMC New Delhi), Dr Naveen Bhardwaj (Consultant Radiologist, Dubai), Dr Manoj Mishra (Renowned Surgery Faculty) and Dr Sahil Batra (Renowned Spine Surgeon in Punjab).

We are also very thankful to Dr Nachiket Bhatia (COO, DBMCI) and Dr Vineet Gupta (Director, MIST) for providing us the platform to interact with the standard and guiding us.

A special thanks to our Radiology Teacher and Colleague who have taught us Radiology so that we can reach to this level and able to bring out this book.

We are very thankful to each and every faculty involved in teaching to PG entrance exam aspirants who have helped us in making this book on preferred book for PG entrance exam with respect to radiology. Few members need special mention include:

1. Dr Thameem Saif
2. Dr Apurv Mehra
3. Dr Ashwani Kumar
4. Dr Praveen Kumar
5. Dr Vineet Gupta

We would like to thank Shri Jitendar P Vij (Group Chairman) of Jaypee Brothers Medical Publishers (P) Ltd. for enabling me to publish this book.

Last but the most important, we would like to thank all our students who have been our inspiration and support for writing this book.

Rajat Jain
Virendra Jain

Contents

Recent Questions and Answers   *xiii–xxviii*

Section A: General Radiology

1. General Radiology   3

Section B: Systemic Radiology

2. Neuroradiology   47
3. Cardiothoracic Radiology   84
4. Gastrointestinal and Genitourinary System   136
5. Musculoskeletal Radiology   184

Section C: Radiotherapy and Nuclear Scans

6. Radiotherapy and Chemotherapy   229
7. Nuclear Scans   257

Section D: Special Section

Few Thumb Rules in Radiology   275

Image-Based Questions   285
AIIMS New Pattern Questions with Answers   311

Recent Questions

GENERAL RADIOLOGY

1. Which of the following investigations can be used in osteoporosis? Multiple completion type:
   1. DEXA
   2. Bone scan
   3. Quantitative CT
   4. Chemical analysis

   Select the answer using following key:
   a. 1, 2
   b. 1, 2, 3
   c. 1, 3, 4
   d. 1, 2, 3, 4

2. A young patient with intermittent pain in the calf is presented to surgery OPD. On examination, a painful ulcer is seen at the tip of great toe surrounded by black colour skin. Best initial investigation in this case would be:
   a. Digital subtraction angiography
   b. Duplex scan
   c. CT angiography
   d. MR angiography

3. A worker who was working with hammer and chisel while he was trying to break a hard stone admitted to hospital after injury to eye. Which among the following investigations done would be detrimental?
   a. CT scan
   b. MRI
   c. X-ray
   d. B mode scan

4. A 63-year-old hypertensive patient presented with chest pain and diaphoresis. On examination he has unequal pulses in both arms. Which of the following is the most useful imaging investigation in emergency in this case?
   a. Cardiac enzymes
   b. TEE
   c. TTE
   d. D Dimer

5. What is the preferred modality for localization of parathyroid adenoma?
   a. Sesta MIBI scan
   b. CT-scan
   c. MRI
   d. FDG-PET

6. In the current scenario, what is the gold standard for diagnosis of myocarditis?
   a. MRI
   b. Endomyocardial biopsy
   c. BNP
   d. Echo

7. Identify the scan given below:

   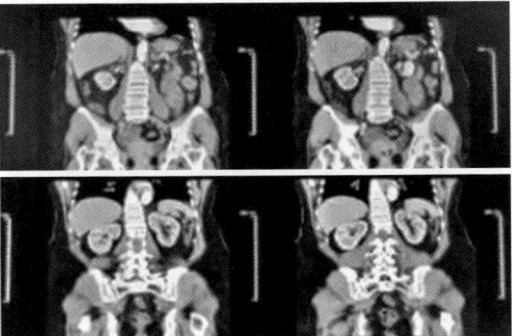

   a. CECT
   b. Contrast (dye) study
   c. MRI
   d. PET scan

NEUROGRADIOLOGY

8. Identify the marked structure shown by the arrow:

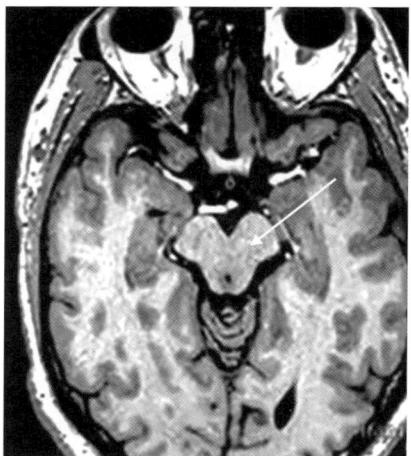

   a. Midbrain
   b. Medulla
   c. Cerebellum
   d. Pons

9. Identify the structure marked as "O" on the CT head image below:

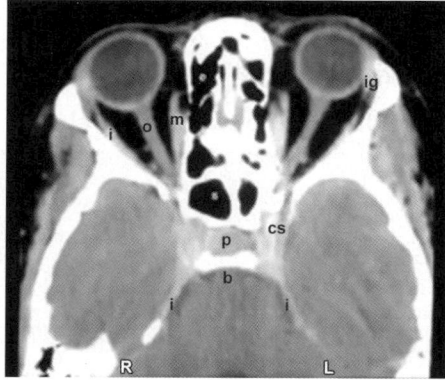

   a. Optic tract
   b. Superior ophthalmic artery
   c. Optic nerve
   d. Optic chiasma

10. A 65-year-old female fell down in the bathroom and sustained head injury, CT scan was performed, what is likely diagnosis?

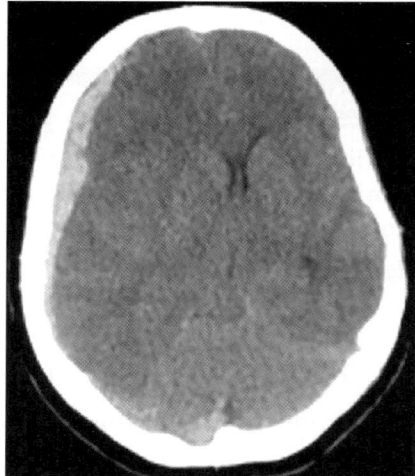

   a. Extradural hematoma
   b. Intracranial bleed
   c. Subdural hematoma
   d. Subarachnoid hemorrhage

11. A 70-year-old hypertensive patient has presented with sudden severe headache. His BP was found to be 220/120. A NCCT of the head was done and shown below. What is the most likely diagnosis?

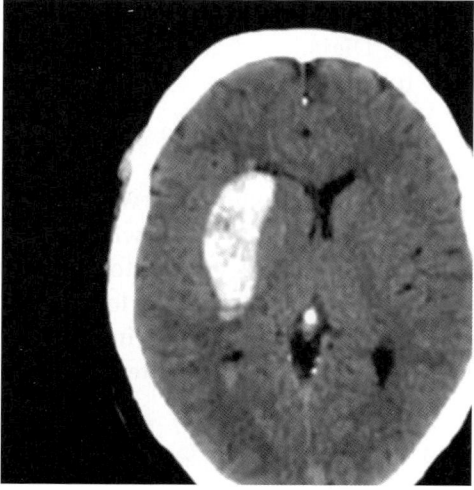

   a. Subarachnoid hemorrhage
   b. Putaminal bleed
   c. Pontine hemorrhage
   d. Intraventricular hemorrhage

12. What is the most likely cause of the finding shown in below Radiograph of Skull?

    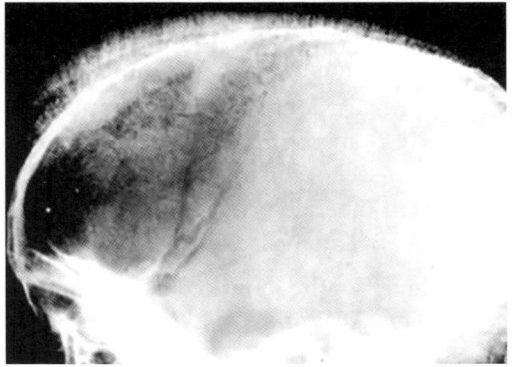

    a. Haemolytic anaemia
    b. Osteopetrosis
    c. Multiple myeloma
    d. Raised intracranial tension

13. Gold standard investigation for FESS:
    a. MRI
    b. PET SCAN
    c. X-ray PNS
    d. CT SCAN

14. A young male met with an RTA and brought to causality with GCS score as e2 v2 m3. He has features of raised ICT. No significant changes were seen on NCCT. The spinal imaging was also normal. What could be the probably diagnosis?
    a. Posterior reversible encephalopathy syndrome
    b. Diffuse axonal injury
    c. Posterior circulation stroke
    d. Post-concussion syndrome

15. The radiograph shown below is done for better assessment of the frontal sinus. What is the common name of this view?

    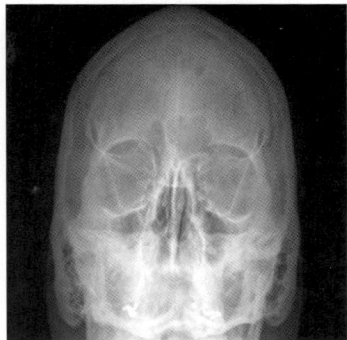

    a. Water's view
    b. Caldwell view
    c. Towne's view
    d. Pierre's view

16. A 12-year-old child with history of fever, headache and chronic ear discharge underwent a CT-scan of brain as shown below. Likely diagnosis is:

    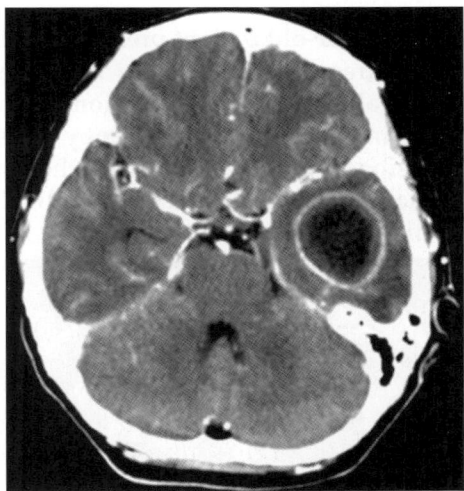

    a. Temporal lobe abscess
    b. Cerebellar abscess
    c. Extradural abscess
    d. Meningitis

17. A 5-year-old child felt difficulty in swallowing when he was playing alone unattended by mother. Radiographs were done and shown below:

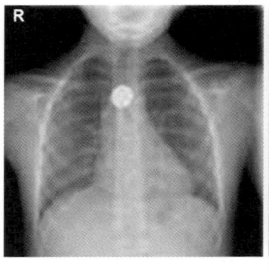
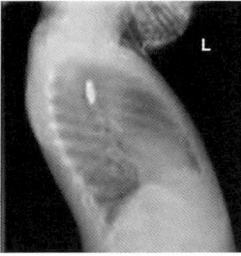

a. Foreign body in the esophagus
b. Foreign body in the trachea
c. Radiological artefact
d. Subcutaneous foreign body

18. A patient presented with loss of vision of the lateral side. MRI image shows an aneurysm compressing the optic chiasma. What is the most likely vessel of origin?
    a. ACOM
    b. ACA
    c. MCA
    d. ICA

19. A 16-year-old patient presented with seizures. An MRI brain was done revealed multiple such lesions in the brain. On MR Spectroscopy these lesions revealed elevated choline, alanine and lactate. The most likely diagnosis is:

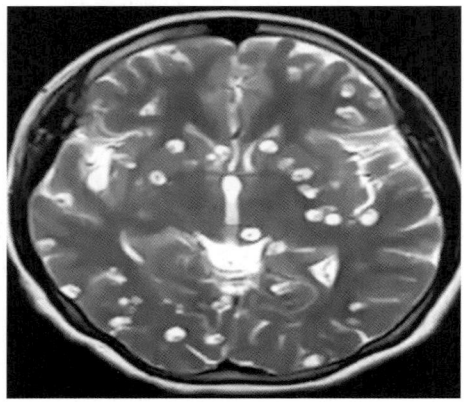

a. Neurocysticercosis
b. Toxoplasmosis
c. Cryptococcosis
d. Tuberculoma

20. A 65-year-old male patient to the causality with right sided hemiparesis and aphasia. His BP was 160/110. His blood sugar was 160 mg/dL. NCCT was normal. What is next step in the management of the patient?
    a. MRI to identify ischemic area
    b. CT angiography to rule out large vessel occlusion
    c. IV labetalol
    d. ABG analysis

21. Identify the marked structure in given CT scan:

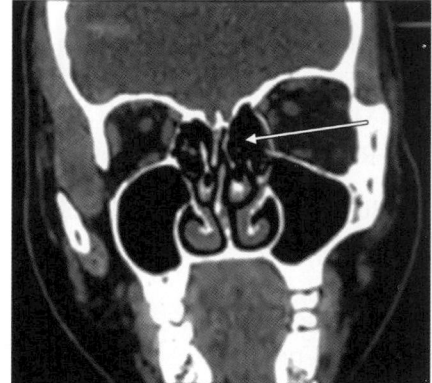

a. Anterior ethmoidal air cell
b. Posterior ethmoidal air cell
c. Cribriform plate
d. Optic nerve

22. Identify the MRI sequence:

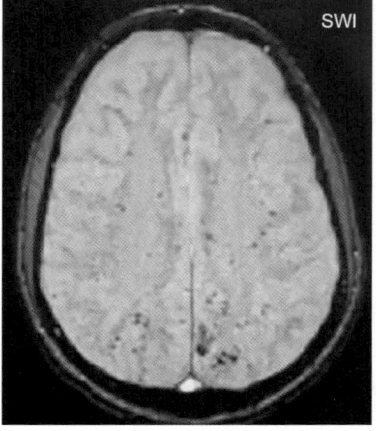

a. Proton density
b. Susceptibility weighted image
c. ADC image
d. DWI

THORAX

23. A chest radiograph of a 45-year-old patient is shown below who has undergone a prior open heart surgery. What is the most likely finding on the given radiograph?

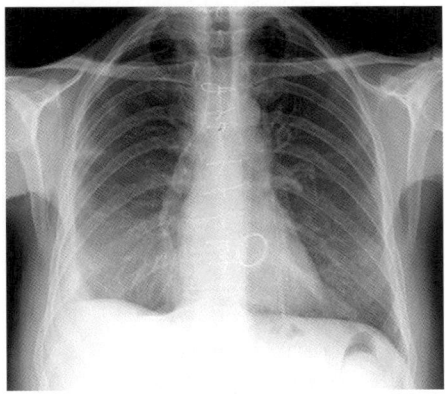

a. Prosthetic mitral valve
b. Prosthetic aortic valve
c. Cardiac pacemaker
d. Pericardial calcification

24. A 55-year-old female came to the OPD for a postsurgery follow-up. A chest radiograph was performed. What is the most likely diagnosis?

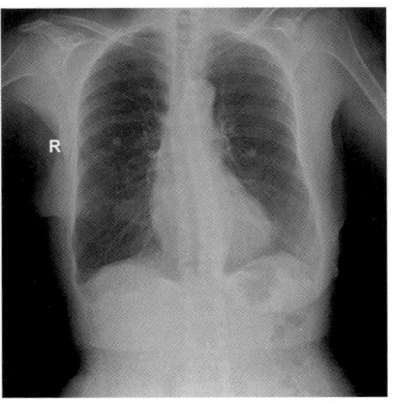

a. Right sided mastectomy
b. Pulmonary metastasis
c. Fibroadenoma
d. Emphysema

25. A 45-year-old patient presents with high grade fever, chills and cough with expectoration. The chest radiographs were taken and shown below. What is the most likely diagnosis?

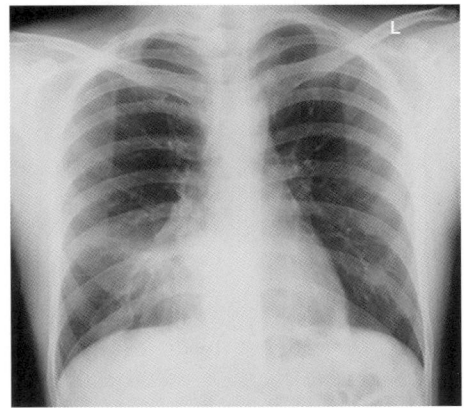

a. Sarcoidosis
b. Right middle lobe consolidation
c. Right lower lobe consolidation
d. Atelectasis

26. What is your interpretation of given chest radiograph?

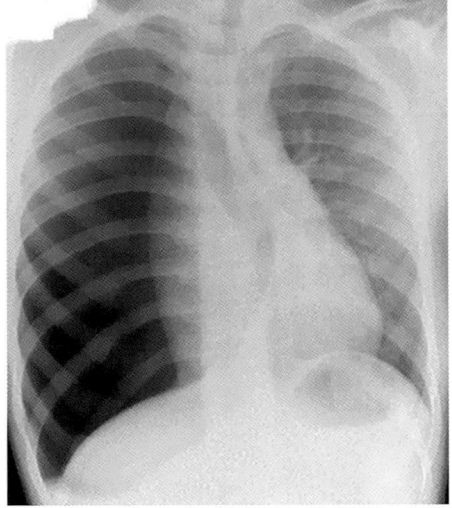

a. Emphysema
b. Pneumothorax
c. Hydropneumothorax
d. Pericardial effusion

27. What is your interpretation of given chest radiograph?

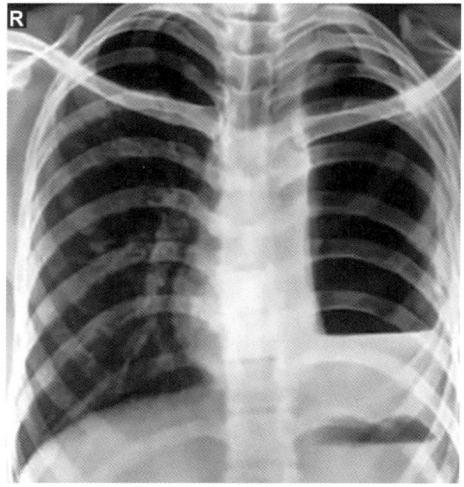

a. Hydropneumothorax
b. Pneumothorax
c. Pneumopericardium
d. Lower lobe pneumonia

28. A 43-year-old female presented with mild fever and weight loss. Her ACE levels were found to be elevated chest radiograph reveals bilateral hilar lymphadenopathy as shown below. What is the most likely diagnosis?

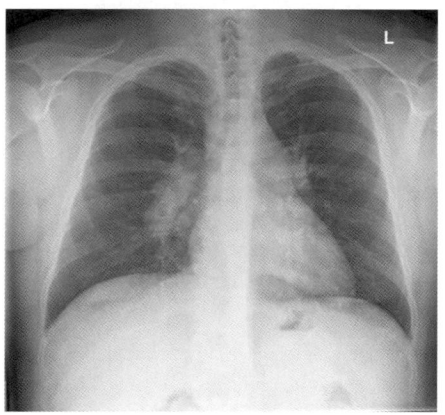

a. Silicosis
b. TB
c. Sarcoidosis
d. Small cell cancer

29. A 35-year-old female with known case of HIV with CD4 <300, presents with fever, dyspnea, cough. A chest radiograph was obtained and shown below. What is the most likely causative organism?

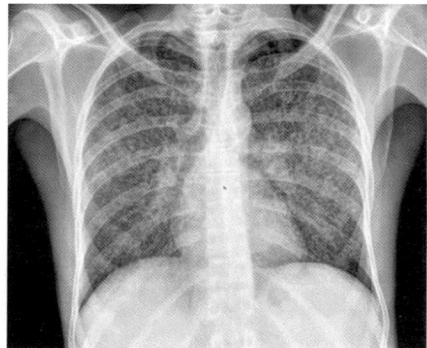

a. Staphylococcus
b. Mycobacterium
c. Histoplasmosis
d. Streptococcus

30. A 3-year-old child while playing develops sudden onset of breathlessness and wheezing. On auscultation significantly decreased breath sounds were seen in right lung. Chest radiograph shows diffusely opaque right hemithorax. What is the probable diagnosis?

a. Pneumothorax
b. Pneumonia
c. Bronchial asthma
d. Foreign body aspiration

31. A 40-year-old patient with history of peptic ulcer disease was having abdominal pain since many days. It gets worse since last two hours. A radiograph was performed and shown here. What is to be done in this patient?

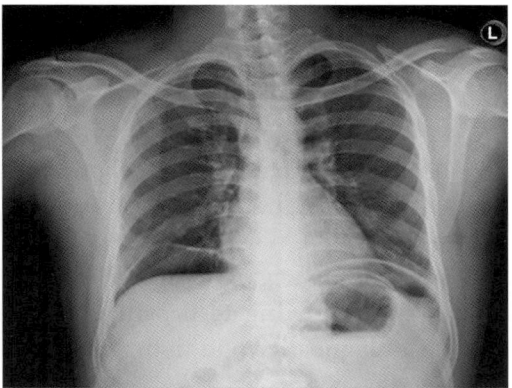

a. IV fluids + Emergency laparotomy
b. Observation
c. USG abdomen
d. CT scan of the abdomen

32. A 25-year-old patient came to emergency after road traffic accident, he was able to speak but not in sentences. On auscultation, hype resonant note is seen on right side. Chest X-ray was given below. What is the most appropriate initial management of this patient?

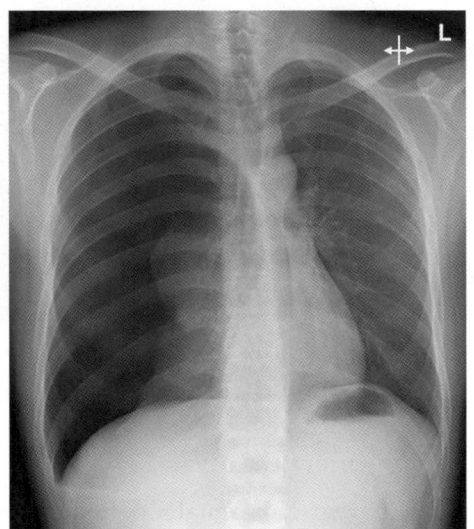

a. Immediately shift the patient to OT for thoracotomy
b. Immediate needle thoracotomy in 5th ICS
c. Put a large bore needle in the 2nd intercostal space and then ICD in 5th intercoastal space
d. HRCT chest

33. A 40-year-old male patient with mucopurulent cough underwent a CT examination. What is the most likely diagnosis?

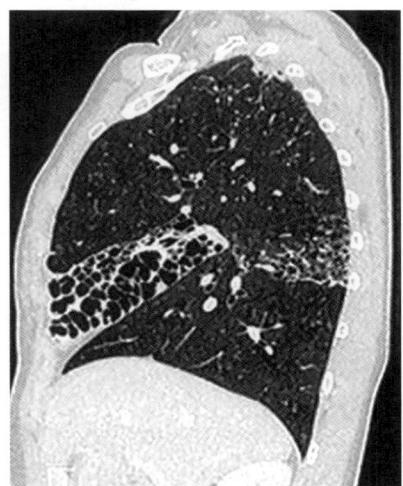

a. Sarcoidosis
b. Cystic fibrosis
c. Bronchiectasis
d. Pulmonary hydatidosis

34. A 12-year-old child was admitted to the hospital with fever. Chest radiograph was given below. What is the correct match?

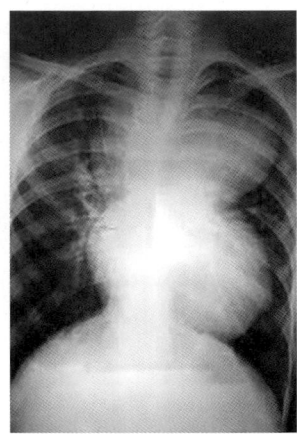

a. Snowman heart – TAPVC
b. BOOT shaped – TOF
c. Egg on string – TGA
d. Cottage loaf heart – Truncus arteriosus

35. A patient presenting with distended abdomen and pain for past 4 days. Radiograph is given below. What is the most likely diagnosis?

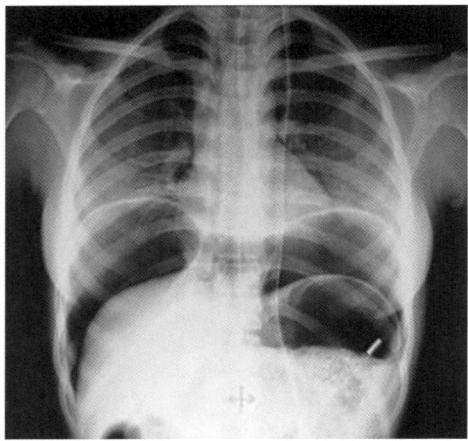

a. Hollow viscus perforation
b. Liver abscess
c. Thoracic empyema
d. Gastric volvulus

36. A patient being mechanically ventilated in the ICU shows signs of worsening respiratory status. A CXR AP view done revealed the following appearance. Most likely diagnosis is:

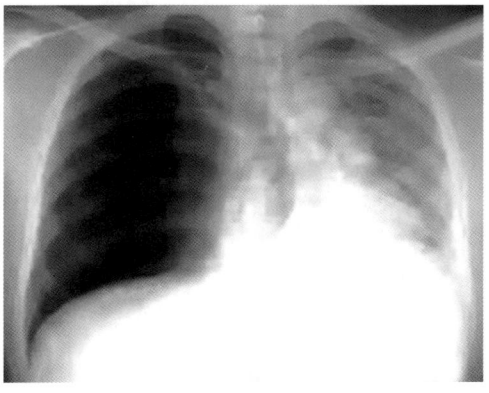

a. Massive pleural effusion
b. Pneumothorax
c. ARDS
d. Loculated pleural effusion

37. A 60-year-old chronic smoker presents with recurrent mild hemoptysis. A CXR PA view is normal and spectrum is negative for AFB. Which of the following tests will give the best diagnostic yield in this patient?
a. Fibro-optic bronchoscopy
b. CE-CT
c. MRI
d. Bronchography

ABDOMINAL RADIOLOGY

38. Identify the structure marked as 9 in the given below image:

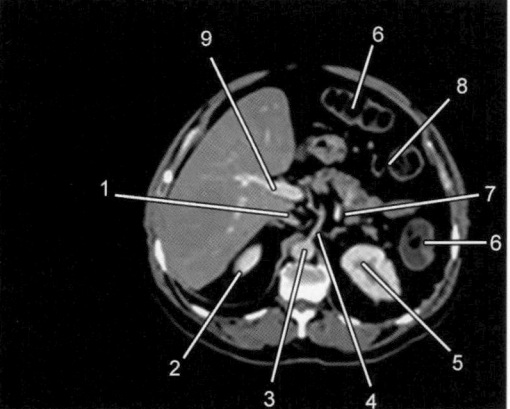

a. Hepatic artery
b. Portal vein
c. Hepatic vein
d. Inferior vena cava

39. A 35-year-old female patient presented with dysphagia which is more marked for liquids. Barium swallow image is shown below. What is the likely diagnosis?

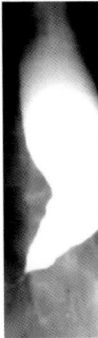

a. Achalasia cardia
b. Esophageal cancer
c. Diffuse esophageal spasm
d. Esophagitis

40. What is the diagnosis of given barium enema image?

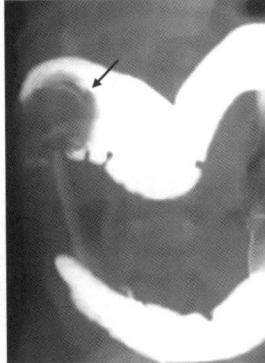

a. Colon cancer
b. Intussusception
c. Ulcerative colitis
d. Ileocecal TB

41. Supine abdominal radiograph of a 2-year-old child is given below. What is the possible diagnosis?

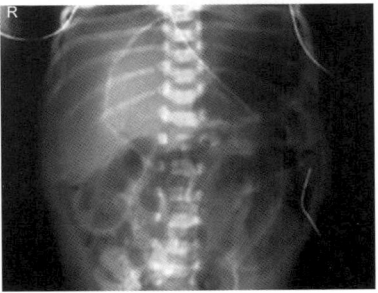

a. Duodenal atresia
b. Subcutaneous emphysema
c. Pneumatosis intestinalis
d. Pneumoperitoneum

42. A 26-year-old patient presented with pain in right hypochondrium region. On USG, water lily sign is seen. What is the most probable diagnosis?
a. Schistosoma
b. Ascariasis
c. Hydatid cyst
d. Entamoeba

43. On 5th postoperative day following Lap cholecystectomy, A patient presented with pain abdomen. On USG, A 5 × 5 cm collection is seen in the Morrison's pouch. A possibility of biliary leak is suspected. What is the most sensitive investigation to detect the leak?
a. ERCP
b. HIDA
c. MRCP
d. CECT

44. A 30-year-old patient with progressive difficulty in swallowing for both solids and liquids for 8 months. Ba swallow was done and shown below. What other investigations should be done in this patient?

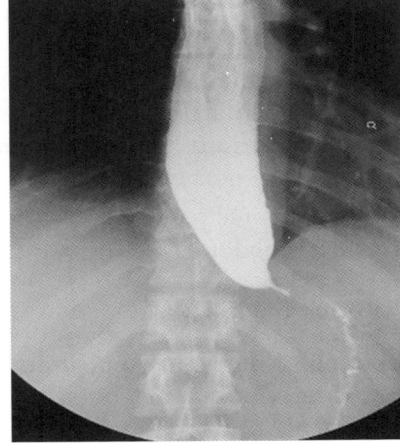

a. UGIE + Manometry
b. UGIE + CECT
c. UGIE + PET
d. UGIE + 24 h pH monitoring

45. In E-FAST, which if the following part of the body is included apart from abdomen?
    a. Thoracic cavity
    b. Pelvis
    c. Peripheral vessels
    d. Dural and subdural vessels

46. In the given radiograph the dilated bowel loops which are marked with arrow represents:

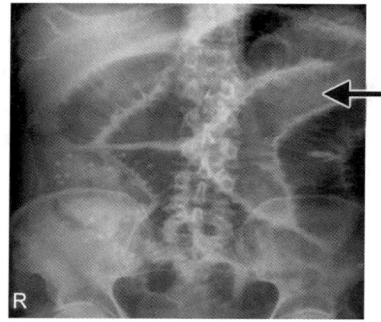

    a. Transverse colon
    b. Ileum
    c. Jejunum
    d. Duodenum

47. A patient met with a road traffic accident. In the causality, he had a feeble pulse with pulse rate of 110 BPM. There is reduced air entry on left side of thorax. Systolic BP is 70. There is bruising in left hypochondrium with ecchymosis. What is the next best shop?
    a. Abdominal paracentesis
    b. X-ray abdomen
    c. FAST
    d. CECT abdomen

48. Which of the following finding is a definite finding of complete large bowel obstruction?

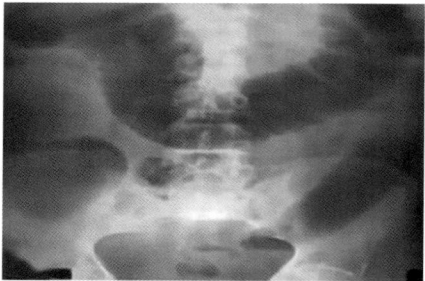

    a. Dilated bowel loops with visible haustrations
    b. Bilious vomiting
    c. Multiple dilated bowel loops with flatulence and increased bowel sounds
    d. Dilated bowel loops with plica circularis

49. USG/FAST is least useful in:
    a. Retroperitoneal hematoma
    b. Pneumothorax
    c. Renal injury
    d. Pericardial effusion

50. This appearance seen on M mode USG of thorax is suggestive of:

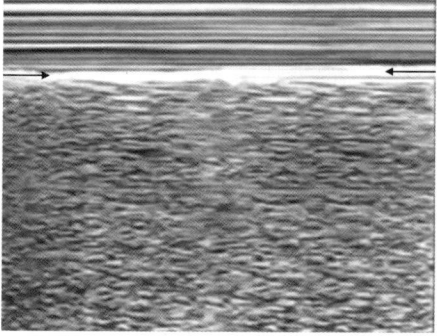

    a. Stratosphere sign
    b. Sea shore sign
    c. A – Line sign
    d. Lung point identification sign

51. A 35-year-old female is found to have a renal mass on USG examination. CT of the patient is done and shown below. What is the most likely diagnosis?

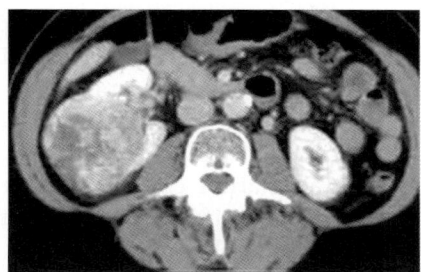

a. Angiomyolipoma
b. Renal cell carcinoma
c. Renal stone
d. Renal cyst

52. A child presented with mild abdominal discomfort with intermittent abdominal pain. There is no other symptom. Radiograph was given below. What is the most likely diagnosis?

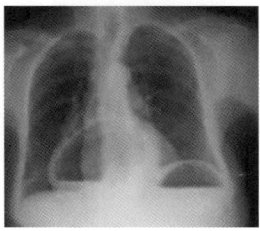

a. Morgagni hernia
b. Bochdalek hernia
c. Gastric volvulus
d. Diaphragmatic eventration

MUSCULOSKELETAL RADIOLOGY

53. The arrow in the below radiograph is pointing to which anatomical structure?

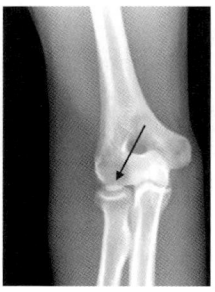

a. Capitellum
b. Medial epicondyle
c. Trochlea
d. Olecranon process

54. A 5-year-old boy is unable to pronate and supinate since childhood. Radiograph of forearm in frontal and oblique projection is given below. What is the most likely diagnosis?

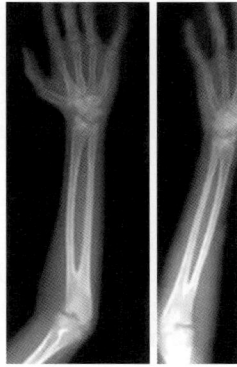

a. Radioulnar synostosis
b. Myositis ossificans
c. Radial head dislocation
d. Monteggia fracture dislocation

55. A 45-year-old patient with tingling, numbness and paresthesias in his lower extremities came for MRI examination which is shown below. Which intervertebral disc is likely to be involved?

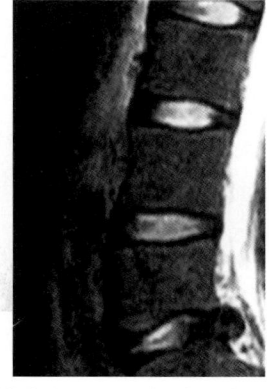

a. L3-L4   b. L4-L5
c. L5-S1   d. S1-S2

56. A 40-year-old male is suffering from increasing difficulty in bending forward with increasing stiffness of the spine. A CT was performed and shown below. Likely diagnosis:

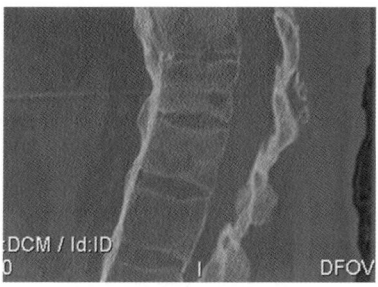

   a. RA
   b. AS
   c. Reiter's
   d. Fluorosis

57. A 10-year-child presented with limb pain with normal Bone Mineralization. Radiograph is shown below. What is the most likely diagnosis?

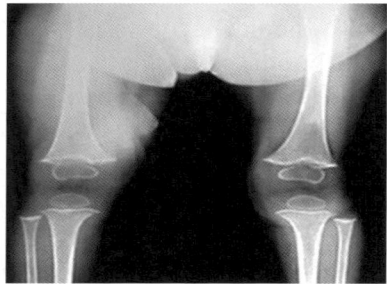

   a. Rickets
   b. Scurvy
   c. Metaphyseal dysplasia
   d. Pyknodysostosis

58. Identify the lesion:

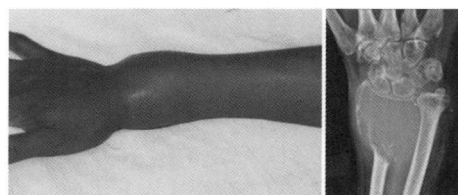

   a. Giant cell tumor
   b. Osteosarcoma
   c. Osteoid osteoma
   d. Osteochondroma

59. A child was brought to the hospital by his father with complaint of fever, low backbone and persistent flexion of the hip joint. He had a history of spine TB in the past. On the examination child has inguinal swilling. Identify the marked muscle responsible to be involved:

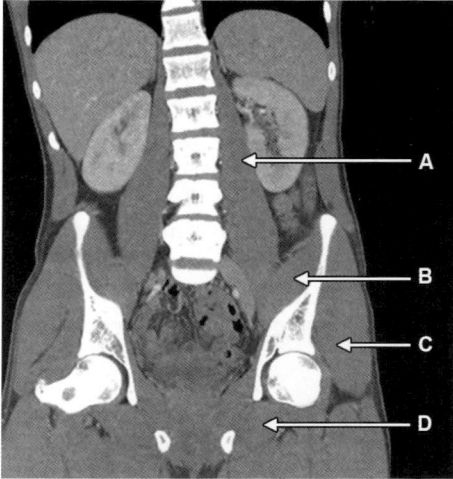

   a. A
   b. B
   c. C
   d. D

60. A 45-year-old male presented with back pain and morning stiffness lasting more than 30 minutes since last 2 years along with redness of eye. Radiograph has been obtained and shown below. Diagnosis:

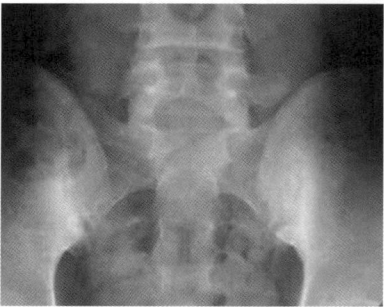

   a. Ankylosing spondylitis
   b. Healed TB spine
   c. Paget's disease
   d. Osteopetrosis

GENITOURINARY RADIOLOGY

61. A 35-year-old patient, with history of recurrent UTI came for the IVP and the image is shown below. On the basis of spot IVP image, location the insertion of ureter of left upper pole moiety:

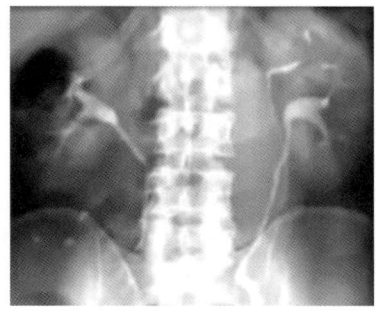

   a. At the trigone
   b. Below and medial to trigone of bladder
   c. Above the dome of the bladder
   d. In the prostatic urethra

62. What is your interpretation of given IVP image?

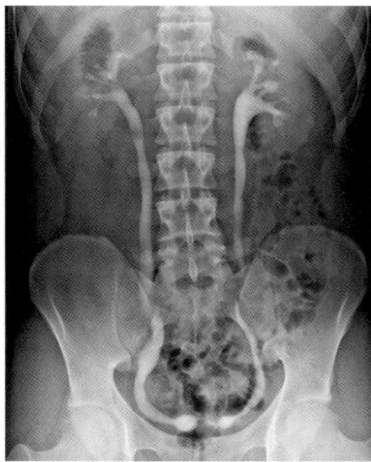

   a. B/L ureterocoele
   b. Bilateral hydronephrosis
   c. Staghorn calculi
   d. Bladder calculi

63. What is your interpretation of given HSG image?

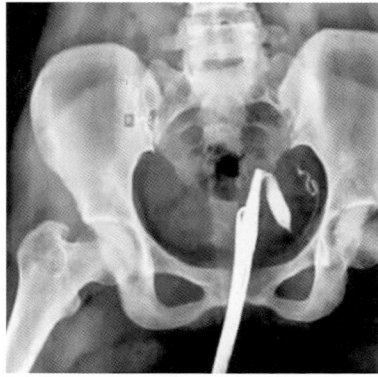

   a. Septate uterus
   b. Bicornuate uterus
   c. Unicornuate uterus
   d. Uterus didelphys

64. A 35-year-old patient present with dull aching pain in the back and sterile pyuria. Radiograph is given. Diagnosis:

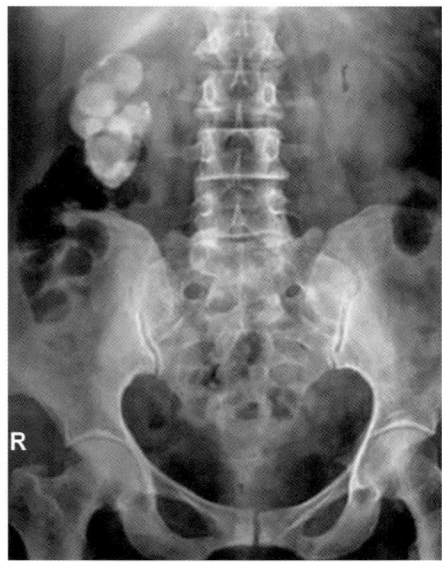

   a. Putty kidney
   b. Nephrocalcinosis
   c. Calcified psoas abscess
   d. Staghorn calculus

65. What is the name of the investigation shows below done in a female who presented with recurrent miscarriage?

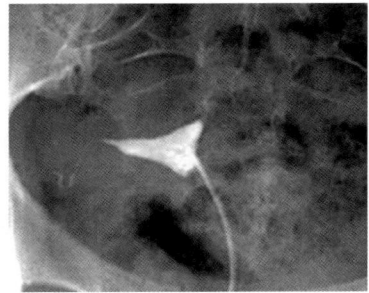

a. Genitogram
b. Saline infusion sonography
c. CT hysterosalpingography
d. Hysterosalpingogram

66. A 23-year-old female came had a history of two stillbirths. Ultrasound reveals of presence of a uterine anomaly. Which of the following investigation will be most helpful in confirming the abnormality?
    a. TVS
    b. Hysteroscopy + Laparoscopy
    c. HSG
    d. MRI

67. Unicornuate uterus can be identified by which of the following investigations?
    A. Laparoscopy B. HSG
    C. X-ray   D. Falloscopy
    a. A & B are true
    b. A & C are true
    c. B & D are true
    d. B & C are true

68. An antenatal USG of a 19 week pregnant female is given below. Identify the likely congenital abnormality:

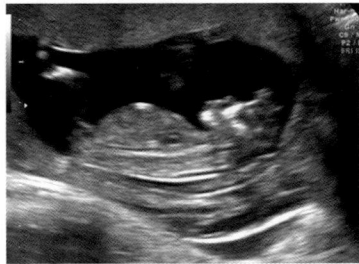

a. Anencephaly
b. Omphalocele
c. Encephalocele
d. Down's syndrome

RADIOTHERAPY

69. Prophylactic craniospinal irradiation is done for which cancer?
    a. Prostate cancer
    b. Seminoma
    c. Small cell cancer of lung
    d. Hodgkin's lymphoma

70. A patient with Brain Metastasis had to undergo head and neck irradiation, what is the most common delayed symptom with head and neck irradiation?
    a. Dysgeusia
    b. Anhidrosis
    c. Xerostomia
    d. Dysphagia

71. A child is suffering from acute lymphoblastic leukemia. He has undergone prophylactic cranial irradiation for the same while waiting for bone marrow transplant. Which of the following will be least affected by radiation exposure?
    a. Neurons in brain
    b. Spermatogonia
    c. Bone marrow
    d. Intestinal mucosa

72. True statement regarding "Acute radiation syndrome" is all *except*:
    a. It presents in 3 stages
    b. GI suppression occurs at a lower radiation dose than that required for bone marrow suppression
    c. Bone marrow suppression occurs earlier than neurovascular effects
    d. Bone marrow suppression occurs at 7.4 Gy

Answers

1. Ans. d. 1, 2, 3, 4
2. Ans. b. Duplex scan
3. Ans. b. MRI
4. Ans. b. TEE
5. Ans. a. Sesta MIBI scan
6. Ans. a. MRI
7. Ans. a. CECT
8. Ans. a. Midbrain
9. Ans. c. Optic nerve
10. Ans. c. Subdural hematoma
11. Ans. b. Putaminal bleed
12. Ans. a. Haemolytic anaemia
13. Ans. d. CT SCAN
14. Ans. b. Diffuse axonal injury
15. Ans. b. Caldwell view
16. Ans. a. Temporal lobe abscess
17. Ans. a. Foreign body in the esophagus
18. Ans. a. ACOM
19. Ans. a. Neurocysticercosis
20. Ans. b. CT angiography to rule out large vessel occlusion
21. Ans. a. Anterior ethmoidal air cell
22. Ans. b. Susceptibility weighted image
23. Ans. a. Prosthetic mitral valve
24. Ans. a. Right sided mastectomy
25. Ans. b. Right middle lobe consolidation
26. Ans. b. Pneumothorax
27. Ans. a. Hydropneumothorax
28. Ans. c. Sarcoidosis
29. Ans. b. Mycobacterium
30. Ans. d. Foreign body aspiration
31. Ans. a. IV fluids + Emergency laparotomy
32. Ans. c. Put a large bore needle in the 2nd intercostal space and then ICD in 5th intercoastal space
33. Ans. c. Bronchiectasis
34. Ans. a. Snowman heart – TAPVC
35. Ans. a. Hollow viscus perforation
36. Ans. b. Pneumothorax
37. Ans. a. Fibro-optic bronchoscopy
38. Ans. b. Portal vein
39. Ans. a. Achalasia cardia
40. Ans. b. Intussusception
41. Ans. d. Pneumoperitoneum
42. Ans. c. Hydatid cyst
43. Ans. b. HIDA
44. Ans. a. UGIE + Manometry
45. Ans. a. Thoracic cavity
46. Ans. c. Jejunum
47. Ans. c. FAST
48. Ans. a. Dilated bowel loops with visible haustrations
49. Ans. a. Retroperitoneal hematoma
50. Ans. b. Sea shore sign
51. Ans. b. Renal cell carcinoma
52. Ans. c. Gastric volvulus
53. Ans. a. Capitellum

54. Ans. a. Radioulnar synostosis
55. Ans. c. L5-S1
56. Ans. b. AS
57. Ans. a. Rickets
58. Ans. a. Giant cell tumor
59. Ans. a. A
60. Ans. a. Ankylosing spondylitis
61. Ans. b. Below and medical to trigone of bladder
62. Ans. a. B/L ureterocoele
63. Ans. c. Unicornuate uterus
64. Ans. a. Putty kidney
65. Ans. d. Hysterosalpingogram
66. Ans. b. Hysteroscopy + Laparoscopy
67. Ans. a. A & B are true
68. Ans. a. Anencephaly
69. Ans. c. Small cell cancer of lung
70. Ans. c. Xerostomia
71. Ans. a. Neurons in brain
72. Ans. b. GI suppression occurs at a lower radiation dose than that required for bone marrow suppression

SECTION A

GENERAL RADIOLOGY

- General Radiology

CHAPTER 1

General Radiology

GENERAL

Radiation: Energy that comes from a source and travel through some material or through space.
Can be:

(1) Ionizing	(2) Non-ionizing
Electromagnetic radiations	(a) UV-rays
(a) X-rays	(b) Visible rays
(b) γ-rays	(c) Infra red-rays
(c) Cosmic rays	(d) Microwaves
Particulate radiations	(e) Radiowaves
(a) α-rays	
(b) β-rays	
(c) Protons	
(d) Neutrons	

Various diagnostic modalities and procedures and radiations

Ionizing Radiations		Non-Ionizing
X-rays are used in	**γ-rays are used in**	MRI
1. CT-scan	PET	USG
2. Radiography	Bone-scan	Thermography
3. DEXA	Radionuclide scan	Doppler
4. IVP/IVU	SPECT	MRCP
5. HSG		
6. Bronchography		
7. ERCP		
8. Fluoroscopy		
9. Barium studies		

> **important**
> Particulate radiations have variable charge and mass where as electromagnetic radiations have no charge and mass.

> **important**
> All electromagnetic rays have same velocity i.e. velocity of light.

> **important**
> X-rays are extranuclear in origin. Gamma rays are intranuclear in origin.

> **important**
> X-rays: Iodinated dye
> ERCP = Diagnostic + Therapeutic but invasive
> MRCP = Only diagnostic but non-invasive

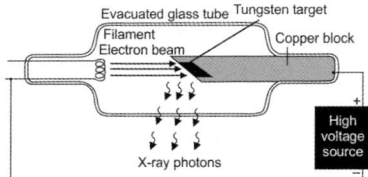

X-ray Tube

Wilhelm Conrad Roentgen, a German physicist, discovered X-rays on **November 8, 1895**.
- Awarded the **first Nobel Prize for Physics in 1901**.
- *Considered as Father of radiology*
- *International radiology day = 8th November*

Type	Mass & Charge	Comment
Electromagnetic		
1. X-ray	0	X-rays and gamma rays do not differ except in the source. Gamma rays are produced intranuclearly, and X-rays are produced extranuclearly (i.e., mechanically).
2. Gamma ray	0	
Particulate		
1. Electron (e)	Variable mass & Charge	—
2. Proton (p)		• **Exhibits a Bragg peak**
3. Neutron (n)		• **Cannot be accelerated by an electrical field**
4. Alpha particle		• **Helium nucleus**

PARTS OF X-RAY TUBE

- **Glass envelope:** Provides protected and vaccumated environment to the tube.
  - **Target window:** It is the thinning of glass in lower part of glass envelope which allows X-ray to come out of tube
- **Cathode:** Negatively charged electrode and consist of filament, supporting wires, and focusing cups
  - **Filament:**
  An electric current is passed through the filament and it gets heated to a very high temperature (approx 2200°C) which makes the metal sufficiently violent to enable a fraction of free electrons to leave the surface despite net attractive pull of the lattice of the positive ions.
- **Anode:** It is the positively charged electrode and the most important part is target, which is usually made of tungsten. The electrons are repelled by the negative cathode and attracted by the positive anode. Because of the vacuum, they are not hindered in any way and bombarded the target with a velocity around half of the velocity of light. X-rays are produced when fast moving electrons

> *i* **mportant**
> - Most important part of cathode is filament.
> - Mostly made up of tungsten
> - Emits electron by thermo-ionic emission.

> *i* **mportant**
> In photoelectric effect maximum photon energy is directly proportional to the atomic no of target material and is independent of KV.

> *i* **mportant**
> In Bremsstrahlung reaction maximum photon energy is numerically equal to the KV.

are stopped by impact on a metal target. The kinetic energy of the electrons is converted into X-rays (1%) and into heat (99%).
- **The production of X-rays is largely because of two processes:**
  - Interaction with the inner shell electron (k shell) a.k.a photoelectric effect resulting in productions of characteristics radiations.
  - Interaction with the nucleus a.k.a Bremsstrahlung reaction. It is the most important reaction (80%) responsible for X-ray production in most of the tube except Mammography where photoelectric effect predominates

Two types of anode are available:
- Stationary
- Rotating

 mportant
The major mechanism of heat dissipation in conventional X-ray tube is via conduction. In modern X-ray tube, heat dissipation is through conduction, convection and radiation, most important being radiation.

 mportant
Note: In majority of cases, rotating anode is used because of better heat tolerant capacity Except: Dental radiography and portable/mobile radiography, where stationary anodes are used.

Filter
- To block the low energy radiation
- To decrease radiation dose to the patient without effecting image quality
- Mostly made up of aluminum
- The target window also acts as an inherent filter in the tube.

Collimator
- Beam – restricting device
- It restrict the scattered radiation
- It also gives direction to the beam.

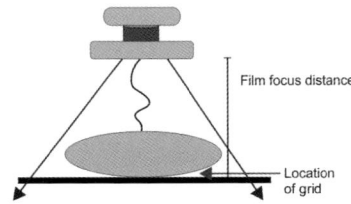

Grid
- Made up of lead
- These are parallel arranged lead stripes placed between patient and cassette
- Blocks scatter radiation from reaching to the film to improve image quality
- Radiation dose to the patient is slightly increased as the useful radiation are also slightly blocked by the grid.

Cassette: In Conventional Radiography, It is a Screen Film System
- **Screen:** Calcium tungstate/rare earth metals.
- It converts X-ray into light.
- Majority of cassette have double screen except mammography which has single screen cassette.

 mportant
Film focal distance: Distance between X-ray tube and cassette. For all radiography, this is 100 cm Except: Chest X-ray (180 cm), to reduce the cardiac magnification.

Film

- Made of photosensitive material, mostly silver bromide
- **Single coated film:** If Agbr is present only on one surface
- Double coated film is used in screen film system and in dental radiography.

Contrast

- It is the ability to see something in relation to the background
- Influenced by both KVP and MAS
- Most important factor to influence contrast is KVP

Kilo volt peak (KVP)	Milliampere second (MAS)
Related with voltage	Current x exposure time
Directly proportional to the energy of the beam	No effect on energy
Directly proportional to penetration	No effect on penetration
Inversely proportional to contrast	Determines the number of photon in a given area
	Determines the background blackening (film density)
	Directly proportional to contrast

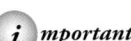

important
- For penetration
  - KVP has to be changed
- For contrast
  - Both KVP and MAS are important
  - ↑ KVP → ↓ contrast
  - ↑ MAS → ↑ contrast

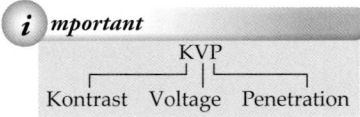

important

KVP

Kontrast   Voltage   Penetration

DIGITAL RADIOGRAPHY

- Digitizing conventional film
- Computed radiography (CR)
- Direct radiography (DR)

Computed Radiography

Conventional X-ray
↓
Phosphor plate (PSP)
↓
Latent image
↓
Laser beam
↓
Emission of light
↓
Ultra-sensitive PMT
↓
Electronic signal (digital)
↓
CRT or Hard copy

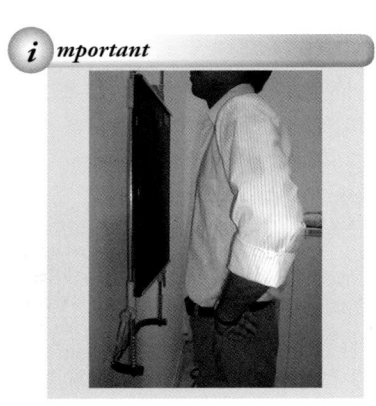

important

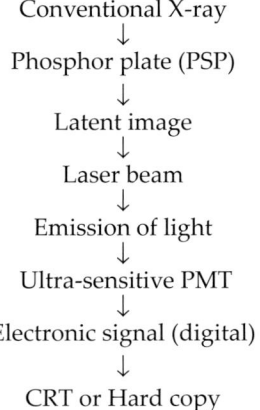

Direct Radiography

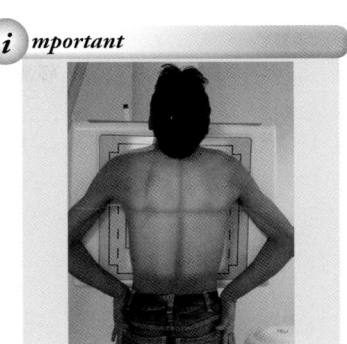

X-ray
↓
Patient
↓
Flat panel detector
↓
Electrical energy
↓
Digital image

	Computed radiography (CR)	Digital radiography (DR)
Steps required	• Load cassette • Position patient • Position tube • Perform exposure • Transport cassette • Process cassette • Assess image quality • End examination	• Position patient • Position tube • Perform exposure • Image is sent to viewing station • Assess image quality • End examination
Advantages	Manipulation and positioning of image receptor for cross table projections is possible (useful in trauma)	• Relatively faster workflow due to elimination of cassettes • Shorter turnaround time for viewing image
Disadvantages	• Slower, more complex workflow • Possibility of repetitive motion injuries due to long-term cassette handling	• Higher costs

MAMMOGRAPHY

Mammography uses lower kV (for higher image contrast) and higher mA (for shorter exposure times) compared with the technique for chest and abdominal examinations.

- Small focal spot size (0.2–0.5 mm)
- Beryllium Window
- Target-Filter combination
    - Molybdenum (preferred); Rhodium; Tungsten
    - Mammography is usually done after 40 years because in Young age, breast has dense glandular

parenchyma. Where it is difficult to see the lesion on mammography and glandular tissue is more sensitive to radiation.

Two Views

- Mediolateral (more important because of the more coverage area)
- Craniocaudal

Note: Mammography has 10–40 times more radiation exposure than CXR.

BIRADS classification for mammography lesion: (Breast imaging Reporting and Data system).

> *important*
> In younger age, MRI is the preferred screening test.
> - **MRI:** Best investigation for breast implant.

Grade	Interpretation	Management
0	Incomplete evaluation	Complete it
1	Normal	None (CRS) continue routine screening
2	Benign fibroadenoma	None (CRS)
3	Probably benign (< 2%)	Short follow-up
4	Suspicious /indeterminate (> 2%)	Biopsy
5	Highly suspicious (> 95%)	Biopsy
6	Biopsy proven malignancy	To look for contralateral breast and multicentric disease in the same breast

RADIATION UNITS

Dose	Conventional	SI Unit
1. Exposure dose	Roentgen	Coulombs/kg
2. Absorbed dose	Rad	Gray
3. Equivalent dose	Rem	Sievert
4. Effective dose	–	Sievert
5. Radioactivity	Curie	Becquerel

Exposure Dose

- The unit of radiation exposure is the Roentgen (R), defined as an amount of X-rays or gamma rays that will liberate a charge of 2.58×10^{-4} C/kg of air, under standard temperature and pressure

- The SI unit for radiation exposure is Coulombs/kg.
- Conventional unit: Roentgen.

Radiation Absorbed Dose
- The unit rad is defined as the radiation necessary to deposit energy of 100 ergs in 1 gram of irradiated material.
- The SI unit for absorbed dose is Gray. One Gray is the amount of radiation necessary to deposit 1 joule of energy in 1 kg of material.
- 1 Gray = 100 rad.

important

S no.	Types of radiations	Quality factor
1	X, gamma, or beta radiation	1
2	Alpha particles and multiple charged particles	20
3	Neutrons	10
4	High energy protons	10

Equivalent Dose
It represents the biological impact of various types of radiation.
- H_T = WR × D, where H_T is the equivalent dose, WR is the quality factor and D is the absorbed dose in Rads or Gray.
- The radiation dose equivalent for which the unit was rem, has now been replaced by 'Sievert' in the SI units (systeme internationale).
- 1 Sievert = 100 rems.

Effective Dose
- It assigns the various tissues/organs the proportional risk of stochastic effect to irradiation, compared to uniform whole body radiation by same equivalent dose.
- It takes into account Tissue Weighting Factor (WT) which depends on the susceptibility of a particular tissue to the stochastic effect by radiation. It is also expressed in Sieverts.
- $H_E = W_T \times H_T$, where H_E is the effective dose, H_T is the equivalent dose, and W_T is the tissue weighting factor. Equivalent dose × Tissue wt-factor = effective dose.

SI unit: Sievert or milli sievert (mSv).

important

Organ/Tissue	ICRP (New)	ICRP (Old)
BREAST	0.12	0.05
Bone marrow	0.12	0.12
Colon	0.12	0.12
Lung	0.12	0.12
Remainder	0.12	0.05
Stomach	0.12	0.12
GONADS	**0.08**	**0.20**
Bladder	**0.04**	0.05
Liver	**0.04**	0.05
Oesophagus	**0.04**	0.05
Thyroid	**0.04**	0.05
Bone surfaces	**0.01**	**0.01**
Brain	**0.01**	–
Salivary glands	**0.01**	–
Skin	**0.01**	0.01

HARMFUL EFFECTS OF RADIATION

- Ionization of molecule- Free radical generation – damage to DNA.
  Note: M/C radiation side effect: Skin erythema.
- Be directly proportional to dose, i.e. deterministic (certainty) effects

- Related with certainty to a known dose of radiation
- Dose threshold exists
- Severity is dose related
- e.g. skin effects, epilation, lens opacities, etc.
- Not directly proportional to dose, i.e. stochastic effects.
  - Random events without threshold
  - Probability increases with dose
  - 'ALL OR NONE' phenomenon
  - Severity may not be dose related
  - e.g. genetic side effects, teratogenity, mutations, etc.

Radiation protection for patient

10-day Rule:
- In a female of reproductive age group, any modality which gives ionising radiation should be performed within first 10 days of menstrual cycle (because there is no ovulation) – to prevent radiation to an undiagnosed pregnancy.

ALARA approach: As low as Reasonably achievable radiation dose.

> **important**
>
> **D**eterministic
> **D**ose Dependent
> **D**irectly proportional to dose
> **D**ose threshold exist

> **important**
>
> Radiation protections aims at eliminating the deterministic side effects and reducing the probability of stochastic side effects.

> **important**
>
> Pregnant occupational worker should not be exposed to more than 2 mSv of radiation applied to surface of her lower abdomen for the declared term of pregnancy which is equivalent to 1 mSv dose to the fetus.

> **important**
>
> - At doses in excess of 20–100 Gy to the total body, death usually occurs within 24 to 48 hrs from neurologic and cardiovascular failure. This is known as the **cerebrovascular syndrome**. Because cerebrovascular damage cause death very quickly, the failure of other systems do not have time to develop.
> - Cerebrovascular syndrome
> - 20–100 gray
> - Death within 24–48 hours
> - Other systems don't have time to develop failure.

	Occupation workers		General public	
	Limit	Annual equivalents	Limit	Annual equivalents
ICRP	20 mSv/yr over 5 years	20 mSv	1 mSv/yr over 5 years	1 mSv
NCRP	Cumulative dose = Age in yrs x 10 mSv	50 mSv	5 mSv for 5-year period	1 mSv
AERB	100 mSv for 5-year period	30 mSv	1 mSv/yr for 5 years	1 mSv

Note: Radiation workers protect themselves from radiation by
- Aprons (made of lead) thickness = 0.5 mm (according to AERB, it should have at least lead equivalance of 0.25 mm), increase thickness, increases the weight of the apron.

- Lead-free apron: Tin, Antimony, and Bismuth.
- **TLD** (thermoluminiscent dosimeter):
  - It is a badge which monitors radiation used by radiation worker.
  - Checked every 3-month.

Amount of radiation exposure in a CT scan is dependent on the body part to be examined for example in CT head, it is 2.3 mSv and in CT abdomen it is 10 mSv.

A CT chest has radiation exposure of almost equal to 400 chest radiographs.

ULTRASOUND

Advantage	Disadvantage
• Real-time image • No radiation • Portable • Easily available • Cheap	• Operator dependent

- Works on the principal of **Piezoelectric effect**: generation of sound waves by passing electricity. The electricity is passed through crystal, vibration of which generates sound waves.
- Most commonly used crystal: Lead zirconate Titanate (PZT)
- Medically used frequency: 2–20 MHz
- A handheld transducer is applied to the body. This transducer both sends US waves into the body and receives reflected sound waves. This information is communicated via cable to the US scanner, and the image is generated on a monitor.
- **Real-time B-scans** allow body structures which are moving to be investigated.
- **Velocity:** The speed at which sound propagates through a given medium. Velocity through a given medium is inversely related to the density and directly related to stiffness of that medium. Ultrasound waves travel faster through a stiff medium, such as bone. In echocardiography, the velocity of sound is assumed to be approximately 1,540 m/sec (or 1.54 m/msec). Sound waves travel through the

> *important*
> At doses between 5 and 12 Gy, death may occur in a matter of days, as a result of the **gastrointestinal syndrome**. The symptoms during this period may include nausea, vomiting and prolonged diarrhea for several days, leading to dehydration, sepsis and death.
> **Gastrointestinal syndrome**
> - 5–12 Gray
> - Death occurs in days
> - Nausea, vomiting of diarrhea leading to dehydration, sepsis of death.

> *important*
> At total-body doses between 2 and 8 Gy, death may occur several weeks after exposure and is due to effects on the bone marrow, which results in the **hematopoietic syndrome**. The full effect of radiation is not apparent until the mature hematopoietic cells are depleted. Death from the hematologic damage occurs at about 20 to 30 days after exposure and the risk of death continues over the next 30 days. Clinical symptoms during this period may include chills, fatigue and petechial hemorrhage.
> **Hematopoietic syndrome**
> - 2–8 Gray
>   - Death occurs in several weeks
> - Usually due to effect on bone marrow
> - Symptoms usually are chills, fatigue and petechial hemorrhage.

> *important*
> USG is done for:
> - Palpable lesion and done to differentiate between solid and cystic lesion and
> - To rule out breast abscess.

> *important*
>
> | A | B |
> |---|---|
> | 2-7 MHz | 7-15 MHz |
> | Low-frequency probe | High-frequency probe |

important
- Lower the frequency of ultrasonography probe more deep it penetrate to see (i.e. more depth).
- More frequency of probe of USG, better will be resolution.

important
Note:
- For all thick and deep body parts: Low-frequency probe is used
- For all thin and superficial body parts: High-frequency.

important
Note: Posterior structure of heart are better seen on transesophageal echocardiography.

important
Note: 5-layer of GIT seen on endoscopic US.

important

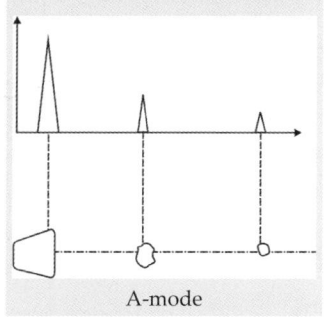

A-mode

important

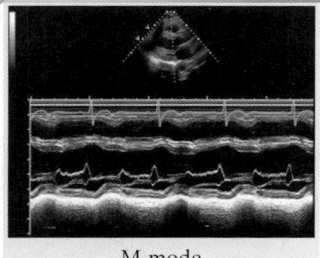

M-mode

air with speed of 330 m/s. The typical velocities for different tissues are provided in the below Table.

Medium	Velocity (m/sec)
Fat	1450
Water	1480
Soft tissue	1540
Kidney	1560
Blood	1570
Muscle	1580
Bone	4080

Clinical Transducer

For thick, deep body parts (Abdomen, obstetric) = 3.5 to 5 MHz.

For small body parts (Orbit, Thyroid, breast) = 7.5 to 10 MHz. As penetration is not a problem, being superficial location.

Intracavitary Transducers (7.5-20 Hz)

Endovaginal—Pelvis

Endorectal—Prostate

Transesophageal—Heart

Intravascular—Blood vessels

Endoscopic ultrasound—Pancreatic lesion, local staging of esophageal cancer, rectal cancer.

Methods of Display

- **A-Mode (AMPLITUDE):** Amplitude of the returning signals is plotted in a graphical form against their distance from transducer/depth. Commonly used for orbital biometry.

- **B-Mode (BRIGHTNESS):** The amplitude of returning signals is given grey scale value based on an scale and is represented in the display to form a image of the scan plane. Most commonly used mode.

- **M-Mode (MOTION):** Detects any rhythmic motion occurring in the scan plane without any amplitude considerations. Used for valvulular morphology and motion.

Nomenclature of USG Images

- Regions which reflect a lot of sound to the transducer are termed as *echogenic* or *hyperechoic* and by convention are viewed as bright or white areas.

- Regions which do not reflect many sound waves are termed as *hypoechoic* and are viewed as dark or black areas.
- The regions which have similar pattern to normal viscera or soft tissue are labeled as isoechoic.

Fat, calculus, bones, and stones are extremely echogenic on USG.

Fluid is absolutely black on USG and is termed as anechoic.

Posterior acoustic enhancement: Increased brightness beyond the objects that transmit a lot of sound waves, e.g. cysts.

Fluid filled structures

Posterior acoustic shadowing has the opposite effect—decreased brightness seen beyond objects that reflect a great deal of sound, e.g. stones (refer to the image shown with B mode USG).

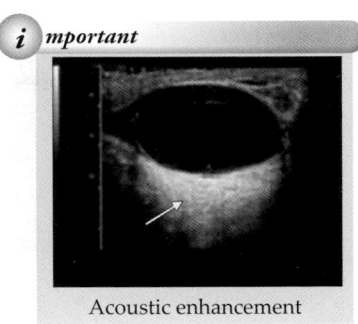

Acoustic enhancement

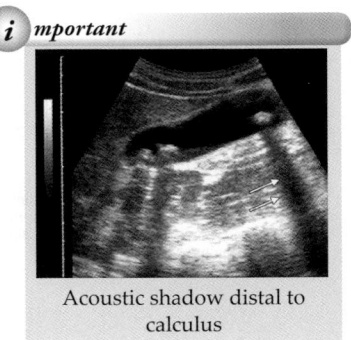

Acoustic shadow distal to calculus

Ultrasonography is Investigation of Choice for

- Hydrocephalus in infants/neonates
- Retinal detachment
- Minimal pleural effusion
- Minimal pericardial effusion
- CHPS
- Gallstones
- Acute cholecystitis (although theoretically HIDA scan is best)
- Screening for Rotator cuff injuries (initial investigation)
- Renal colic in pregnancy
- Minimal ascites
- Pararenal fluid collection post renal transplant
- Obstetrics indications
- Scrotal pathologies
- Varicose veins
- DDH (developmental dysplasia of hip) (screening investigation)

ADVANCE APPLICATIONS OF USG DOPPLER

Doppler US: For moving structure, i.e. blood. It can be used for
1. **Presence/absence of flow**
2. **Direction of flow**
   Note: Blood flow toward the probe = Red
   Blood flow away from probe = Blue

important

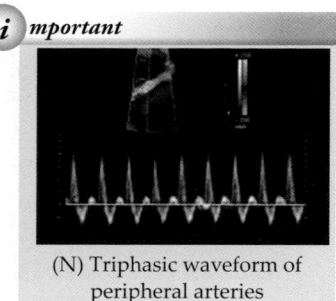

(N) Triphasic waveform of peripheral arteries

| Triphasic signal Normal | Biphasic - Arterial Vasoconstriction | Monophasic (Tardus parvas) - distal to occlusion |

important

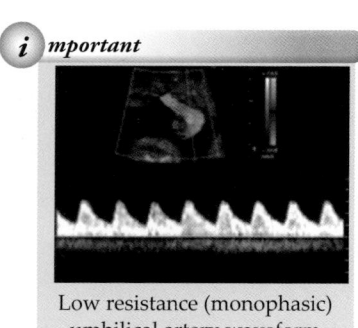

Low resistance (monophasic) umbilical artery waveform

important

Note: Hepatic veins have triphasic pattern due to the pressure change in the RA and its continuity with it without any valve.

Note: Green color in Doppler is seen in turbulent blood flow due to mixing of red and blue

3. **Velocity of flow**

Doppler can be used to asses velocity of the blood flow which is important in assessing the stenosis in a vessel. As there is a stenosis, velocity increases at the point of stenosis.

Note: The vessel transducer angle should be less than 60 degree for proper velocity calculation on USG.

4. **Pattern of flow–Spectral pattern/waveform**

Every vessel in the body has a specific pattern of flow which can be detected on Doppler

- The peripheral arteries in the body has high resistance due to peripheral vascular resistance and commonly shows triphasic pattern.
  - In case of arterial vasoconstriction, the peripheral resistance increase and flow becomes biphasic.
  - In case of peripheral vasodilation, the peripheral resistance decreases and flow becomes monophasic with pulsatility.
  - In case of arterial obstruction, there is significant loss of pressure and the flow distal to obstruction becomes monophasic (tardus pavus) with ↑ acceleration time.
- The visceral arteries (hepatic artery, renal artery, umbilical artery) in the body has low resistance and usually has low resistance flow, which is monophasic pattern with pulsation.
  - In cases of IUGR, as there is increase in the placental resistance, diastolic flow decreases and the S/D ratio increases (normal S/D ratio is < 2.5. It is increased to > 3.0 in IUGR).
  - When the placental resistance increases further, diastolic flow decreases further and a time comes when the diastolic force becomes equal to the placental resistance and no flow is seen in Doppler, this is called as absent diastolic flow and is a sign of severe IUGR.
  - When the placental resistance is increased further, there is reversal of flow in diastole and it is the sign of impending fetal death.
- The veins in the body has continuous flow without pulsation, a.k.a monophasic pattern without pulsations.

ELASTOGRAPHY

Elastography is a new method which applies a distorting force (stress) to a tissue to move it by few millimetres, and create an image of the tissue's response (strain) by comparing the two. In principle, any imaging method can be used: ultrasound has the advantage that the transducer can be used to apply the stress and of working in real time while magnetic resonance has also been used successfully.

For ultrasound, the transducer is usually used to apply the stress manually and the strain is detected by tracking the speckle pattern as it changes during probe-induced distortion. The information used to create the images is similar to that gained from clinical palpation except that it is much more sensitive, especially to deeper structures. It has already found clinical applications in the breast, liver, and prostate, and is an active research area. The important uses of elastography include:
- Assessment of degree of fibrosis in liver
- To differentiate benign lesion from malignant lesion in liver, breasts, and prostate.

CT SCAN

The first CT machine used for clinical purposes, developed by the late Sir Godfrey Hounsfield, was installed at the Atkinson Morley Hospital, London, in the early 1970s. In the initial days only sequential acquisition was possible. In 1980s, the development of slip-ring technology enabled continuous revolution of the X-ray unit, which not only reduced the acquisition time per axial image to 1 sec, but also allowed helical data to be acquired. The next step of development occurred in the late 1990s, when detectors were split into multiple thin rows along the z-axis to permit acquisition of multiple sections simultaneously (multidetector CT). This decreased acquisition time yet further and made it possible to routinely use thin sections. As a result, multi-detector CT is nowadays able to provide near isotropic volumetric data sets in which spatial resolution is similar in all planes. 2000s saw the introduction of cardiac CT which is based on ECG-synchronization to freeze cardiac motion. The number of detector rows increased from 4 to somewhere between 64 and 320 rows, depending on the manufacturer. Rapid tube rotation (<0.3 s) and dual-source systems with two X-ray tubes were developed to optimize cardiac imaging.

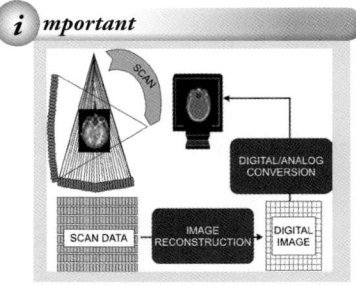

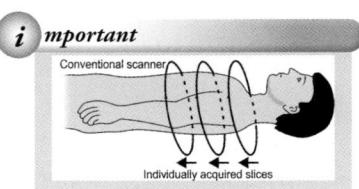

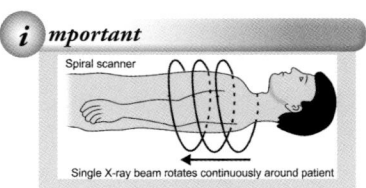

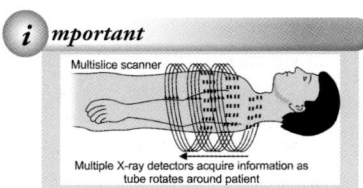

Basic Principle of CT is Linear Attenuation of X-rays
- **CT No./HU value:** Numerical value, given to a tissue depending on degree of attenuation of X-ray by that tissue

The linear attenuation coefficient (µ)
- The linear attenuation coefficient (µ) describes the fraction of a beam of X-rays or gamma rays that is absorbed or scattered per unit thickness of the absorber. This value basically accounts for the number of atoms in a cubic cm volume of material and the probability of a photon being scattered or absorbed from the nucleus or an electron of one of these atoms

Substance	HU value
Air	–1000
Fat	–50 to –100
Water	0
Muscle	10–40
Blood	~60
Contrast	130
Bone	>400

> ***important***
> **Note:**
> - More HU value causes more white (Hyperdense)
> - Less HU value cause more black (Hypodense)
> - $HU = 1000 \times \dfrac{\mu - \mu_{water}}{\mu_{water} - \mu_{air}}$

- **Slice thickness:** Thickness of tissue scanned in one rotation

$$\text{Pitch} = \dfrac{\text{Table movement per rotation}}{\text{Beam collimation or slice thickness}}$$

Scan length = Table movement during entire scan

$$= \dfrac{\text{Table movement}}{\text{Rotation}} \text{ no. of rotation}$$

$$= \text{Pitch beam collimation} \dfrac{\text{Total duration of scan}}{\text{Time taken in 1 rotation}}$$

- Increase in the pitch leads to decrease in the scan duration and radiation but reduces the scan quality.
- Decrease in the pitch leads to increase in the scan duration and radiation but improves the scan quality.

Advantage of Multislice CT/Multidetector C7
- Faster acquisition
- Coverage of larger area
- Less movement artefacts
- Isotropic multiplanar reformats
- Improved vascular and cardiac imaging
- Potential for faster throughput of patients.

> ***important***
> As you increase the number of detectors, the scan quality improves and time taken to complete the scan reduces.

DUAL SOURCE CT

Two X-ray sources are used operating at different potential (Kv). The interaction between the two with tissues in the body is different and by comparing those differences in the two images, radiologists can differentiate, characterize, isolate and distinguish body tissues and fluid, leading to breakthroughs in medical imaging.

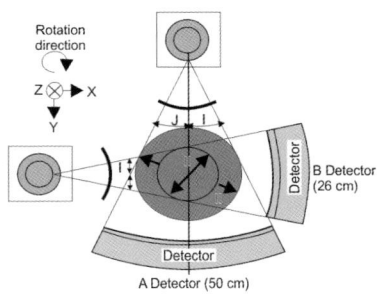

Applications	Bottom-line inference
• Pulmonary nodule characterization	• Not useful
• Fatty liver quantification for liver donors	• Useful, present application
• Characterization of liver lesions	• Limited data
• Characterization of an adrenal mass	• Useful (more validation needed)
• Coronary in-stent stenosis	• Further data needed
• Bone subtraction for CTA post processing	• Few data available
• Kidney-stone differentiation	• Useful results from initial patient studies More data needed
• Iron deposition in liver	• MRI is superior to CT in this respect
• Bone densitometry	• Better tests are available

 mportant
Beam hardening artifact is seen is posterior fossa in CT scan images due to increase in average kVp of the beam as it passes through dense petrous bone.

Advantage

- Ability to scan at any heart rate
- No need to use beta-blockers
- Better temporal resolution - 83 ms
- Trauma, oncology, obese patient

HIGH RESOLUTION CT SCAN (HRCT)

It is a type of CT technique done for some specific diseases like
- Interstitial lung disease
- Bronchiectasis
- Miliary tuberculosis
- Temporal bone evaluation
- CSF leaks

mportant
MR cisternography is the IOC to identify CSF leak whereas HRCT is done to assess bony defect.

Principle

- Thin slice-thickness or collimation
- Narrow field of view
- Bone algorithm for image reconstruction

RADIATION DOSE IN A CT SCAN

CTDI (CT Dose Index): CT dose index (CTDI) is a standardized measure of radiation dose output of a CT scanner which allows the user to compare radiation output of different CT scanners.

CTDI represents the average absorbed dose, along the z-axis, from a series of contiguous irradiations. It is measured from one *axial* CT scan (one rotation of the X-ray tube), and is calculated by dividing the integrated absorbed dose by the nominal total beam collimation. The CTDI is always measured in the axial scan mode for a single rotation of the X-ray source, and theoretically estimates the average dose within the central region of a scan volume consisting of multiple, contiguous CT scans [Multiple Scan Average Dose (MSAD)] for the case where the scan length is sufficient for the central dose to approach its asymptotic upper limit.

Dose Length Product (DLP)

DLP (mGy-cm) = *CTDI*vol (mGy) × *scan length* (cm)

The DLP reflects the total energy absorbed (and thus the potential biological effect) attributable to the complete scan acquisition. Thus, an abdomen-only CT exam might have the same CTDIvol as an abdomen/pelvis CT exam, but the latter exam would have a greater DLP, proportional to the greater z-extent of the scan volume.

> *important*
> Radiation dose depends on tube current (amperage), slice scan time, and tube peak kilovoltage.

MRI

Magnetic resonance imaging (MRI) is a non-invasive method of mapping structure and various aspects of function within the body by producing images by the virtue of *gyromagnetic property* of protons, with the greatest advantage of not using ionizing radiation for imaging.

Principle of MRI: i.e. NMR (Nuclear magnetic resonance): given by Purcell and Bloch (1952)

Invention of MRI: Lauterbeur and Mansfield (2003)

Functional MRI: Ogawa and Rosen

General Radiology

Magnetic resonance is a phenomenon whereby the nuclei of certain atoms, when placed in a magnetic field, absorb and emit energy at a specific or resonant frequency.

Nuclei suitable for MRI contain odd no of protons and/or neutrons. Almost all clinical MR images are produced using the simplest of all nuclei, that of hydrogen (comprising a single proton), which is present in virtually all biological material and exhibits relatively high MR sensitivity.

Parts of MRI

- Maxwell Coil: Gradient coil used to create magnetic field gradients along the direction of the main magnetic field
- Radiofrequency coils: To generate stronger magnetic field along the scan field.
- Faraday cage/shield/Hoffman Box: Blocks out external static electric fields. Made up of copper [Cu]
- Superconductors: Electromagnets (determines the strength of magnet) measured in tesla.

How Image is Acquired in MRI

- In the absence of magnetic field all protons have random movement
- Under the influence of magnetic field, alignment of proton takes place
- Realignment occurs under the influence of radiofrequency pulse
- After switching off the radiofrequency pulse, the atoms return to their original position and release energy in the form of electrical voltage signal
- When proton releases energy to surrounding lattice, it is called as spin lattice relaxation or T1 relaxation
- When proton releases energy to the surrounding spin, it is called as spin-spin relaxation or T2 relaxation
- This electrical signal (produced in receiver coil) is **digitized and analyzed** in a **computer**, to produce **MR images.**

Using T1 and T2 relaxation time, two types of images are broadly acquired using this principal; T1 weighted MR and T2 weighted MR.

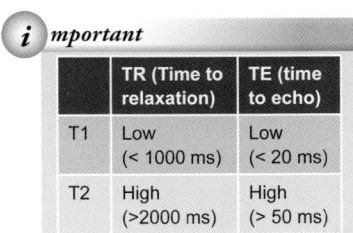

important

	TR (Time to relaxation)	TE (time to echo)
T1	Low (< 1000 ms)	Low (< 20 ms)
T2	High (>2000 ms)	High (> 50 ms)

Contraindications of MRI

It is a common saying that MRI means "metal results in injury" however it is not true in current scenario and there are many metallic devices compatible with MRI and students should be aware of those, particularly devices made up of TITANIUM which are very much compatible with MRI.

Few important devices or conditions where MRI is usually contraindicated are:
- Cardiac pacemakers
- Cochlear implants
- Intraoccular Metallic foreign body
- Electronically, magnetically, and mechanically activated implants
- Ferromagnetic or electronically operated active devices like defibrillators
- Aneurysmal clips
- Prosthetic heart valves—metallic
- Insulin pumps and nerve stimulators
- Stapedial implants
- Claustrophobia
- First trimester of pregnancy

Note: Even in the devices mentioned above, MRI can be performed depending upon the make of the device, e.g. some pacemakers are MRI compatible at lower strength magnet, i.e. up to 1.5 Tesla so it is always advised to check the compatibility of the device before saying NO to MRI.

MRI can be Safely Performed in

- Orthopedic implants (usually made of titanium). In cases of implants made of stainless steel, MRI can still be done however, heating is a problem so it is usually recommended for a shorter time and on a lower strength magnet. In permanent tattoos also because of the heavy metal dyes, heating may be an issue.
- Pregnancy after 1st trimester. Safety profile of MRI is not established in first trimester so, should not be done in 1st trimester.
- Cholecystectomy clips, sternal sutures
- IUCD
- Non metallic foreign bodies
- Breast implants (investigation of choice is MRI)

important

	T1-weighted MR	T2-weighted MR
Information	Anatomical Information	Pathological information
CSF	Black	White World war 2 (WW2) Water is white on T2
Brain	Gray matter-gray White matter-white	Gray matter-white White matter-gray
Pathologies	Mostly black (Hypointense)	Mostly white (Hyperintense)

important

Things bright on T1W	Dark on both T1W & T2W
Fat	Air
Hemorrhage	Flowing-(Flow void) blood (on SE/FSE images)
Proteinaceous substances	Cortical bone
Melanin	Ligaments, tendons, and other dense fibrous tissues
Paramagnetic agents (gadolinium)	

- Pediatric patients (MRI is usually preferred because of lack of ionising radiation however, it is usually done under sedation due to uncooperative behavior)
- Coronary stents. Usually drug eluting stents are used and MRI can be done after 3 months.

SPECIAL SEQUENCES OF MRI

FLAIR: Fluid Attenuated Inversion Recovery Sequence
(Flair = T_2 minus water)

It is type of T2 weight MRI where the water is suppressed to make pathology more visible. It is predominantly used at places where water is the confounding factor and limiting the contrast, e.g. brain.

Uses

- For better appreciation of pathologies in brain (most of the pathology being white.
- To differentiate arachnoid cyst from epidermoid cyst (arachnoid is a CSF filled cyst and becomes black on FLAIR, where as epidermoid is not).

STIR (Short Tau Inversion Recovery Sequence)

STIR can be easily remembered as T2– Fat means pathology will remain white whereas Fat will become black.

It is predominantly used at places where fat is the confounding factor and limiting the contrast, e.g. rest of the body and musculoskeletal imaging.

Uses

- Identification of bone marrow edema in diseases like stress fracture, avascular necrosis (image), Perthes disease, etc.
- For better appreciation of diseases in body where presence of Fat is reducing the contrast due to background whiteness.

Contrast Enhanced MRI (CEMRI)

Gadolinium containing compunds are most commonly used contrast agents in MRI.

Presence of gadolinium causes reduction in both T1 and T2 relaxation time which leads to increases in signal on T1-weighted MRI and decreases in signal on T2 weighted MRI. As human eyes appreciate white color better, post contrast MRI images are always acquired as T1-weighted MRI.

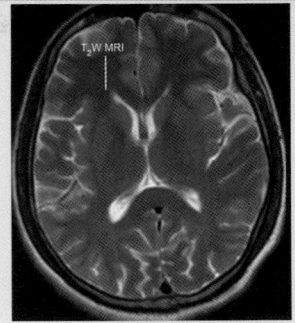
T2W axial image of brain

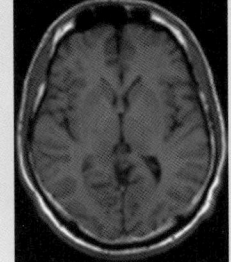
T1W axial image of brain

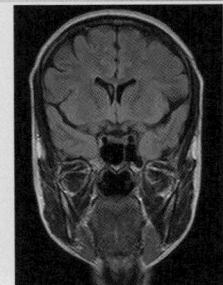
FLAIR coronal image of brain

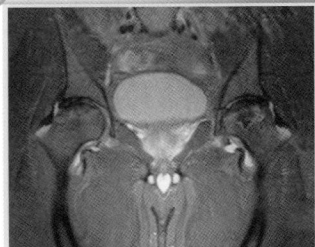
STIR coronal image of pelvis

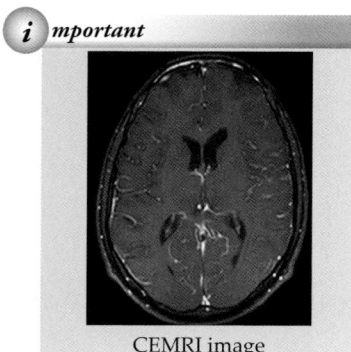
CEMRI image

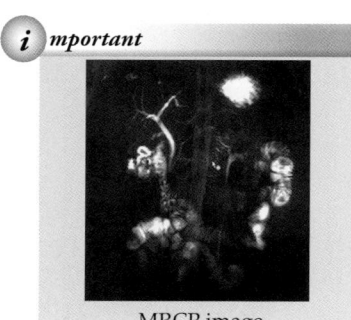
MRCP image

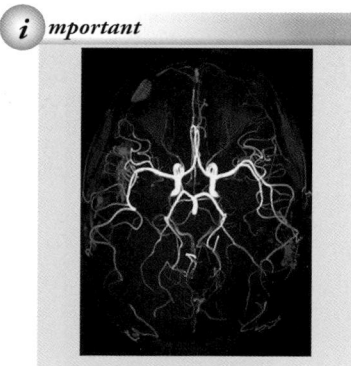
TOF MR angio image

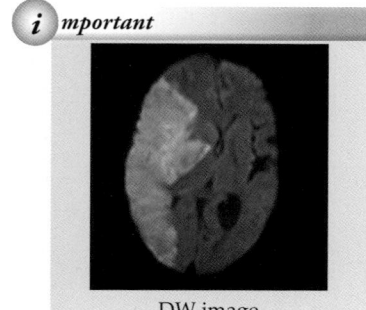
DW image

MRCP (Magnetic Resonance Cholangio-pancreatography)

MRCP images are heavily T2-weighted sequences which demonstrate fluid-filled structures as areas of very high signal intensity and are very commonly used to show the biliary and pancreatic ducts in magnetic resonance cholangiopancreatography (MRCP). Being non-invasive and no need of external contrast, it is considered as a preferred investigation to diagnose pathologies of biliary duct and pancreatic duct in comparison to diagnostic endoscopic retrograde cholangiopancreatography (ERCP).

MR Angiography

Visualization of vessels using MRI.

This technique is unique due to the fact that the beautiful angiographic images can be obtained without external administration of contrast. The technique used in MRI for angiography is called **TOF (time of flight)**. It is a very commonly used angiographic technique now days and is the preferred imaging technique to assess renal artery stenosis and an intracerebral aneurysm. It is also preferred investigation to look for carotid artery stenosis.

Diffusion Weighted MRI (DWI)

It is a special type of MRI technique which assesses the random (brownian) motion of the water molecule, which is a normal phenomenon. In some disease, there is reduction in the brownian motion of the water molecule, which is called as restricted diffusion. Areas of restricted diffusion are seen as white on DWI.

Common Causes of Restricted Diffusion

- Acute ischemic infarct (most common cause)
- Abscess
- High cellular tumors
- Epidermoid cyst
- Encephalitis

Gradient Echo Images

Used to see calcification and hamorrahge on MRI which show blooming on gradient images.

Spectroscopy

It is a new technique of MRI to assess certain metabolites in the body tissues. Metabolic changes occur earlier than the structural changes and since routine MRI picks up

structure changes, new techniques have been developed for the early diagnosis of the diseases. Commonly studied metabolites are:
- N acetyl aspertate (NAA)
  - Neuronal marker
  - Assess neural integrity
  - Decrease in most of the brain disorders except Canavan's disease
- Choline
  - Present in cell membrane
  - Marker of cell membrane turnover
  - Increased in malignancies
- Creatine
  - Present in ATP
  - Marker of energy stores
  - Reference marker, used to see the relative concentration of metabolites as it is a stable marker and doesn't change much during diseases.
- Lipid peak. Tuberculomas are rich in caseous necrosis and presence of lipid peak is a useful way to differentiate tuberculoma from cysticercosis which will be seen in tuberculoma and not in neurocysticercosis.

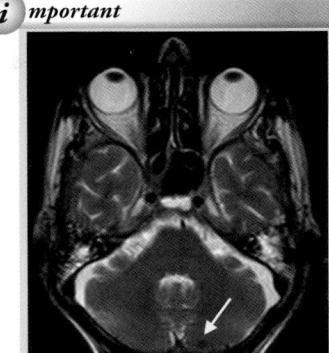

Axial T2 image showing a hypointense lesion in (L) cerebellar hemisphere

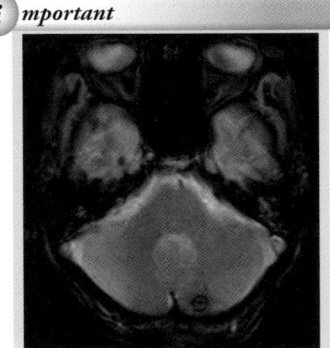

The lesion becomes enlarged in size on Gradient echo images and is much better appreciated

Functional MRI

Functional MRI (FMRI) is based on the principle that cerebral blood flow and neuronal activation are coupled. It measures brain activity by detecting changes associated with blood flow. Blood flow to a particular region of the brain increases once that area is put into use.

FMRI uses blood-oxygen-level dependent (BOLD) sequence. This sequence map neural activity in the brain by assessing the hemodynamic response (change in blood flow) related to energy use by brain cells. The technique is used to measure eloquent cortex of the brain like motor cortex, language area, visual cortex etc. by asking the subject to perform specific task. These task activates the specific area in the brain leading to hemodynamic changes which are picked up on these imaging sequences. The technique can localize activity to within millimeters and has lot of use in patients in preoperative workup to assess for postoperative outcomes.

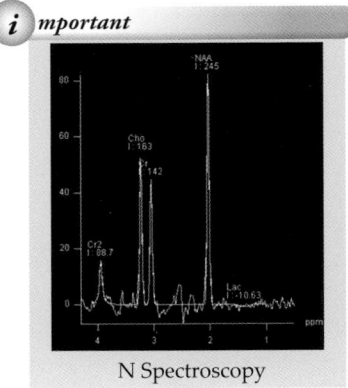

N Spectroscopy

MRI is Usually a Preferred Investigation for

- For all brain tumors (contrast enhanced MRI)
- For extent of pancoast tumor (due to neural involvement)

- Ventricular function (most accurate investigation)
- Posterior mediastinal mass (neurogenic in origin)
- Bony metastais in spine (bone scan is preferred at other places)
- Chronic subarachnoid hemorrahge
- Traumatic paraplegia due to neural involvement
- Extent of Pott's spine (for diagnosis Bx is the best)
- Stress fracture, Perthe's disease, avascular necrosis, early osteomyelitis (bone marrow edema)
- Pregnancy after first trimester (not for obstetrics problem but for other abdominal pathologies). For antenatal scanning, USG is still preferred over MRI
- Spinal cord pathologies
- Gynecological malignancies
- Uterine anomalies

important

Best MRI sequences to differentiate Epidermoid cyst/Arachnoid cyst
- DWI
- FLAIR

(DWI> FLAIR)

	MRI	CT Scan	USG
Ionizing radiation	No	Yes Moderate - high radiation	No
Principal	Magnetic moment of protons (gyro magnetism)	Linear attenuation of X-rays	Piezoelectric effect
Time for scanning	10 minutes to hour	Less than a minute	Variable
Bony details	Cortical bone is not well seen but bone marrow is very well seen	Cortical bone is very well seen	Not well seen. Structure posterior to bone are not seen due to acoustic shadowing
Soft tissue structure	Very well seen and differentiated	Seen but not well characterized	Very well seen
Multiplanar capability	Images can be acquired in any planes	Scans are acquired in axial planes and later can be reconstructed in any planes on MDCT	Yes depending on the position of the probe
Real time imaging	Mostly not	No	Yes
Portable	Usually not	Usually not	Yes
Cost	Very costly	Costly	Cheap

Contd...

General Radiology

	MRI	CT Scan	USG
Uses	• For neural tissues • For bone marrow • Cartilage • Ligaments • Tendons • Soft tissues	• Cortical bone • Acute hematoma in brain • Calculi • Calcifications • Air • Guiding biopsies in lung	• Fluid containing structures • Guiding biopsies

CONTRAST AGENTS IN RADIOLOGY

MRI CONTRAST AGENTS

Gadolinium chelates are most commonly used contrast agents in MRI studies. Due to lack of iodine, these compounds are relatively safe without any significant risk of anaphylaxis or allergic reactions unlike iodinated contrasts.

Being paramagnetic in nature, they predominantly acts by reduction of the T1 and T2 relaxation time.

The most common side effects of these agents are mild headache and a metallic taste.

Pregnant patients should not receive gadolinium chelates. Many of the agents are known to be able to cross the blood-placental barrier, and their effect on the fetus is unknown.

Nephrogenic systemic fibrosis is a scleroderma like dermatopathy that is known to precipitate due to use of gadolinium chelates in patients with compromised renal function.

Risk factors are:
- Increased dose of gadolinium
- Repeated doses
- Use of linear gadolinium chelates particularly gadodiamide (omniscan).

European Guidelines for Prevention of Nephrogenic Systemic Fibrosis

Patients at a high risk for nephrogenic systemic fibrosis
- Chronic kidney disease (CKD) and (GFR <30 mL/min), including those who require dialysis and those who have reduced renal function who have had or are awaiting renal transplant.

Low risk
- CKD 3 (GFR 30–59 mL/min) and
- Children younger than 1-year-old, because of their immature renal function.

> **important**
> Paramagnetic substances reduces both T1 and T2 relaxation time on MRI. Hence given oral for MRCP acquisition for better delineation of biliary system.

> **important**
> Gadolinium does not cross BBB.

> **important**
> Risk of Nephrogenic systemic fibrosis due to gadolinium is seen only in patients suffering from chronic kidney disease.

> **important**
> Gadolinium containing compounds are considered more nephrotoxic than iodinated compounds in equimolar concentration; however, the amount of gadolinium given is much less than iodinated contrast agents; hence, nephrotoxic side effects are not seen.

Not at risk
- Normal renal function

Contrast agents with highest risk for NSF
- Gadodiamide
- Gadopentetate dimeglumine
- Gadoversetamide

The use of these agents is contraindicated in patients who have CKD4 and 5 (GFR <30 mL/min), including those who require dialysis and patients who have reduced renal function who have had or are awaiting kidney transplantation.

They should be used with caution in patients who have CKD 3 (GFR 30–59 mL/min) and children younger than 1-year-old.

Serum creatinine (eGFR) levels should always be measured before using these three agents.

The intermediate-risk group includes the following agents:
- Gadobenate dimeglumine
- Gadofosveset trisodium
- Gadoxetate disodium

The determination of eGFR levels is not mandatory before using these agents.

The low-risk group includes the following agents:
- Gadobutrol
- Gadoterate meglumine
- Gadoteridol

The measurement of eGFR levels before administration is not mandatory.

USG CONTRAST AGENTS
- Gas filled microbubbles with diameter ranges from 0.1 to 10 μm.
- Inert gas enclosed in a phospholipidic, albumin, or polymer shell.

MOA
- Increases the backscattering echo intensity, proportional to the change in acoustic impedance between the blood, and the gas making the bubbles.
- Seen as an increase in color, power and spectral Doppler signal strength or gray scale image intensity, e.g. Albumex, levovist, echogen.

Uses
- In the liver
    - Characterization of focal liver lesions (most important role)

- Can detect flow in portal vein or collaterals in patients with cirrhosis
- Improves evaluation of TIPSS stent for patency and stenosis
- Small intrahepatic collaterals in patients with Budd-Chiari syndrome
• Better visualization of vessels in doppler.

IODINATED WATER SOLUBLE CONTRAST MEDIA

Name of the contrast agent	Iodinated water soluble contrast agents			
	Ionic monomers	Ionic dimers	Non-ionic monomers	Non-ionic dimers
Iodine particle ratio	3:2	6:2	3:1	6:1
Osmolality	HOCM	LOCM	LOCM	IOCM
e.g.	(UROGRAFFIN, GASTROGRAFFIN)- Diatrizoate -Iothalamate	-Ioxaglate	-Iohexol (IOHEXOL) -Iomeron -Iopamidol -Ipromide -Ioversol -Xenetix	-Iodixanol (VISIPAQUE)
Uses	Preferred for non vascular use	Not available	Most preferred contrast for vascular administration	-The best for patients with associated renal disease

> **important**
> Note: At least 100 mL of air required to cause air embolism but in USG-contrast we give only 0.5 mL air.

Contrast Reactions
• Idiosyncratic anaphylactoid reactions (DOC is adrenaline)
• Non-idiosyncratic reactions.

Contrast-induced Nephropathy
Contrast-induced nephrotoxicity (CIN) is a sudden deterioration in renal function following the recent intravascular administration of iodinated contrast medium in the absence of another nephrotoxic event.

> **important**
> Adrenaline is usually given through I/M or deep S/C route in patients of anaphylaxis because of risk of arrhythmia with I/V adrenaline unless patients is in severe hypotension when I/V adrenaline is given.

Diagnosis
There are no standard criteria for the diagnosis of CIN; criteria used in the past have included percent change in

the baseline serum creatinine (an increase of variously 25% to 50%) and absolute elevation from baseline serum creatinine (e.g., an increase of variously 0.5 to 2.0 mg/dL). One of the most commonly used criteria has been an absolute increase of 0.5 mg/dL.

Pathogenesis

The exact pathophysiology of CIN is not understood and the Nephrotoxicity of contrast media is likely to be due to decreased renal perfusion due to renal vasoconstriction due to high osmolality of the contrast media.

Symptoms: Usually asymptomatic. Creatinine peaks in 3–5 days. In severe oliguric patients: peaks in 5–7 days.

Risk Factors for CIN

- Pre-existing renal impairment (S.creat > 1.3 mg/dL, GFR < 60 mL/min)
- Dehydration
- CHF
- Use of nephrotoxic drugs (NSAID, aminoglycosides)
- Hypersensitivity disease (multiple myeloma)
- Hypertension
- Hyperuricemia (as in active gout)
- Proteinuria (> 0.5 gm/dL)
- DM, age > 70 years

Prevention of Contrast-induced Nephropathy in High Risk Patients

- *Avoidance of Iodinated Contrast Medium:*
- *Contrast media selection: Increased osmotic overload on the diseased kidney is considered to be the major etiology of CIN so; these can be significantly reduced by substituting IOCM/LOCM for the very hypertonic HOCM.*
- ***Hydration: Adequate hydration is considered to be the single most effective way to prevent CIN.*** *The ideal infusion rate and volume is unknown. One possible protocol would be 0.9% saline at 100 mL/hr, beginning 6 to 12 hours before and continuing 4 to 12 hours after intravascular iodinated contrast medium administration. Oral hydration has also been utilized, but with less demonstrated effectiveness.*
- *Sodium bicarbonate: It has been found to be useful in prevention from CIN according to some studies.*
- *N-acetylcysteine: The role is controversial. There is evidence that it reduces serum creatinine in normal volunteers without changing cystatin-C (cystatin-C is*

> **important**
> As per Harrison, CIN is defined as increase in S.Cr by > 1.0 mg/dL. *Ref: P.440e-2*

> **important**
> Most effective way to prevent CIN is adequate hydration of the patients with I/V normal saline.

reported to be a better marker of GFR than serum creatinine). This raises the possibility that N-acetylcysteine might be simply lowering serum creatinine without actually preventing renal injury. N-acetylcysteine should not be considered a substitute for appropriate pre-procedural patient screening and adequate hydration.
- **Diuretics: Mannitol and Furosemide:** There is no reported benefit and neither mannitol nor furosemide is recommended for CIN risk reduction.
- **Other Agents:** The evidence for other theoretically renal-protective medications, such as theophylline, endothelin-1, and fenoldopam is even less convincing. Use of these agents to reduce the risk of CIN is not recommended.
- Hemodialysis has not shown to be of much effect in prevention from CIN. Hemofiltration has some benefit.

Patient on Metformin

Remember: Metformin + Chronic Renal Insufficiency + I/V contrast = Lactic Acidosis

Category 1	Category 2	Category 3
Normal renal function with no known co-morbidities No reason to discontinue Metformin	Normal renal function with known co-morbidities +, then suspend Metformin for 48 hrs If the patient had normal renal function at baseline, was clinically stable, and had no intercurrent risk factors for renal damage (e.g. treatment with aminoglycosides, major surgery, heart failure, sepsis, repeat administration of large amounts of contrast media), metformin can be restarted	Renal dysfunction then suspend Metformin for 48 hrs and restart only if repeat KFT is normal

BARIUM STUDIES

Barium sulfate is commonly used for evaluation of GIT because it is an inert substance and not absorbed from the GIT. It also causes mucosal coating and helps in assessing mucosal details.

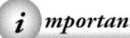

Important

For suspected esophageal perforation, though $BaSO_4$ is the best contrast agent. However, iodinated water soluble contrast agents are usually the agent of choice and once a large perforation is ruled out using these, dilute $BaSO_4$ may be used to assess small perforation.

- **Barium swallow:** Done for dysphagia to rule out stricture or mass. Replaced by endoscopy for these indications. Now commonly done for motility disorder.
- **Barium meal:** Abdominal pain (to rule out gastric or duodenal ulcer disease), replaced by endoscopy.
- **Small bowel follow-through:** Diarrhea or constipation (to rule out Crohn's disease or other small bowel pathologic conditions). Replaced by barium enteroclysis commonly called as small bowel enema and now a days with another technique called as CT enterography.
- **Barium enema:** Rectal bleeding (to rule out a polyp or mass). Still performed but at some places, CT virtual colonoscopy is done.

Contraindications of Barium Sulfate in GIT Studies

- Small bowel obstruction (ionic contrast are preferred)
- Intestinal perforation (ionic contrasts are preferred)
- Tracheoesophageal fistula (non-ionic contrasts are preferred because of the risk of pulmonary edema with ionic contrast due to very high osmolarity).

Myelography

- Contrast agent is injected into the SUBARACHNOID space following a lumbar puncture.
- Non-ionic contrast agents are preferred due to the risk of arachnoiditis with previously used contrast agents.
- Most common side effect of myelography is headache
- Most severe side effect is arachnoiditis.

QUESTIONS

1. CT or Hounsfield numbers depend upon:
   a. Mass density
   b. Electron density
   c. Atomic number
   d. Atomic mass

2. Which of the following statement is true?
   a. By reducing KVP by 50% radiation dose is reduced to half
   b. In pediatric patients dose should be reduced
   c. CT dose index is not useful for control exposure in multislice CT
   d. kV has no control over CT dose index

3. Which artery is dissected most commonly following arteriography by femoral route?
   a. Celiac trunk
   b. Superior mesenteric artery
   c. Inferior mesenteric artery
   d. Gastroduodenal artery

4. Earliest investigation for diagnosis of Ankylosing spondylitis:
   a. MRI STIR sequence
   b. Bone scan
   c. CT scan
   d. X-ray
   e. USG

5. How much area is covered by spiral CT in 30 seconds?
   a. Entire organ
   b. Entire abdomen
   c. Entire trunk
   d. Whole body

6. In CT scan, Hounsfield units depends on:
   a. Electron density
   b. Mass density
   c. Effective atomic number
   d. Linear attenuation coefficient

7. X-ray view of choice for lumbar spondylosis is/are:
   a. PA view
   b. PA view
   c. Lateral view
   d. Left oblique view
   e. Right oblique view

8. High resolution CT of the lung is a specialized CT technique for greater detail of lung parenchyma and it utilizes:
   a. Special lung filters
   b. Thick collimation
   c. Bone algorithm for image reconstruction
   d. Large filed of view

9. Which of the following is non-ionising radiation?
   a. X-ray   b. β-rays
   c. α-rays   d. Microwave
   e. γ-rays

10. Time sector scanning of neonates is preferred because of the following reason. Most practical reason:
    a. Open fontanelles
    b. Inexpensive
    c. Children more co-operative
    d. Better resolution

11. PET stands for:
    a. Positive electron tomography
    b. Proton-electron therapy
    c. Positron emission tomography
    d. Photon emitting tomography

12. What modification is needed for proper radiographic image in a heavy bony built person?
    a. ↑ed ma   b. ↑kvp
    c. ↑ed exposure time
    d. ↑ed developing time

13. Maximum radiation exposure occurs in:
    a. Bone scan   b. X-ray
    c. MRI   d. CT scan
14. USG is definitive investigation of:
    a. Vasa previa
    b. Abruption placenta
    c. Placenta previa
    d. Imperforate hymen
15. Investigation of choice in whole body imaging in metastasis is:
    a. Magnetic resonance imaging
    b. Angiography
    c. Venography
    d. PET scan
16. Gyromagnetic property of proton is seen in:
    a. MRI   b. CT
    c. PET scan   d. USG
17. Most reliable test for spinal tuberculosis:
    a. Raised ESR
    b. PPD skin test
    c. CT guided biopsy
    d. MRI
18. In magnetic resonance imaging, paramagnetic substances cause:
    a. Shortening of both T1 and T2 relaxation times
    b. Shortening of T2 relaxation time only
    c. Shortening of T1 relaxation time only
    d. No effect on T1 or T2 relaxation times
19. SI unit of absorbed dose of radiation is:
    a. Roentgen   b. Gray
    c. Sievert   d. Coulomb
20. Frequency of ultrasound waves in USG:
    a. 2000 Hz   b. 5000 Hz
    c. <2 MHz   d. >2 MHz
21. Which of the following is a non-Iodine containing contrast?
    a. Gadolinium   b. Visipaque
    c. Iopamidol   d. Diatrizoate
22. In computed tomography (CT), the attenuation value are measured in Hounsfield units (HU). An attenuation value of '0' (zero) HU corresponds to:
    a. Water
    b. Very dense bone structure
    c. AIR
    d. Fat
23. The best contrast to perform an IVU in the contemporary era is:
    a. Iodinated ionic water soluble contrast
    b. Iodinated nonionic water soluble contrast
    c. Gadolinium based contrast
    d. Lipidol
24. All of the following are true about iodinated intravascular contrast media except:
    a. They are used in digital subtraction angiography
    b. They are radio-opaque
    c. They can cause anaphylactic reactions
    d. They are used in magnetic resonance imaging
    e. They are excreted mainly by the kidneys
25. BIRADS stands for:
    a. Breast imaging reporting and data system
    b. Best imaging reporting and data system
    c. Brain imaging reporting and data system
    d. Breast investigation reporting and data system

26. Doppler effect is due to:
    a. Change in frequency in relation to the movement of source or observer
    b. Change in attenuation
    c. Change in absorption
    d. Change in reverberation
27. Diagnosis of pulmonary embolism is primarily made by:
    a. Multidetector CT contrast
    b. Angiography
    c. Ventilation perfusion scan
    d. CXR
28. Alpha particle is similar to:
    a. Electron   b. Proton
    c. Neutron   d. Helium nucleus
29. Neural tube defect is best detected by:
    a. USG
    b. Chromosomal analysis
    c. Amniocentesis
    d. Placentography
30. Light rays and X-rays have same:
    a. Velocity
    b. Wavelength
    c. Energy
    d. Frequency
31. The magnetic field in a MRI machine is measured in:
    a. Hounsfield unit
    b. Tesla
    c. Watt/sec
    d. None of the above
32. The basic principle behind ultrasound probe technology is:
    a. Piezoelectric effect
    b. Photoelectric effect
    c. Calorimetric effect
    d. Raman effect
33. PACS in medical imaging stands for:
    a. Portal archiving common system
    b. Photo archiving computerized system
    c. Picture archiving communication system
    d. Planning archiving communication scheme
34. Wavelength of light is:
    a. 400–700 nm   b. 700–800 nm
    c. 700–900 nm   d. 300–600 nm
35. CAT was invented by:
    a. Hounsfield   b. Roentgen
    c. Cormack   d. Tesla
36. The study using barium for small intestine is known as:
    a. Barium meal follow through
    b. Barium swallow
    c. Barium enema
    d. None of the above
37. Which is not echogenic while doing ultrasonography?
    a. Bile   b. Gas
    c. Bone   d. Gallstones
38. The dark areas in a conventional radiographic film are due to particulate deposits of:
    a. Carbon   b. Iron
    c. Silver   d. Copper
39. IV contrast is not used in:
    a. CECT   b. MRI
    c. IVP   d. Myelography
40. Maximum scattering in X-ray plate occurs in:
    a. Carbon   b. Mercury
    c. H$^+$ d. Ca^{++}
41. Radiation produced by nuclear decay/disintegration:
    a. Gamma rays
    b. X-rays
    c. Proton beam
    d. Cosmic rays
42. Contrast used in CT:
    a. Gadolinium
    b. Technetium
    c. Iodine
    d. Chromium

43. Investigation of choice to see gallbladder:
    a. CT
    b. USG
    c. Plain X-ray
    d. Oral cholecystogram
44. Radiocontrast is contraindicated in all except:
    a. Renal failure
    b. History of previous severe allergic reaction
    c. Dehydration
    d. Morbid obesity
45. The wavelength of X-ray is:
    a. Greater than that of light
    b. Lesser than that of light
    c. Equal to that of light
    d. None of the above
46. Slice of tissue X-rays is:
    a. Tomography
    b. Mammography
    c. Contrast studies
    d. All of the above
47. Contrast agent used in PET scan is:
    a. FDG
    b. Gallium
    c. Gadolinium
    d. Iodine
48. In which of the following form of imaging, harmonic imaging is related:
    a. Sonography
    b. Digital radiography
    c. MRCP
    d. Nuclear imaging
49. Not a contraindication to MRI is:
    a. Cochlear prosthesis
    b. Foley's catheter
    c. Penile implants
    d. Metallic intraocular implants
50. The CT scanner room are coated with:
    a. Lead
    b. Glass
    c. Tungsten
    d. Iron
51. "Time of Flight" technique is employed in:
    a. Spiral CT
    b. MR angiography
    c. CT angiography
    d. Digital radiography
52. Which of the following is not ionizing?
    a. Beta radiation
    b. Alpha radiation
    c. Gamma radiation
    d. UV radiation
53. USG wave travel in human body at the rate of:
    a. 1500 m/s
    b. 2500 m/s
    c. 3500 m/s
    d. None of above
54. Rad is burned to produce:
    a. 10 ergs/g
    b. 100 ergs/g
    c. 0.1 erg/g
    d. 1000 ergs/kg
55. Ultrasound frequency used for diagnostic purposes in obstetrics:
    a. 1–20 MHz
    b. 20–40 MHz
    c. 40–60 MHz
    d. 60–80 MHz
    e. 80–100 MHz
56. All of them use nonionizing radiation except:
    a. Ultrasonography
    b. Thermography
    c. MRI
    d. Radiography
57. Most important interaction for X-ray production in mammography:
    a. Characteristic radiation
    b. Thermography
    c. Campton effect
    d. Bremsstrahlung effect
58. X-rays are modified:
    a. Protons
    b. Electrons
    c. Neutrons
    d. Positrons

59. Contrast in X-rays is predominantly dependent on:
    a. kV
    b. MA
    c. Duration of exposure
    d. Distance between source and object
60. Negative contrast medium is:
    a. Difficult for X-rays to penetrate
    b. Easily penetrated by X-rays
    c. High in atomic number
    d. Opaque to X-rays
61. The contract used for MRI includes:
    a. Perfluorocarbons
    b. Ferric ammonium citrate
    c. Gadolinium diethylmethylamine
    d. All of the above
62. NMR based in the principle of:
    a. Electron beam
    b. Proton beam
    c. Magnetic field
    d. Neutron beam
63. MRI is not better than CT for detection of:
    a. Ligament injury
    b. Soft tissue tumors
    c. Meningeal pathology
    d. Calcified lesions
64. All of the following about MRI are correct except:
    a. MRI is contraindicated in patients with pacemakers
    b. MRI is useful for evaluating bone marrow
    c. MRI is better for calcified lesions
    d. MRI is useful for localizing small lesions in the brain
65. Patient with a metallic foreign body which investigation is not done:
    a. MRI
    b. USG
    c. X-ray
    d. CT
66. The EEG cabins should be completely shielded by continuous sheet of wire mesh of copper to avoid the noise from external electromagnetic disturbances. Such a shielding is called as:
    a. Maxwen cage
    b. Edison's cage
    c. Faraday cage
    d. Ohm's cage
67. Ionizing radiation is the substance which ionizes the atoms when it passes. It is harmful for biological matter. Which of the following is non-ionizing modality?
    a. Conventional X-rays
    b. Computerized tomography
    c. Magnetic resonance imaging
    d. Isotopic scanning
68. Investigation of choice for focal neurologic deficit in emergency room is:
    a. CT
    b. MRI
    c. Lumbar puncture
    d. USG
69. Fracture of nose, which view X-ray taken:
    a. Waters view
    b. Caldwell's view
    c. Lateral view
    d. Occlusive anterior view
70. Which of the following statements about contrast in radiography is true?
    a. Ionic monomers have three iodine atoms per two particles in solution
    b. High osmolar contrast agents may be ionic or nonionic
    c. Gadolinium may cross the blood brain barrier
    d. Iohexol is a high osmolar contrast media

71. Doppler effect results from change in:
    a. Amplitude of sound
    b. Frequency of sound
    c. Direction of sound
    d. None of the above
72. Investigation of choice for subdural hemorrhage is:
    a. Angiography
    b. NCCT
    c. CECT
    d. MRI
73. Which of the following contrast agents is preferred in a patient with decreased renal function to avoid contrast nephropathy?
    a. Acetylcysteine
    b. Fenoldopam
    c. Mannitol
    d. Low osmolar contrast
74. High resolution computed tomography of the chest is the ideal modality for evaluating:
    a. Pleural effusion
    b. Interstitial lung disease
    c. Lung mass
    d. Mediastinal adenopathy
75. Investigation of choice in congenital uterine anomaly is:
    a. MRI   b. CT
    c. HSG   d. Hysteroscopy
76. Best investigation for pericardial effusion is:
    a. MRI
    b. CT
    c. X-ray
    d. Echocardiography
77. Barium swallow is used for:
    a. Colon   b. Esophagus
    c. Duodenum   d. Jejunum
78. Rhese view is used for:
    a. Superior orbital fissure
    b. Inferior orbital fissure
    c. Optic foramen
    d. Sella turcica
79. Becquerel is equal (disintegration/sec) to:
    a. 3.7×10^{10} b. 2.7×10^{10}
    c. 1.7×10^{10} d. 3.7×10^{-2}
    e. 1
80. Which one of the following has the maximum ionization potential?
    a. Electron   b. Proton
    c. Helium ion   d. Gamma-Photon
81. Which of the following techniques uses Piezo-electric effect?
    a. MR spectroscopy
    b. Xeroradiography
    c. Ultrasonography
    d. Conventional tomography
82. Investigation of choice in choledocholithiasis:
    a. CT   b. PET scan
    c. USG   d. MRCP
83. Investigation of choice for DVT is:
    a. Doppler USG
    b. Angiography
    c. CT scan
    d. MRI
84. An 8-year-old child was injected contrast in hand for CECT chest. Immediately he developed swelling in the arm which gradually increased. After 4 hours, there was numbness and pain, and he was not allowing the doctor to flex the hand. Pulse is present. What should be done?
    a. High dose prednisolone
    b. Arterial thrombectomy
    c. Immediate fasciotomy
    d. Angiography
85. Use of water-soluble contrast medium is done for:
    a. Constipation
    b. Perforation
    c. Ileocecal tuberculosis
    d. Gastroesophageal reflux

86. Which of the following liver metastasis appears hypoechoic on ultrasonography?
    a. Breast cancer
    b. Colon cancer
    c. Renal cancer
    d. Mucinous adenocarcinoma
87. X-ray artifact is:
    a. A radiolucent area
    b. Any abnormal opacity in the radiograph
    c. Produced when patient moves while taking the shoot
    d. Any of the above
88. Decubitus view is useful in diagnosing:
    a. Pleural effusion
    b. Pleural effusion with dependent hemithorax
    c. Pericardial effusion
    d. Middle lobe consolidation
89. X-rays were discovered by:
    a. Godfrey Hounsfield
    b. Roentgen
    c. Coulomb
    d. Sievert
90. Grid is a device used for:
    a. Reducing scattered radiation
    b. Reducing patient's exposure time
    c. Reducing the contrast of the X-ray
    d. All of the above
91. The active ingredient of X-ray film is:
    a. Silver chloride
    b. Silver bromide
    c. Silver nitrate
    d. Gold chloride
92. The best X-ray view for minimal pleural effusion:
    a. AP   b. PA
    c. Lateral   d. Lateral decubitus
93. Half life of Tc99 is:
    a. 6 hours   b. 3 days
    c. 10 months   d. 12 years
94. Interlobar pleural effusion can be detected in best way in:
    a. Lateral decubitus
    b. Reverse lordotic
    c. Lateral oblique
    d. Posterior oblique
95. Piezoelectric crystals are made use of in which modality that is safe from radiation also?
    a. MRI   b. US
    c. CT   d. All of above
96. Radioisotope used in PET scan is:
    a. Technetium 99m
    b. Iodine 123
    c. Iodine 131
    d. Fluoride 18
97. Most common radiological feature of sarcoidosis in Indian patients:
    a. Normal chest X-ray
    b. Bilateral hilar lymphadenopathy
    c. Bilateral hilar lymphadenopathy with parenchymal infiltrate
    d. Only parenchymal infiltrate
98. Which one of the following imaging modalities is most sensitive for evaluation of extra-adrenal Pheochromocytoma?
    a. Ultrasound
    b. CT
    c. MRI
    d. MIBG scan
99. The diagnostic procedure not done in case of pheochromocytoma:
    a. CT scan   b. MRI
    c. FNAC   d. MIBG scan
100. True about electromagnetic radiations are all except:
    a. Pair production occur for low energy
    b. Infrared is an EM radiation
    c. Compton scattering occur for intermediate energy
    d. X-ray is EM radiation

101. Earliest diagnosis of cerbral infarct can be done by:
    a. NCCT
    b. CECT
    c. Diffusion weighted MRI
    d. FLAIR MRI
102. Best investigation for diagnosing abdominal aortic aneurysm is:
    a. USG
    b. CT angiography
    c. Classical radiography
    d. Noncontrast CT scan
103. Fluorescein angiography is used to examine:
    a. Ciliary vasculature
    b. Retinal vasculature
    c. Corneal vasculature
    d. Conjunctival vasculature
104. Hounsfield unit of fat ranges from:
    a. 1 to 20   b. 100–1000
    c. −10 to −100   d. 100–300
105. Chest X-ray, most common view is:
    a. AP   b. PA
    c. RAO   d. LAO
106. Which of the following is the gold standard for imaging of swallowing disorders?
    a. Dynamic MRI
    b. Barium swallow
    c. Video fluoroscopy
    d. X-ray
107. 1 Gray is equal to:
    a. 1 Roentgen   b. 1 Rad
    c. 100 Rad   d. 1 Rem
108. Inferior rib notching is seen in:
    a. Coarctation of aorta
    b. SLE
    c. RA
    d. Scleroderma
109. Most sensitive test for ureteric stone is:
    a. CECT   b. MRI
    c. USG   d. NCCT
110. Contrasts used in USG:
    a. Urograffin   b. Ultragraffin
    c. Sonavist   d. Conray
    e. Barium
111. Best view for collapse of middle lobe lung is:
    a. Lateral
    b. AP
    c. Oblique
    d. Lordotic
112. On imaging diffuse axonal injury is characterized by:
    a. Multiple small petechial hemorrhage
    b. Patch ill, defined low density lesion mixed with small hyperdense petechial hemorrhage
    c. Crescentic extra-axial hematoma
    d. White matter lucencies
113. Miliary nodules are seen in all except:
    a. Silicosis
    b. TB
    c. Aspergillosis
    d. Anthracosis
114. Hour glass appearance of stomach is seen in:
    a. Linitis plastica
    b. Gastric ulcer
    c. Duodenal ulcer
    d. Gastric carcinoma
115. Which of the following is the investigation of choice for dissecting aortic aneurysm?
    a. CECT   b. PET
    c. MRI   d. TEE
116. Ultrasonogram is the primary modality of choice in obstetrics and in surgery. Frequency of the ultrasound used to image the breast, thyroid and testis are:
    a. 2–5 MHz   b. 5–10 MHz
    c. 1–2 MHz   d. 20–25 MHz

117. In a 90-year-old man with pyonephrosis and with pacemaker and Sr. creatinine of 3 mg/dL, which of the following should be used:
    a. CECT b. NCCT
    c. MRI   d. X-ray

118. Endoscopic ultrasound is not very useful for:
    a. Evaluating the extent of disease in GI malignancy
    b. Choledocholithiasis
    c. Evaluation of severity of enteritis
    d. Drainage of pancreatic pseudocyst

119. Duplex ultrasonography combines:
    a. A-mode imaging and pulse-wave Doppler examination
    b. B-mode imaging and pulse-wave Doppler examination
    c. M-mode imaging and power Doppler examination
    d. M-mode imaging and waveform analysis

120. What would be the contrast of choice in esophageal perforation?
    a. Barium sulphate
    b. Gadolinium
    c. Iohexol
    d. Tc99m

121. Bragg's peak effect is due to:
    a. Proton   b. Neutron
    c. Electron d. X-rays

Multiple Correct Questions

122. Energy linear acceleration used in:
    a. X-ray   b. Cathode rays
    c. Photon rays d. α-rays
    e. γ-rays

123. Which of the following do not use radiation?
    a. MRI b. CT
    c. USG d. SPECT
    e. PET

124. True about virtual colonoscopy are A/E:
    a. Provide endoluminal view
    b. Biopsy can be taken
    c. CT and MRI used
    d. Used even when conventional colonoscopy fails
    e. Used for screening of carcinoma-colon

125. Radiological findings of eosinophilic granuloma is/are:
    a. Hilar involvement
    b. Miliary shadowing
    c. Honey comb appearance
    d. White out lung
    e. Splitting of pleura

126. Tracheal bifurcation on X-ray corsponds to:
    a. T5T6
    b. T4T5
    c. Sternal angle
    d. Thoracic inlet

127. Radiation hazard is absent in:
    a. MRI
    b. Doppler USG
    c. Digital substraction angiography
    d. Tc 99 scan

128. Attenuation value (Hounsfield unit) of < zero (i.e. negative) on CT is seen in:
    a. Muscle b. Bone
    c. Fat   d. Air
    e. Blood

129. Which of the following statements about stochastic effects of radiation is true?
    a. Severity of effect is a function of dose
    b. Probability of effect is a function of dose
    c. It has a threshold
    d. Erythema and cataract are common examples

Recently Asked Questions

130. Colour flow Doppler study of femoral vein shows?
    a. Biphasic flow
    b. Monophasic flow
    c. Triphasic flow
    d. Turbulent flow

131. What would be the contrast of choice in esophageal perforation ?
    a. Barium sulphate
    b. Gadolinium
    c. Iohexol
    d. Tc99m

132. Which of the following Ix does not have ionising radiation:
    a. X-ray
    b. MRI
    c. Angiography
    d. CT

ANSWERS

1. **Ans. a.** Mass density
2. **Ans. b.** In pediatric patients dose should be reduced
3. **Ans. c.** Inferior mesenteric artery
4. **Ans. a.** MRI STIR sequence
5. **Ans. d.** Whole body
6. **Ans. d.** Linear attenuation coefficient (d > b)
7. **Ans. c.** Lateral view
8. **Ans. c.** Bone algorithm for image reconstruction
9. **Ans. d.** Microwave
10. **Ans. a.** Open fontanelles
11. **Ans. c.** Positron emission tomography
12. **Ans. b.** ↑kvp
13. **Ans. d.** CT scan. *Its a wrongly framed question friends, idealy the body part of CT should have been mentioned.*
14. **Ans. c.** Placenta previa
15. **Ans. d.** PET scan
16. **Ans. a.** MRI
17. **Ans. c.** CT guided biopsy
18. **Ans. a.** Shortening of both T1 and T2 relaxation times
19. **Ans. b.** Gray
20. **Ans. d.** >2 MHz
21. **Ans. a.** Gadolinium
22. **Ans. a.** Water
23. **Ans. b.** Iodinated nonionic water soluble contrast
24. **Ans. d.** They are used in magnetic resonance imaging
25. **Ans. a.** Breast imaging reporting and data system
26. **Ans. a.** Change in frequency in relation to the movement of source or observer
27. **Ans. a.** Multidetector CT contrast
28. **Ans. d.** Helium nucleus
29. **Ans. a.** USG
30. **Ans. a.** Velocity
31. **Ans. b.** Tesla
32. **Ans. a.** Piezoelectric effect
33. **Ans. c.** Picture archiving communication system
34. **Ans. a.** 400–700 nm
35. **Ans. a.** Hounsfield
36. **Ans. a.** Barium meal follow through
37. **Ans. a.** Bile
38. **Ans. c.** Silver
39. **Ans. d.** Myelography
40. **Ans. b.** Mercury

As we all know that Scattering of the radiation is the function of Compton effect and Compton effect is proportional to the no of electron per unit volume which is equal to no of electron/ volume = physical density (m/v) × electron density (number of electrons per unit mass).

Electrone density is proportional to Z/A (as number of atoms per unit mass is proportional to 1/A and number of electrons per atom is proportional to Z)

A- is atomic mass, Z is atomic number.

Electrone density is maximum for H^+ (Z/A = 1/1), while rest of the elements have Z/A ~ 0.5.

Physical density of various elements are as follows:

Mercury	–	13.5 gm/cm^3
Hydrogen	–	0.000082
Carbon	–	3.513 (diamond); 2.2 (graphite)
Calcium	–	1.54

So if we look at the combine picture, though hydrogen has most favorable Z/A ratio for Compton effect, the difference in mass density is so much that virtually,

Compton effect become proportional to the mass density.
Hence the answer should be Mercury (Hg).

41. **Ans. a.** Gamma rays
42. **Ans. c.** Iodine
43. **Ans. b.** USG
44. **Ans. d.** Morbid obesity
45. **Ans. b.** Lesser than that of light
46. **Ans. a.** Tomography
47. **Ans. a.** FDG
48. **Ans. a.** Sonography
49. **Ans. b.** Foley's catheter
50. **Ans. a.** Lead
51. **Ans. b.** MR angiography
52. **Ans. d.** UV radiation
53. **Ans. a.** 1500 m/s
54. **Ans. b.** 100 ergs/g
55. **Ans. a.** 1-20 MHz
56. **Ans. d.** Radiography
57. **Ans. a.** Characteristic radiation
58. **Ans. b.** Electrons
59. **Ans. a.** kV
60. **Ans. b.** Easily penetrated by X-rays
61. **Ans. c.** Gadolinium diethylmethylamine
62. **Ans. b.** Proton beam
63. **Ans. d.** Calcified lesions
64. **Ans. c.** MRI is better for calcified lesions
65. **Ans. a.** MRI
66. **Ans. c.** Faraday cage
67. **Ans. c.** Magnetic resonance imaging
68. **Ans. a.** CT
69. **Ans. c.** Lateral view
70. **Ans. a.** Ionic monomers have three iodine atoms per two particles in solution
71. **Ans. b.** Frequency of sound
72. **Ans. b.** NCCT
73. **Ans. d.** Low osmolar contrast
74. **Ans. b.** Interstitial lung disease
75. **Ans. a.** MRI
76. **Ans. d.** Echocardiography
77. **Ans. b.** Esophagus
78. **Ans. c.** Optic foramen
79. **Ans. e.** 1
80. **Ans. c.** Helium ion
81. **Ans. c.** Ultrasonography
82. **Ans. d.** MRCP
83. **Ans. a.** Doppler USG
84. **Ans. c.** Immediate fasciotomy
85. **Ans. b.** Perforation
86. **Ans. a.** Breast cancer
87. **Ans. c.** Produced when patient moves while taking the shoot
88. **Ans. b.** Pleural effusion with dependent hemithorax
89. **Ans. b.** Roentgen
90. **Ans. a.** Reducing scattered radiation
91. **Ans. b.** Silver bromide
92. **Ans. d.** Lateral decubitus
93. **Ans. a.** 6 hours
94. **Ans. b.** Reverse lordotic
95. **Ans. b.** US
96. **Ans. d.** Fluoride 18
97. **Ans. b.** Bilateral hilar lymphadenopathy
98. **Ans. d.** MIBG scan
99. **Ans. c.** FNAC
100. **Ans. a.** Pair production occur for low energy
101. **Ans. c.** Diffusion weighted MRI
102. **Ans. b.** CT angiography
103. **Ans. b.** Retinal vasculature
104. **Ans. c.** −10 to −100
105. **Ans. b.** PA
106. **Ans. c.** Video fluoroscopy
107. **Ans. c.** 100 Rad
108. **Ans. a.** Coarctation of aorta
109. **Ans. d.** NCCT
110. **Ans. c.** Sonavist

111. **Ans. d.** Lordotic
112. **Ans. b.** Patch ill, defined low density lesion mixed with small hyperdense petechial hemorrhage
113. **Ans. c.** Aspergillosis
114. **Ans. b.** Gastric ulcer
115. **Ans. a.** CECT
116. **Ans. b.** 5–10 MHz
117. **Ans. b.** NCCT
118. **Ans. c.** Evaluation of severity of enteritis
119. **Ans. b.** B-mode imaging and pulse-wave Doppler examination
120. **Ans. c.** Iohexol
121. **Ans. a.** Proton

Multiple Correct Answers

122. **Ans. a.** X-ray, **b.** Cathode rays
123. **Ans. a.** MRI, **c.** USG
124. **Ans. b.** Biopsy can be taken
125. **Ans. a.** Hilar involvement, **b.** Miliary shadowing, **c.** Honey comb appearance, **d.** White out lung, **e.** Splitting of pleura
126. **Ans. b.** T4T5

   Most of the standard radiology textbooks and 40th edition of Gray's anatomy says the bifurcation is at T4T5 level which however descend to T6 level on deep inspiration.

   41st edition of Gray's anatomy says that bifurcation is at upper half of T6 vertebra level which however descend to T6 level on deep inspiration which looks like a controversial statement.

127. **Ans. a.** MRI, **b.** Doppler USG
128. **Ans. c.** Fat, **d.** Air
129. **Ans. b.** Probability of effect is a function of dose

Answers of Recently Asked Questions

130. **Ans. b.** Monophasic flow
131. **Ans. c.** Iohexol
132. **Ans. b.** MRI

SECTION B

SYSTEMIC RADIOLOGY

- Neuroradiology
- Cardiothoracic Radiology
- Gastrointestinal and Genitourinary System
- Musculoskeletal Radiology

CHAPTER 2

Neuroradiology

NCCT-Non-contrast CT	SAH-Subarachnoid hemorrhage
SDH-Subdural hemorrhage	EDH-Extradural hemorrhage
IOC-Investigation of choice	D/d-Differential diagnosis

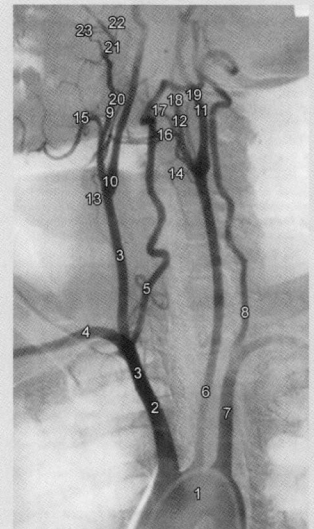

1. Arch of aorta
2. Brachiocephalic trunk
3. Right common carotid artery (superimposed upon the subclavian artery)
4. Right subclavian artery
5. Right vertebral artery
6. Left common carotid artery
7. Left subclavian artery
8. Left vertebral artery
9. Right external carotid artery
10. Sinus of right internal carotid artery
11. Left internal carotid artery
12. Left external carotid artery
13. Right superior thyroid artery (arising from the external carotid artery)
14. Left superior thyroid artery (arising from common carotid artery)
15. Right lingual artery
16. Left lingual artery
17. Left facial artery
18. Left ascending pharyngeal artery
19. Left posterior auricular artery
20. Right posterior auricular artery
21. Right maxillary artery
22. Middle meningeal artery (branch of right maxillary artery)
23. Right superficial temporal artery

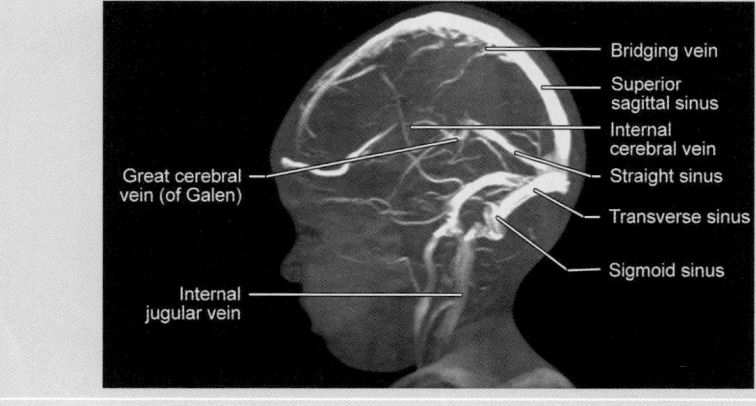

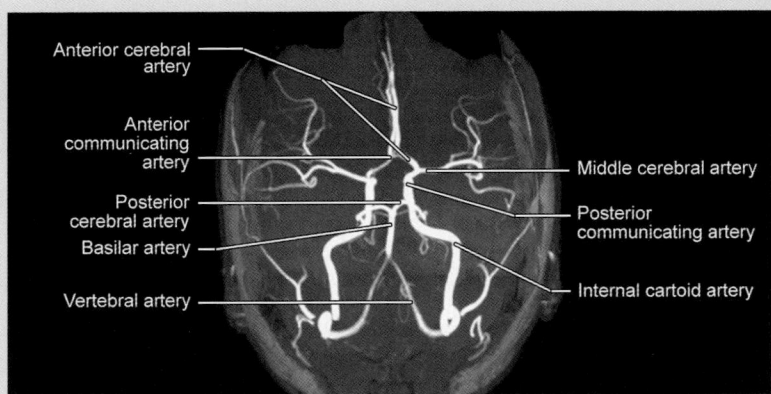
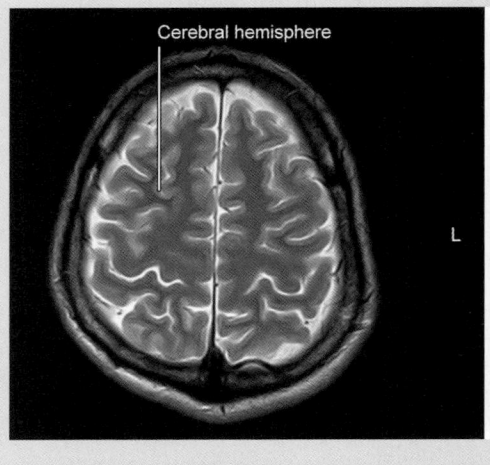
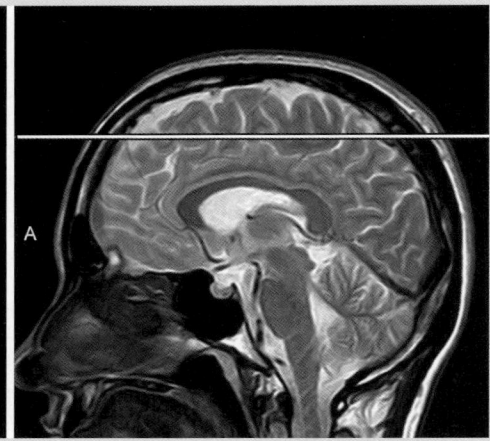
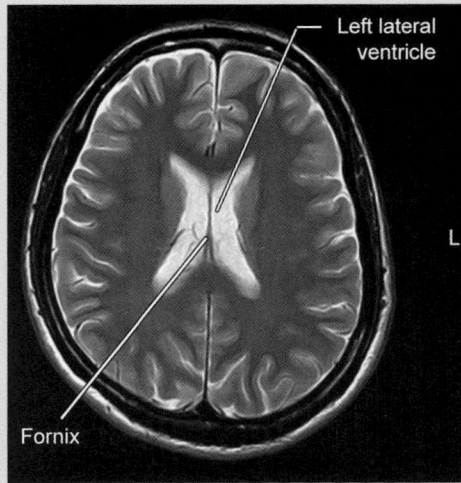
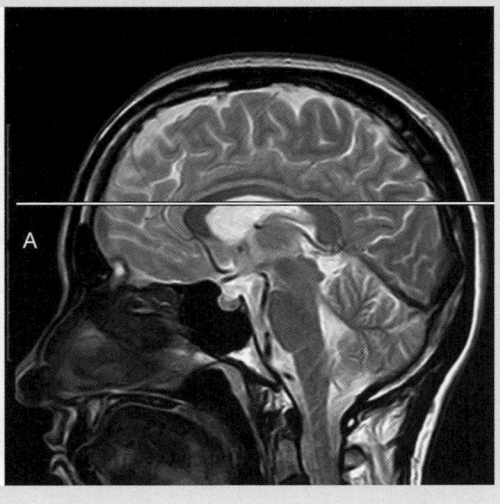

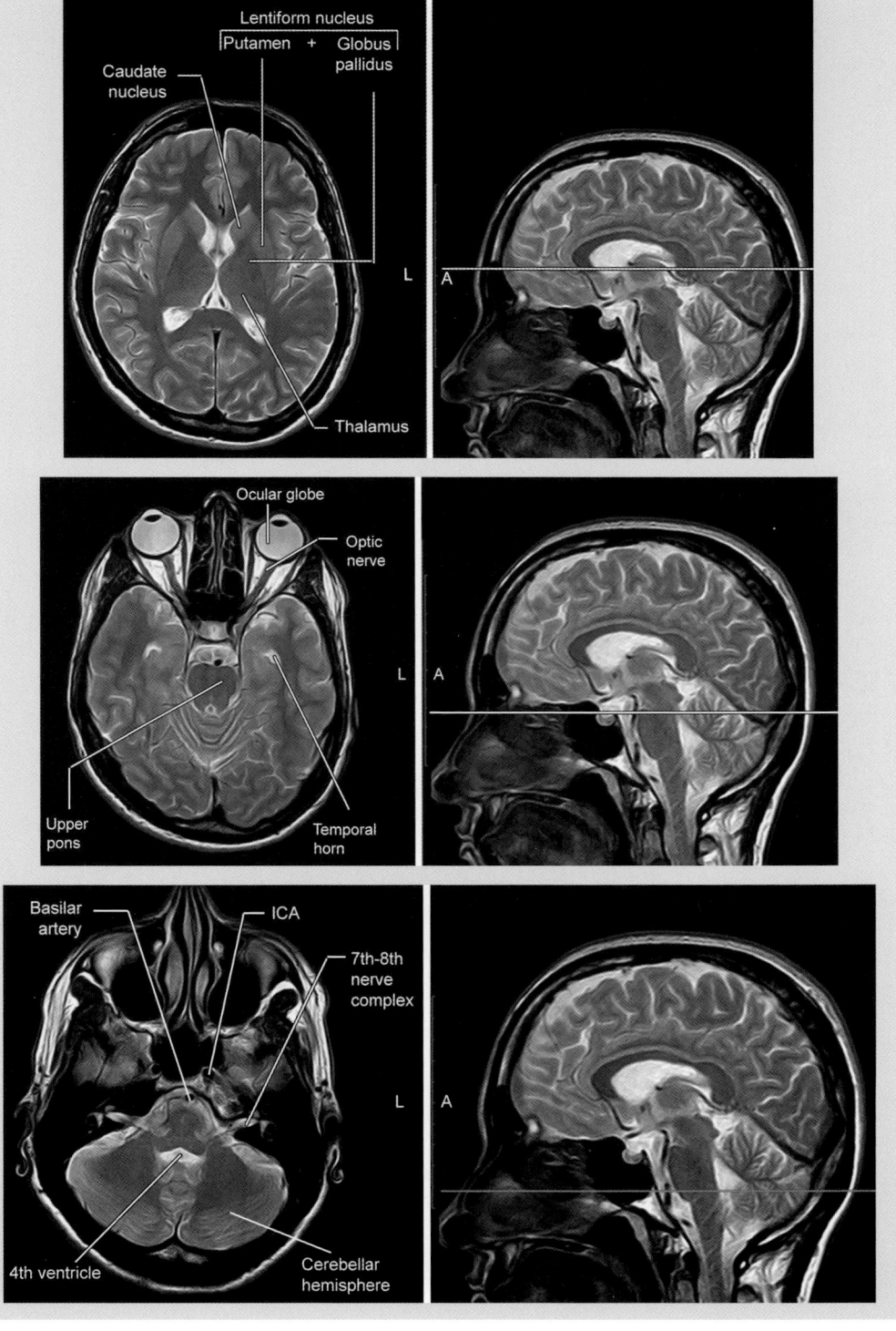

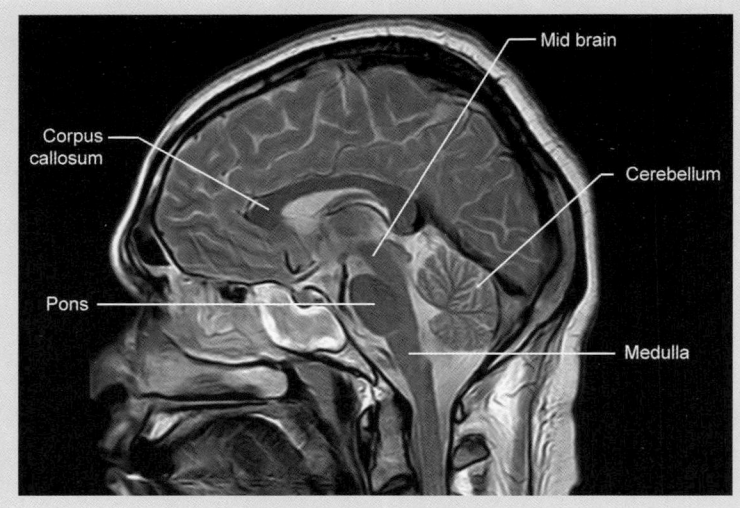
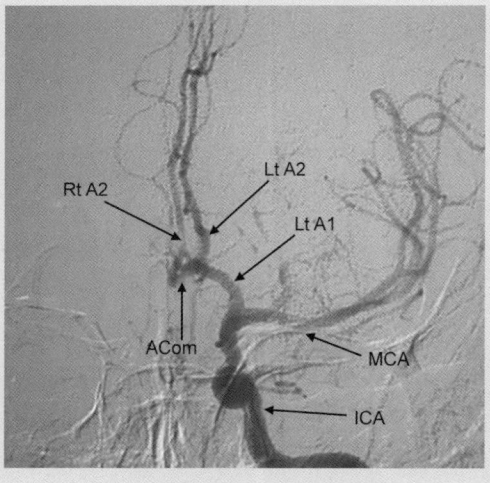

TRAUMA/STROKE

- IOC for suspected intracranial bleed in case of trauma—NCCT Head
- IOC for acute SAH–NCCT Head (MC cause is trauma)
- **IOC for cause of acute SAH (nontraumatic)**– Angiography (MC cause is aneurysm)
- **MC-cause of nontraumatic SAH** → Rupture of berry aneurysm (IMAGE)
- **MC-cause of SAH** → trauma
- IOC for diagnosis of chronic Intracranial bleed → MRI (>48 hrs) → As it can pick hemorrhagic products like hemosiderin even if they are not visible on CT (on gradient images of MRI)
- In unconscious patients IOC for stroke → NCCT Head as it rules out acute bleed or hemorrhagic infarct (which is a contraindication for thrombolysis).
- IOC for Nonhemorrhagic infarct/stroke—MRI (**Diffusion weighted images**)
- 1st investigation for TIA → USG Doppler of carotid vessels-**best modality to visualize small atherosclerotic plaque**.
- **Screening modality** for **atherosclerotic brain** disorder standard MR angiography.

Signs of Hyperacute Infarct on NCCT

- Hyperdense MCA sign
- Cortical ribbon/insular ribbon sign
- Ill-marginated lentiform nuclei
- Sulcal effacement due to edema.

Acute Infarct on NCCT

- Wedge shaped cortical based hypodense area involving both grey and white matter
- Fogging effect in subacute stage of infarct due to reopening of capillaries and leak leads to increase attenuation of brain of acute infarct.
- As hyperacute infarct can be missed on NCCT
  - IOC for Hyperacute Infarct → MRI-[best sequence –DWI]

important
IOC for acute intracranial bleed is NCCT as it appears hyperdense on CT and CT can be performed in unstable patients unlike MRI as it is very fast.

important

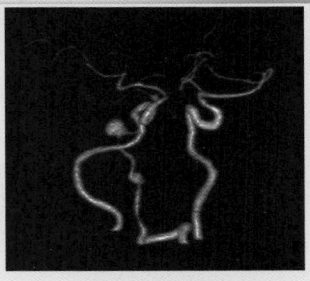
Berry aneurysm

important
Restricted diffusion appears hyperintense on DW images and hypointense on ADC images.

important

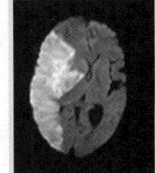 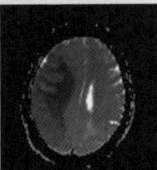
DWI, ADC- showing restricted diffusion

important

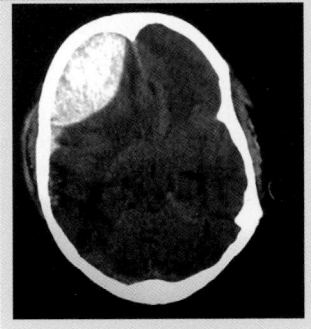
Acute EDH

> ***important***
> Active bleed can be iso to hypodense if
> - Clotting pathway abnormality
> - Severe anemia

> ***important***
> **Subclavian Steal Phenomenon**-Can cause Stroke due to reversal of blood flow in I/L vertebral artery due to thrombosis in proximal SCA. **(Initial IOC-USG Doppler)**

> ***important***
>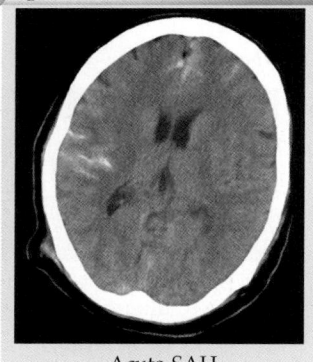
> Acute-SAH

> ***important***
> Swirl Sign- due to active bleed in EDH seen as **hypodense area in hyperdense bleed on NCCT.**

- Acute/hyperacute infarcts shows restricted diffusion
- NCC1-CTA-CT Perfusion protocol can be performed if mechanical thrombectomy is planned.

Bleeds	
Intra-axial	Extra-axial
• Hemorrhagic contusion	• SAH-Linear collection along sulci
• DAI	• SDH-concavo convex-(cres centric)
	• EDH-Biconvex (lentiform) **(IMAGE)** due to torn MMA

Acute bleed → **Hyperdense**
Subacute bleed → Isodense to brain parenchyma
Chronic bleed → **Hypodense**

SDH	EDH
• Shear type injury	• Associated with skull fractures
• *Crescent shaped collection*	• **Biconvex collection**
• **Not limited by sutures**	• **Limited by sutures**
• **Limited by dural reflection–does not cross the midline**	• **Not limited by dural reflection–can cross the midline**
• **Bridging veins (source)**	• **Middle meningeal artery (source)**

Acute SAH—Linear Hyperdensities along Sulci, (IMAGE) Fissure or any other CSF Space

DAI—Best sequence to pick DAI → **Gradient sequence/ susceptibility imaging**

Uncal herniation → compression of C/L cerebral peduncle against tentorium → (Kernohan's notch)

Deep Venous sinus Thrombosis—Nonenhancing hypodense triangular density- Empty Delta sign-(Only on Contrast Enhanced CT and MRI of Superior Sagittal Sinus) **Delta sign**-hyperdense triangular shadow in superior sagittal sinus. (IMAGE) on non-contrast CT.

Common Skull Appearances on X-ray

Hemolytic anemia (most common Thalassemia)	– Hair on end appearance

Neuroradiology

Raised ICT — Silver/copper beaten appearance

Growing fracture — Skull in pediatric patient with trapped leptomeninges (the leptomeninges does not let fracture unite and with formation of leptomeningeal cyst cause expansion of fracture- growing fracture)

Eosinophilic granuloma — Geographic lytic lesion with bevelled edge

Multiple myeloma — Punched out lytic lesions

Hyperparathyroidism — Salt and pepper/mottled skull

Craniolacunia (lacunar skull) — defect in ossification of the bones (membranous) (no significance) but generally associated with Myelomeningocele or encephalocoele

Cotton wool skull — Paget's disease (IMAGE)

- **Wormian bones:**
  - Cleidocranial dysostosis
  - Osteogenesis imperfecta
  - Hypothyroidism
  - Pyknodysostosis

Physiological Intracranial Calcification

- **Pineal gland (MC)**
- Habenular commissure → 'c'-shaped open posteriorly
- Choroid plexus
- Interhemispheric falx
- Anterior petroclinoid ligaments
- Basal ganglia/dentate nucleus (5% of normal population)
- Pacchionian bodies

**pituitary/lens

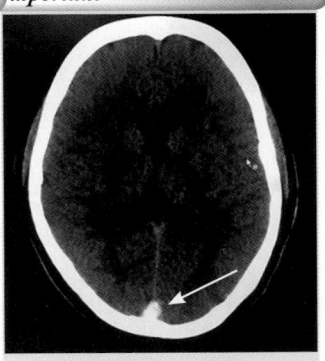
Delta sign on NCCT

i **mportant**
Pseudodelta sign is seen in acute SAH on non-contrast CT scan due to outline of the venous sinus.

i **mportant**
Double delta sign- bucket handle tear of meniscus (MRI).

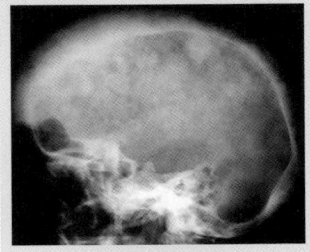
Cotton wool skull

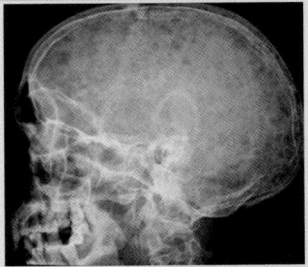
Punched out lytic lesions-MM

> **important**
> - Vein of Galen Malformation
>   - Child with hydrocephalus with congestive cardiac failure
>   - Large arc like calcification in the region of pineal gland
>   - Midline Hypoechoic tubulocystic lesion with high velocity turbulent bidirectional Flow on cranial USG in pediatric population.

> **important**
> *Gold standard for evaluation of SAH → four vessel angiography [by transfemoral catheterization of both ICA and one vertebral with other fills by reflex].

> **important**
> Six Vessel Angiography
> - B/L ICA
> - B/L ECA
> - B/L VA
> - [Via puncture of R femoral artery]

> **important**
>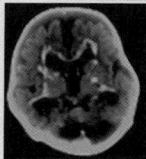
> Periventricular calcification in CMV infection

> **important**
> Rich focus → small subpial subependymal cortical focus of infection (TB).

> **important**
>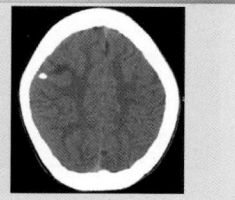
> Nodulo calcific stage of NCC

Abnormal Calcification

Periventricular calcification	– Cytomegaloviral infection
Diffuse nodular pattern Subependymal calcified nodules	– Toxoplasmosis – Tuberous sclerosis (candle dripping appearance)
Bracket calcification Tram track pattern or gyral calcification Starry sky pattern	– Corpus callosal lipoma – Sturge Weber syndrome – Neurocysticercosis

Basal Ganglia → Calcification

- Idiopathic
- Thyroid dysfunction
- CO/lead poisoning
- Toxoplasmosis
- Cockaynes
- Fahr's

INFECTIONS

Triad of acute tubercular meningitis
- Basilar/basal meningitis (IMAGE)
- Hydrocephalus
- Vasculitic infarcts

Chronic tubercular meningitis → en plaque dural thickening and popcorn-like dural calcification

Peripheral/Ring Enhancing Lesions (MAGIC DRT)

- M → Metastasis
- A → Abscess [with Restricted diffusion]
- G → glioma/high grade glioma
- I → Infection-Tuberculomas/toxoplasmosis
- C → cysticerci → NCC
- D → Demyelination → acute phase with incomplete rim (MS)
- R → Radiation necrosis
- Thrombosed aneurysm

Pachymeningitis

- TB
- Meningioma
- Lymphoma
- Sarcoidosis

NCC Escobar's Four Pathologic Stages

- 1st vesicular stage—Non-enhanicng/**no edema**
- IInd colloid vesicular—Thick Rim enhancement/edema/enhancing eccentric mural nodule
- IIIrd granular nodular—Thick Rim enhancement/calcified mural nodule/large edema
- IVth nodular calcified → calcified nodule/ no edema, **may be seen in context of seizure activity** [Stary sky on NCCT]

Encephalitic form—multiple small enhancing lesions with diffuse cerebral edema. (IMAGE)

Intraventricular NCC → MC in 4th ventricle.

Racemose variety–cisternal location with **lack of mural nodule**, multilobulated large cysts of CSF signal + hydrocephalus

- Because no host response in basal cisterns [Scolex never being formed]
- **Peas in a pod appearance** → cysticercosis in extra-ocular muscles.

Hydatid

Calcification of wall is rare in brain.

HSV-1

- Basifrontal (orbital surface) and temporal lobe [Inferomedial]
- Cingulate gyrus
- Hemorrhagic encephalitis
- Relative sparing of basal ganglia/thalami/posterior fossa structures.

Cryptococcus [AIDS] →

- Non-enhancing dilated perivascular spaces (**cryptococcomas**)
- Gelatinous pseudocyst
- Basal exudates present **(Basal meningitis)**

JE → Japanese Encephalitis

- Isolated T2W Hyperintensity in the substantia niagra and B/L thalami
- Hemorrhage in the B/L thalami.

---

important
Cryptococcal meningitis can also show basal meningitis however differentiating feature from tubercular meningitis is prominent Virchow-Robin spaces.

important

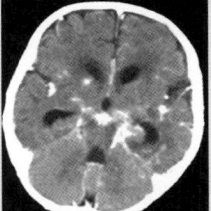

Basilar meningitis and hydrocephalus in TB

important
Pineal gland is most common site of normal calcification in the brain but if >1 cm can be due to Pinealoblastoma.

important
HIV can involve basal ganglia, periventricular and subcortical white matter, but no involvement of cingulated gyrus.

important

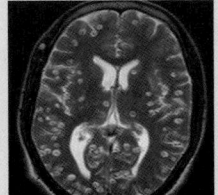

Encephalitic form of NCC (T_2W MRI—Cyst c hypointense mural nodule.)

important
- No inflammatory reaction if the parasite is live as in vesicular stage and hence no inflammatory reaction—no edema
- Nodular calcified lesion can have residual edema

HIV encephalitis	Progressive multifocal leuko-encephalopathy (PML)
• *Dementia*	• *Focal deficit/cognitive/speech*
• *Symmetric*	• *Asymmetric*
• *Cortical atrophy (MC)*	• *Periventricular and subcortical*
• *Periventricular* **Diffuse** *Mild T1W hypointense*	• **Multifocal-** *Scalloped lesion Mild to severe T1W, hypointense*

PML–involvement of subcortical white matter
With Grey-White interface (Scalloped appearance)
- No mass effect in (PML or HIV)
- **Relative sparing of cortical ribbon**
- "Heart of the Gyrus Sign"

LEUKODYSTROPHIES OR WHITE MATTER DISEASES

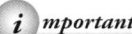

Number and size of lesions increase with increase in dose of contrast in MS.

Multiple Sclerosis Relapsing-remitting (McDonald's Criteria)

1. Demyelinating lesions disseminated in space
2. Demyelinating lesions disseminated in time
3. Exclusion of alternative explanation for clinical presentation.

MRI features
- **Dawson's fingers**
  - [along periventricular veins] right angle to lateral ventricles
  - Focal areas along calloso-Septal interface [highly sensitive and specific] Specifically at inferior margin of Corpus Callosum Earliest indication of MS
  - Spared in ischemic demyelination
- Dot and dash sign on FLAIR MRI
- In acuate phase → Homogenous enhancement → ring like enhancement (also in acute on chronic reactivation)
- **Black hole** → T2W hyper and T1W hypo → **(severely injured white matter)**
- Atrophy (severely injured brain)

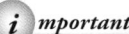

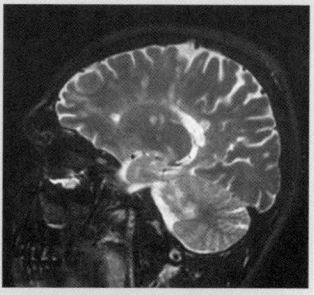

Dawson's fingers in MS

Other Leukodystrophies
- **Adreno-cortico-leukodystrophy** → Splenium and peritrigonal white matter (Triple layers on post gado)

- **Alexander's disease** → frontal and periventricular white matter and involvement of caudate nuclei/Macrocephaly
- **Krabbe's disease:**
  - Increase density in **basal ganglia and Thalamus**
  - Cerebellar white matter and pyramidal tracts.
- **Pelizaeus-Merzbacher disease** → Diffuse periventricular and subcortical white matter with atrophy (**tigroid pattern**)
- **Metachromatic leukodystrophy** → (MC) confluent symmetric B/L peripheral supratentorial white matter (Relative sparing of subcortical 'U')
- **MLC (Megaloencephalic leukodystrophy with subcortical cysts)** → B/L symmetrical Globus pallidus with sparing of rest (also seen in Kernicterus and Kearn-Sayre syndrome)
- **Glutaric aciduria** → subcortical 'U' fibers and basal ganglia involvement and spare thalami
- **Schilder's disease** (diffuse sclerosis) from corpus collosum to B/L parieto occipital region
- **Marchiafava-Bignami** → mainly corpus callosum
- **Central pontine Myelinolysis** → pontine white matter only
- **Extrapontine Myelinolysis** → Midbrain, thalami and subcortical white matter
- **Canavan's disease** → Diffuse white matter involvement/macrocephaly/↑↑**NAA on spectroscopy**.
- **Leigh's disease** (Mitochondrial)
  - Brainstem
  - Deep cerebellar grey matter
  - Subthalamic nucleus
  - Basal ganglia

Wilson's Disease 'Panda face' → Due to involvement of substantia nigra and tegmentum.

> *important*
> Hallervorden-Spatz Disease
> **Eye of tiger appearance**, involvement of B/L globus pallidus.
> **Humming bird sign**-progressive supranuclear palsy d/t atrophy of midbrain
> **Bat wing and molar tooth appearance**-Joubert's syndrome.

> *important*
> **Double panda sign**
> Face of giant panda - mid brain
> Face of miniature Panda- pons
> on (T2W) MRI- Wilson disease

> *important*
> Globus Pallidus involvement seen in:
> - MLC
> - Kernicterus
> - Kearns Sayre syndrome
> - Hallervarden Spatz disease

Causes of Macrocephaly
- **Canavans (only disease which shows raised NAA peak on Spectroscopy)**
- GM2 Gangliosidosis
- MLC
- Alexander's
- Glutaric acid urea

EPILEPSY

MTS (mesial temporal sclerosis) Most Common Cause of Medically treatable Seizures [surgical resection possible]

Primary MRI features →
- Atrophy, Hippocampal (**IMAGE-R**)
- ↑ T2W signal

Secondary Features

Excitotoxicity induced neuronal death (as hippocampus is most sensitive structure in brain to ischemia)
- Temporal horn dilatation (IMAGE-R)
- Loss of hippocampal signal on T1 W images.
- **Loss of hippocampal head digitations. (IMAGE-R)**
- Loss of collateral white matter
- Poor parahippocampal grey-white matter differentiation
- I/L atrophy of temporal lobe, thalamus, fornix and mammillary body

> *i important*
> Intracarotid amobarbital test [Wada's Test] → to test hemispheric functions in patients undergoing epilepsy surgery → helps in language lateralization and predicts for global amnesia.

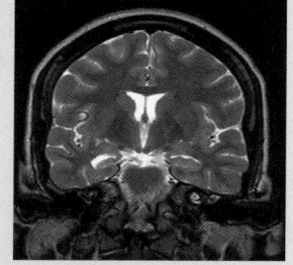
Right hippocampal sclerosis

> *i important*
> Meningioma bone-en plaque type invade bone-causing hyperostosis thickening and sclerosis.

> *i important*
> MIS ME lesions
> NF-2 → Multiple inherited schwonnoma, meningioma, Ependyoma)

TUMORS

- Most common primary brain tumor — Meningioma (35%)
- Most common primary intraparenchymal brain tumor — Glioma (30%)
- Most common brain tumor to show calcification — Craniopharyngioma
- Most common intraparenchymal brain tumor to show calcification — Oligodendroglioma (highest propensity to calcify)
- Most common brain tumor — Metastasis
- Hemorrhagic metastasis → Choriocarcinoma/Kidney
- Leptomeningeal metastasis → Breast/lung/melanoma
- Calvarial metastasis → Breast > lung
- Dural metastasis → Breast/lung/kidney
- Solitary metastasis → Lung > Kidney
- T1W hyperintense metastasis → Melanoma

Meningioma → MC Tumor Brain (IMAGE)

If Multiple → neurofibromatosis-II
- X-ray:
  - Hyperostosis (MC)/erosion (unlikely) of overlying bones

- Tumor calcification (Psammoma/sand bodies)
- Enlarged vascular grooves
- Pneumosinus dilatans
- **Angio:**
    - Dual vascular supply—[spoke wheel sunburst pattern of enlarged dural feeders]
    - Mother in law lesions—contrast comes early and stays for long
- **CT:**
    - Hyperdense
    - Enhance intensely
    - Calcification [20–30%]
    - Degenerative perilesional cyst/trapped arachnoid
    - 60% perilesional edema
- **MRI:**
    - Buckling of Grey-white matter interphase
    - CSF cleft/or pseudocapsule
    - Pseudocapsule due to vessels surrounding mass and CSF
    - Dural tail (60%) [not pathognomonic]
    - Iso intense to grey matter on all pulse sequences

Pineal Germinoma

- Hypedense on CT with homogenous contrast enhancement
- Engulf calcified masses

Schwannoma

- MC-8th > 5th > 7th CN
    - Ist and IInd nerve not involved (lack Schwan sheath)

Meningioma	Schwannoma
Obtuse angle with dura	Acute angle with dura
Ca^{++} common	Ca^{++} Rare
Homogenous	Heterogenous usually
Not common at CP angle	**MC CP angle mass**
Hyperostosis of IAC	Widening of IAC comma shaped or ice cream cone appearance
Homogeneous with broad dural base enhancement	Heterogenous enhancement

i mportant

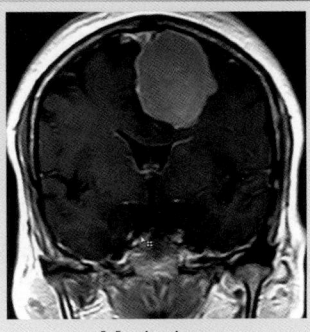

Meningioma

i mportant
Spinal meningioma →
Myelography → Intradural-extramedullary mass

i mportant
- Vestibular schwannoma from inferior vestibular nerve
- Ice cream cone appearance

i mportant
Spectroscopy -to differentiate rim enhancing lesions
- Necrotic tumor → only lactate peak
- Tuberculoma → only lipid lactate [cho/cr>1]
- Pyogenic abscess → Lactate + other amino acids
- NCC → Non-specific/very Less lipid

i mportant
Spectroscopic findings
- Myoinositol peak → low grade tumors/Gliomatosis cerebri
- Tumors → choline
- Meningioma- Alanine peak

i mportant

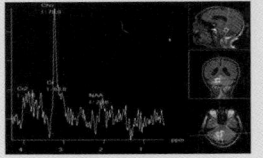

Choline peak- malignancy

important

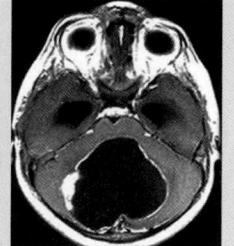

Pilocytic astrocytoma

important

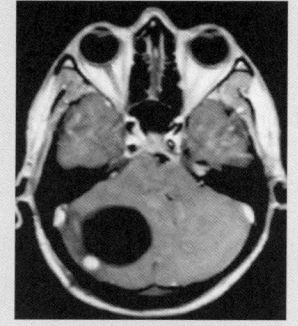

Hemangioblastoma

important
- IOC for microadenoma- dynamic MRI
- If no microadenoma on MRI in pituitary
- Next IOC → Inferior petrosal sinus venous sampling

important
- Pituitary Hypoplasia → kissing carotid sign
- Tuber cinereum Hamartoma → gelastic seizures

Pilocytic Astrocytoma
- Associated with NF-1
- Cystic lesion with intensely homogenously enhancing mural nodule but no enhancement of cyst wall

Hemangioblastoma
- Associated with VHL
- Large avascular posterior fossa mass with a small highly vascular mural nodule (pial nodule) showing prolonged stain (mother in law phenomenon)
- Prominent serpentine flow voids due to enlarged vessels in the wall

Craniopharyngioma
- From Rathke's pouch
- Solid cystic – suprasellar mass
- Most common variant - admantimatous (90%)
- 80% cases – calcification
- [papillary variety usually does not calcify and is solid in adults].

Petrous/CP Pangle Paraganglioma
- Salt and pepper appearance (salt- blood, pepper- flow void)

Pituitary Macroadenoma
- > 1 cm
- **Figure of '8' (ballooning of sella)**

Pituitary Microadenoma
- (< 1 cm) - most common is prolactionoma
- IOC dynamic CEMRI where microadenoma shows delayed enhancement

Medulloblastoma	Ependymoma
From vermis	*From 4th ventricle*
Solid-hyperdense on CT	Solid cystic-Hypo on CT
Necrosis/Ca^{++} -not common	**Common**
Foraminal extention-not common	**Common**
Subependymal spreads/drop metastasis	

Brain Tumors which Spread Along CSF Flow/ Drop Metastasis

- Medulloblastoma
- Germ cell tumor/Germinoma)
- Lymphoma
- Ependymoma (after local recurrence)
- Pineoblastoma
- Primitive neuroectodermal tumor (PNET)
- Anaplastic glioma/glioblastoma multiforme

Epidermoid cyst	Arachnoid cyst
• FLAIR- Mixed Iso/Hypo signal	• Follow CSF signal on all sequences
• **DWI (diffusion weighted)- High**	• Low
• ADC- low	• High
• Show restricted diffusion	• No restricted diffusion
• Encase vessels	• Displace vessels

Raised ICT

Earliest
- **Adults** → Erosion of dorsum sella.
  - Loss of lamina dura (later)
  - Pineal displacement
- **Pediatric population** → sutural diastasis [as unfused bones give way]
  - Copper beaten skull (later)
  IOC for hydrocephalus → MRI
  Ist IOC for hydrocephalus in child → USG [open fontanelle].

Retinal Detachment

- **Posterior hyaloid detachment** → fluid-fluid level
- **Retinal Detachment** → 'V' shaped with apex at optic disk
- **Hemorrhagic choroidal detachment** → Lentiform
- **Serous choroidal detachment** → Crescent/Ring

Graves Ophthalmology

- Enlargement of extraocular muscle but sparing tendinous insertion (MRI) (Cock bottle appearance)
- Order of involvement of muscles –IMS (Inferior, medial and superior rectus)

> *important*
> *Double ring sign on CT around cochlea otosclerosis.
> *Optic foramen projection Rhese projection.

> *important*
> PET-IOC to differentiate b/w tumor recurrence vs radiation changes.

> *important*
> Butterfly Glioma—Glioblastoma multiforme- due to spread along corpus callosum to opposite side

> *important*
> • Heavy/streaky/ribbon like Ca++ → oligodendroglioma (70-90% cases)
> • Dense punctate Ca++ → Ependymoma

> *important*
> Tumors to calcifiy
> COME Ca++
> C-craniopharyngioma
> O-oligodendroglioma
> M-Meningioma
> E-Ependymoma
> C-Choroid plexus papilloma
> A-astrocytoma

> *important*
> Popcorn Pattern
> Mammo → Fibroadenoma
> CX-ray → Pulmonary hamartomas
> MRI Brain → Cavernous angioma

> **important**
> MRI is IOC for
> - **Juvenile angiofibroma** → To assess Intracranial extension
> - Laryngeal Malignancy

Pseudotumor

- Involve both muscle and tendinous insertion

Jaw Cysts

- Radicular cyst
  - Cyst near root of carious tooth
- **Dentigerous cyst**
  - Cyst related to crown of unerupted tooth
- **Ameloblastoma**
  - Thinning of cortex in buccolingual cortex
  - Multilocular cystic/soap bubble/honey comb lesion

Initial IOC

OPG – orthopantomogram X-ray

NEUROCUTANEOUS SYNDROMES

VHL

- Heart → rhabdomyoma
- Pancreas → Islet cell tumor
- Endolymphatic sac neoplasm
- Hemangioblastoma
  - Cerebellar
  - Spinal
  - Retinal
  + cystic lesions of kidney, pancreas, liver, and epididymis
  + Pheochromocytomas
  + RCC

Gorlin's syndrome

- [basal cell nevus syndrome] → Medulloblastoma

Li-Fraumeni syndrome

- Medulloblastomas, gliomas APC,

Gardner's syndrome

- Medulloblastomas' Glioblastoma, Craniopharyngioma, **osteomas**

MEN-1 (Werner's syndrome)

- Malignant schwannoma, pituitary adenoma parathyroid and pancreatic islet cell tumor

NF-1

- Schwannoma, astrocytoma, meningioma's, optic nerve gliomas, Neurofibromas (Dumbbell tumors), neurofibrosarcomas.

Osseous Lesions of NF-1

- Widening of neural foramina
- Hypoplastic sphenoid wing
- Sutural defects
- Kyphoscoliosis
- Dural ectasia
- Meningoceles
- Ribbon ribs
- Tibial bowing
- Pseudoarthrosis
- Focal overgrowth of digit
- Multiple ossifying fibroma
- Absent/small fibula
- Scalloping of post border of vertebral body

Eye in NF-1 →

- Optic glioma
- Lisch nodule of iris
- Buphthalmos
- Plexiform neurofibroma
- Empty orbit/Bare orbit
- Harlequin appearance of orbit
- Concentric enlargement of optic foramen [sclerosis in optic N. Sheath meningioma]

NF-2 (MISME)

- **MIS** → Multiple Inherited Schwannomas
- **M** → Meningiomas
- **E** → ependymomas
- **Misnomer** → as No neurofibromas

Cowden's Syndrome

- Dysplastic cerebellar gangliocytoma (Lhermitte duclos disease), Meningioma, Astrocytoma

Sturge-Weber/Encephalotrigeminal Syndrome

- Capillary/cavernous hemangioma
- Tram track calcification
- Atrophy
- Scleral/choroidal angioma

> *important*
> Blood oxygenation level dependent contrast mechanism-BOLD For functional imaging of brain.

> *important*
> Cavernous angioma → popcorn like lesion (MR)
> venous angioma → medusa head appearance (venous phase)

> *important*
> Tram track pattern in MCQs
> - MPGN-II (pathology)
> - CRAO (angio)
> - Optic nerve sheath meningioma (MRI)
> - Bronchiectasis (HRCT)
> - Sturge-Weber synd (X-ray)
> - AS (X-ray)
> - H Ducreyi (Microscopy)

> **important**
> Lateral Meningoceles are seen in
> - NF-1
> - Marfan's syndrome
> - Ehlers -Danlos syndrome

> **important**
> Angiomyolipoma- kidney
> (Lesions of mean attenuation -50 to -100 HU on CT)

> **important**
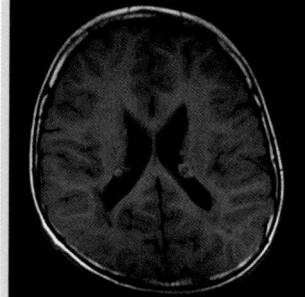
Subependymal nodules -TS

> **important**
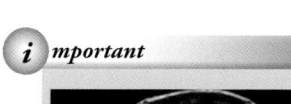

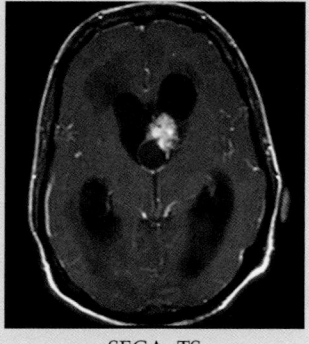
SEGA- TS

Tuberous Sclerosis

EPi- loi-a → epilepsy/low IQ/Adenoma sebaceum
- Cortical tubers
- Subependymal nodules in lateral ventricles
- Retinal phakomas
- Subependymal giant cell astrocytoma at foramen of Monro
- Skin → facial angiofibroma, shagreen patch
- Kidneys → Renal cysts and angiomyolipoma
- Cardiac rhabdomyomas, honeycomb lung (cysts)
- Adenomas

SEGA–Subependymal Giant Cell Astrocytoma

- At foramen of Monro
- In patients with tuberous sclerosis
- Heavy intratumor calcification common
- Strong heterogeneous contrast enhancement
- (obstructive hydrocephalus with dialated lateral and normal 3rd and 4th ventricles)

Crouzon Syndrome →

- Brachycephaly
- Parrot beak, maxillary hyperplasia, proptosis
- Ocular hypertelorism
- Hydrocephalus
- Chronic tonsillar herniation (MRI)

Apert Syndrome →

(Acrocephaly syndactyly)
- Brachycephaly
- Small cranial base
- Syndactyly [IInd–IIIrd and IVth finger] [Mitten hand]
- Radially deviated broad thumb.
- Toe syndactyly [sock toes]
- Fusion of C5-C6 bodies
- Low IQ

Histiocytosis [LCH]

- Geographical lytic lesion with bevelled edges
- Button Sequestrum (Skull)
- Floating teeth if (mandible)

- Vertebra plana
- Cysts in lung (bizarre) – honeycomb lesion

Malformations of Cortical Development

- **Abnormal neuronal-glial proliferation or apoptosis**
  - Microcephaly
  - Megalencephaly
- **Abnormal neuronal migration**
  - Periventricular nodular heterotopia
  - Lissencephaly/subcortical band heterotopia
  - Cobblestone cortex/congenital muscular dystrophy
- **Abnormal cortical organization**
  - Polymicrogyria
  - Focal Cortical Dysplasia

  Five outcomes are possible in the MCDs:
1. Fewer or more than normal neurons are produced (microcephaly, megalencephaly).
2. Neurons do not migrate at all from the ventricles (periventricular heterotopia) or migrate half way (subcortical band heterotopia).
3. Some neurons reach the cortex but large numbers do not. No normal cortical layers are formed (lissencephaly, pachygyria, cobblestone cortex).
4. Neurons over-shoot the cortex and end up in the subarachnoid space (marginal-leptomeningeal glio-neuronal heterotopia, cobblestone cortex).
5. The late stage of migration and cortical organization is disrupted (polymicrogyria).

> **important**
> SEGA-Causes obstructive hydrocephalus with dilatation of bilateral lateral ventricles and normal 3rd and 4th ventricles.

Craniosynostosis (Fusion of)

- **Brachycephaly:** Bicoronal and/or bilamboid sutures
- **Scaphocephaly/dolichocephaly:** Sagittal suture
- **Plagiocephaly:** Unilateral coronal and lambdoid sutures
- **Trigonocephaly:** Metopic suture
- **Pachycephaly:** Lamdoid suture
- **Oxycephaly/turricephaly:** Sagittal, coronal and lambdoid sutures (tower-like skull) combined synostosis
- **Cloverleaf skull:** Intrauterine sagittal, coronal, lambdoid sutures (most severe).

CJD

MRI findings may be bilateral or unilateral and symmetric or asymmetric, and include:
- **T2:** Hyperintensity
  - Basal ganglia (putamen and caudate)
  - Thalamus (hockey stick sign and pulvinar sign)
  - Cortex: most common early manifestation
  - White matter
- **DWI/ADC:** Persistent restricted diffusion (**considered the most sensitive sign**)

Review of sequential studies also typically demonstrates rapidly progressive cerebral atrophy.
- Nuclear Medicine: Hypometabolism on ^{18}FDG-PET studies.

Spinal Cord Tumors

Intramedullary Tumors	Intradural-extramedullary Tumors	Extradural Tumors
Single: Ependymoma, myxopapillary ependymoma, astrocytoma, ganglioglioma, hemangioblastoma, subependymoma, paraganglioma *Multiple:* Hemangioblastomas, metastases, lymphoma	*Single:* Meningiomas, nerve sheath tumors, intradural metastases, lymphoma/leukemia, paraganglioma *Multiple:* Any of the preceding except paraganglioma	*Single:* Aneurysmal bone cyst, giant cell tumor, osteoblastoma, osteochondromas, chordoma, chondrosarcoma, chondroblastoma, metastasis, hemangioma, solitary plasmacytoma, lymphoma *Multiple:* Metastatic disease, hemangiomas, multiple myeloma, lymphoma *Epidural Lesions:* Angiolipoma and angiomyolipoma, epidural lipomatosis, lymphoma

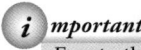
Important
Empty thecal sac sign is seen in arachnoiditis.

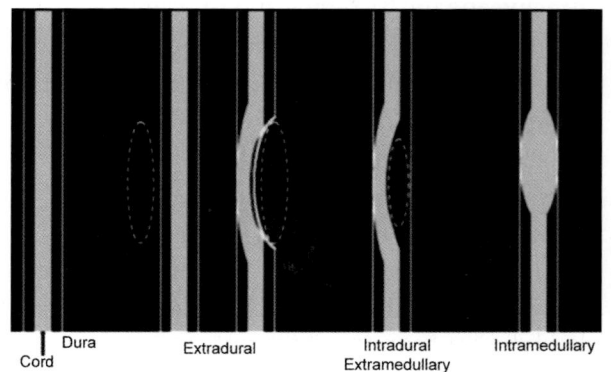

Neuroradiology

Myelographic Appearance for Various Spinal Lesion

- Extradural block → feathered appearance
- Intradural extramedullary → meniscus sign (widening of CSF space)
- Intramedullary → trouser leg appearance.

LE FORT FRACTURES

Le Fort fractures are fractures of the midface, which collectively involve separation of all or a portion of the midface from the skull base.

Classification

The commonly used classification is as follows:

Le Fort type 1

- Horizontal maxillary fracture, separating the teeth from the upper face
- Fracture line passes through the alveolar ridge, lateral nose and inferior wall of maxillary sinus

Le Fort type 2

- Pyramidal fracture, with the teeth at the pyramid base, and nasofrontal suture at its apex
- Fracture arch passes through posterior alveolar ridge, lateral walls of maxillary sinuses.

Le Fort type 3

- Craniofacial disjunction
- Fracture line passes through nasofrontal suture, Maxillo-frontal suture, orbital wall and zygomatic arch

A memory aid is

- Le Fort 1 is a floating palate
- Le Fort 2 is a floating maxilla
- Le Fort 3 is a floating face

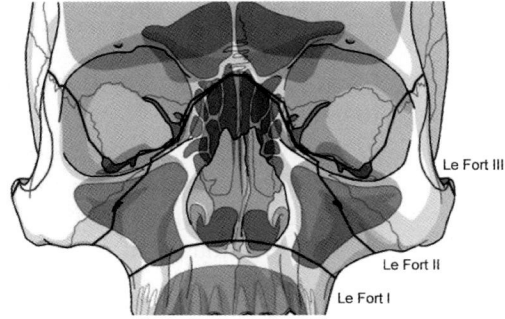

QUESTIONS

1. Bracket calcification on skull X-ray is seen in:
   a. Tuberous sclerosis
   b. Sturge-Weber Syndrome
   c. Corpus callosum lipoma
   d. Meningioma

2. Puff of smoke appearance on cerebral angiography is seen in:
   a. ACA aneurysm
   b. Cavernous sinus thrombosis
   c. Moyamoya disease
   d. Vein of Galenmalformation

3. A 7-year-old patient presents with severe headache, paralysis of upward gaze, loss of light perception and accommodation, nystagmus and failure of convergence. CT scan showed homogenous hyperdense lesion above the sella and in the posterior part of the third ventricle. MRI showed that the lesions were homogenous and isointense on T1 weighted imaging, and isointense onT2 weighted imaging with intense contrast enhancement. The most likely diagnosis is:
   a. Teratoma
   b. Germinoma
   c. Dermoid
   d. Choroid plexus carcinoma

4. Which of the followings is used to differentiate between the epidermoid cyst and arachnoid cyst?
   a. Contrast enhancement
   b. Restricted diffusion
   c. CSF signals on FLAIR
   d. Smooth margin

5. Investigation of choice for leptomeningeal carcinomatosis:
   a. PET
   b. SPECT
   c. Gadolinium enhanced MRI
   d. CT scan

6. A middle aged female presents with slowly progressive weakness of lower limbs, spasticity and recent onset hesitancy of Micturition. On neurological examination there is evidence of dorsal myelopathy. MRI scan of spine reveals mid dorsal intradural contrast enhancing mass lesion. Diagnosis is:
   a. Intradural lipoma
   b. Dermoid cyst
   c. Meningioma
   d. Epidermoid cyst

7. A patient was diagnosed with intracranial cavernous angioma on MR scan. MRI finding characteristic of the lesion is:
   a. Well defined nidus
   b. Well defined arterial feeders
   c. Phlebectasis
   d. Reticulated 'popcorn-like configuration'

8. Which of the following is the investigation of choice for evaluation of acute head injury?
   a. NCCT Head   b. CECT Head
   c. MRI Brain   d. PET scan

9. Posterior scalloping of vertebral bodies is seen in:
   a. Aortic aneurysm
   b. Neurofibromatosis
   c. Lymphadenopathy
   d. Cretinism

10. Meningiomas occur at all the following site except:
    a. Lateral cerebral convexities
    b. Basal ganglia
    c. Cerebello pontine angles
    d. Foramen magnum

11. On MRI, the differential diagnosis of spinal cord edema is:
    a. Myelodysplasia
    b. Myelomalacia
    c. Myeloschisis d. Cord tumors
12. Insult during neuronal migration results in delayed neuronal migration and organization, which results in certain disorders. The least likely possibility is:
    a. Polymicrogyria
    b. Schizencephaly
    c. Lissencephaly
    d. Focal cortical dysplasia without balloncells
13. A middle aged man presents with progressive atrophy and weakness of hand and forearms. On examination he is found to have slight spasticity of the leg, generalized hyperreflexia and increased signal in the corticospinal tracts on T2 weighted MRI. The most likely diagnosis is:
    a. Multiple sclerosis
    b. Amyotrophic lateral sclerosis
    c. Subacute combined degeneration
    d. Progressive spinal muscularatrophy
14. All are true about MS except:
    a. Corpus callosum lesions are characteristic
    b. Periventricular white matter distribution with decreased CT attenuation
    c. T1 WI are most diagnostic for acute plaques
    d. 4th ventricle, 5th nerve entry site-and brachium pontis are involved
15. The MRi imaging in multiple sclerosis will show lesions in:
    a. White matter b. Grey matter
    c. Thalamus   d. Basal ganglia
16. A child presented with clinical features of demyelination. The chances of progression to MS is least with which of the following:
    a. Absent oligoclonal band
    b. Bilateral visual loss
    c. Poor recovery
    d. Cord complete transaction
17. Extensive involvement of deep white matter with bilateral hyperdense thalami on non-contrast CT scan of the brain is virtually diagnostic of:
    a. Alexander's disease
    b. Krabbe's disease.
    c. Canavan's disease
    d. Metachromatic leukodystrophy
18. Which of the following is not a MRI feature of mesial temporal sclerosis:
    a. Atrophy of mammillary body
    b. Atrophy of fornix
    c. Blurring of grey and white matter junction of ipsilateral temporal lobe
    d. Atrophy of hippocampus
19. A newborn presents with congestive heart failure resistant to treatment, on examination has bulging anterior fontanelle with a bruit on auscultation. Transfontanellar USG shows hypoechoic midline mass with dilated lateral ventricles. Most likely diagnosis is:
    a. Encephalocele
    b. Medulloblastoma
    c. Arachnoid cyst
    d. Vein of Galen malformation
20. All are the characteristics of raised ICP on plain radiology except:
    a. Erosion of dorsum sella
    b. Ballooning of sella
    c. Increased convolutions
    d. Sutural diastasis
21. A male was brought unconscious to the hospital with external injuries. CT shows no midline shift, but basal cisterns were compressed with multiple small hemorrhages. The most probable diagnosis is:

a. Brain contusion
b. Diffuse axonal injury
c. Subdural hemorrhage
d. Multiple infarct

22. A 15-year-old boy had 10-12 partial complex seizures per day inspite of adequate 4 drug antiepileptic regime. He had history of repeated high grade fever in childhood. MRI for epilepsy protocol revealed normal brain scan. What should be the best non-invasive strategy to make a definite diagnosis so that he can be prepared to undergo epilepsy surgery:
    a. Interictal scalp EEG
    b. Video EEG
    c. Interictal 18F-FDgPET
    d. Video EEG with Ictal 99m Tc-HMPAO Brain SPECT

23. Basal exudates, infarcts and hydrocephalus on computed tomography are seen in:
    a. Tuberculous meningitis
    b. Viral meningitis
    c. Herpes simplex encephalitis
    d. Cerebral malaria/neurocysticercosis

24. Focal cerebral lesion with ring enhancement on CT scan is caused by:
    a. Toxoplasmosis
    b. Intracranial hemorrhage
    c. Cysts
    d. Hamartoma

25. Suprasellar calcification is characteristic of:
    a. Medulloblastoma
    b. Craniopharyngioma
    c. Meningioma
    d. Ependymoma

26. Which of the following is the most common mixed cystic and solid suprasellar mass seen on scan of a 10-year-old child:
    a. Pituitary adenoma
    b. Craniopharyngioma
    c. Optic chiasmaglioma
    d. Germinoma

27. A 6-year-old boy has been complaining of ignoring to see the objects on the side of examination, he is not mentally retarded, school are good and visual acuity is diminished visual charting showed significant field scan of the head showed supra sellar mass with calcification. Which of the following is the most probable?
    a. Astrocytoma
    b. Craniopharyngioma
    c. Pituitary adenoma
    d. Meningioma

28. Tumor associated with extracranial spread:
    a. Ependymoma
    b. Medulloblastoma
    c. Glioblastomamultiforme
    d. Choroid plexuspapilloma

29. In 7-year-old boy presented with posterior fossa mass with cyst formation, hypodense on CT, hyperintense on T2WI and showing post gadolinium nodule enhancement is:
    a. Medulloblastoma
    b. Ependymoma
    c. Astrocytoma d. Cysticerosis

30. A 35-year-old patients presents with complaints of headache, vomiting (raised ICT) and ataxia. MRI findings are well demarcated cystic lesion with a mural nodule in the right cerebellar hemisphere with homogenous contrast enhancement. The most likely diagnosis is:
    a. Ependymoma
    b. Hemangioblastoma
    c. Pilocytic-astrocytoma
    d. Medulloblastoma

31. Which of the following tumor is typically associated with VHL?
    a. Hemangioblastoma
    b. Hemangioendothelioma
    c. Neurofibroma
    d. Glioma

32. All is true about von Hippel Lindau syndrome except:
    a. Hemangioblastomas seen in craniospinal axis
    b. Multiple tumors common
    c. Tumors of Schwann cells are common
    d. Supratentorial lesions are uncommon

33. A child presents with raised ICT. On CT scan, a lesion is seen around foramen of Monro with multiple periventricular calcific foci. What could be probable diagnosis?
    a. Subependymal giant cell astrocytoma (SGCA)
    b. Subependymoma or ependymoma
    c. Pilocytic astrocytoma
    d. Neurocytoma

34. Investigation of choice for a lesion of temporal bone:
    a. CT   b. MRI
    c. USG   d. Plain X-ray

35. Wide neural foramina is associated with:
    a. Neurofibromatosis type 1
    b. Sturge-Weber syndrome
    c. Von Hippel Lindau disease
    d. Tuberous sclerosis

36. True about MRI/CT appearance of lateral meningocele are all except:
    a. Solid dural masses
    b. Usually outside the spinal canal
    c. Widened neural foramen
    d. Generally there is no spinal cord compression and deformity

37. Mesencephalo-oculo-facial angiomatosis is seen in:
    a. KTW syndrome
    b. NF-l and 2
    c. Sturge-Weber syndrome
    d. Wyburn-Mason syndrome

38. Tram-track appearance on CT scan of head is seen in:
    a. Sturge-Weber syndrome
    b. Von Hippel Lindau syndrome
    c. Tuberous sclerosis
    d. Neurofibroma

39. Vertical linear striations are typically seen in on X-ray:
    a. Vertebral myeloma
    b. Vertebral lymphangiomas
    c. Vertebral metastasis
    d. Vertebral hemangiomas

40. Earliest sign of raised ICT is:
    a. Erosion of dorsum sella
    b. Copper beaten appearance
    c. Silver beaten appearance
    d. Displacement of pineal gland

41. Intracranial calcification with cystic lesion in plain X-ray skull is seen in:
    a. Meningioma
    b. Glioma
    c. Craniopharyngioma
    d. Medulloblastoma

42. Basal ganglia calcification is seen in all except:
    a. Hypoparathyroidism
    b. Wilson's disease
    c. Perinatal hypoxia
    d. Fahr's syndrome

43. In children raised ICT is manifested by:
    a. Lytic lesions in skull
    b. Rarefaction of dorsum of sella
    c. Sutural diastasis
    d. None of the above

44. Finding in meningioma are all except:
    a. Vascular markings around falx

b. Calcification
c. Erosions
d. Osteosclerosis

45. Characteristic featurs of meningioma are all except:
   a. Dural tail sign
   b. Hyperostosis
   c. Prominent vascularity
   d. Intra-axial tumor

46. A 20-year male patient with 6th cranial nerve palsy on T2 weighted MRI shows a markedly hyperintense lesion in cavernous sinus which shows intense homogenous contrast enhancement. Most probable diagnosis is:
   a. Schwannoma
   b. Meningioma
   c. Cavernous sinus hemangioma
   d. Astrocytoma

47. Periventricular calcification is often due to:
   a. Toxoplasmosis
   b. CMV infection
   c. Congenital syphilis
   d. All of the above

48. Subdural hematoma most commonly results from:
   a. Rupture of intracranial aneurysm
   b. Rupture of cerebral AVM
   c. Injury to cortical bridging veins
   d. Hemophilia

49. Which of the following is classic CT appearance of acute subdural hematoma?
   a. Lentiform-shaped hyperdense lesion
   b. Crescent-shaped hypodense lesion
   c. Crescent-shaped hyperdense lesion
   d. Lentiform-shaped hypodense lesion

50. CT scan of a patient with history of head injury shows a biconvex hyperdense lesion displacing the grey-white matter interface. The most likely diagnosis:
   a. Subdural hematoma
   b. Diffuse axonalinjury
   c. Extradural hematoma
   d. Hemorrhagic contusion

51. Which tumor is suggested by "Trouser leg Appearance" on an ascending myelogram?
   a. Extradural
   b. Extramedullary
   c. Intramedullary
   d. Vertebral

52. The first investigation of choice in a patient with suspected subarachnoid hemorrhage should be:
   a. Non-contrast computed tomography
   b. CSF examination
   c. Magnetic resonance imaging (MRI)
   d. Contrast-enhanced computed tomography

53. The best investigation to diagnose a case of acoustic neuroma is:
   a. Gadolinium enhanced MRI
   b. CT scan
   c. Audiometric analysis
   d. PET scan

54. Which of the following is the best choice to evaluate radiologically a posterior fossa tumor?
   a. CT scan   b. MRI
   c. Angiography d. Myelography

55. Parameningeal Rhabdomyosarcoma is best evaluated by:
   a. MRI   b. CT scan
   c. SPECT   d. PET

56. Cerebral blood flow in an asphyxiated child is best measured by:
   a. NIRS
   b. PET
   c. Radionuclide imaging
   d. MlU angiography

57. Investigation which should not be done in a patient with brain tumor:
    a. CT Scan
    b. Lumbar puncture
    c. MRI
    d. X-ray
58. All are X-ray findings of retinoblastoma except:
    a. Widening of optic canal
    b. Intracerebral calcification
    c. Intraocular calcification
    d. Secondaries in cranial bones
59. Best view for visualizing sella turcica on X-ray:
    a. AP View
    b. Town's view
    c. Lateral view
    d. Open mouth view
60. A 30-year-old man presents with 6 month history of nasal discharge, facial pain and fever. On antibiotic therapy, fever subsided. After 1 month again had symptoms of mucopurulent discharge from the middle meatus and the mucosa of the meatus appeared congested and oedematous. Next best investigation would be:
    a. MRI of the sinuses
    b. Non-contrast CT of the nose and para-nasal sinuses
    c. Plain X-ray of the paranasal sinuses
    d. Inferior meatus puncture
61. Basal skull view (submentovertical view) X-ray is best to visualize:
    a. Ethmoid sinus
    b. Frontal sinus
    c. Sphenoid sinus
    d. Maxillary sinus
62. Rabbit ear sign is seen in:
    a. Bilateral subdural hematoma in CT
    b. Unilateral subdural hematoma in CT
    c. Bilateral subarachnoid hemorrhage
    d. Unilateral subarachnoid hemorrhage
63. bat wing deformity of cerebral ventricles on CT/MRI is seen in:
    a. Bilateral subdural hematoma
    b. Bilateral subarachnoid hemorrhage
    c. Agenesis of corpus callosum
    d. Agenesis of cerebral ventricles
64. "Face of giant panda" sign on MRI brain is seen in:
    a. Wilson's disease
    b. Japanese encephalitis
    c. Rasmussen's encephalitis
    d. Wernicke's encephalopathy
65. The markedly hypointense globus pallidus on T2W MRI surrounding a higher-intensity center due to excess iron accumulation and central gliosis is characteristic of:
    a. Krabbe's disease
    b. Joubert syndrome
    c. Lhermit Duclos disease
    d. Hallervorden-Spatz disease
66. Abnormal signals in bilateral thalami on MRI brain is seen in:
    a. Wilson's disease
    b. Japanese encephalitis
    c. Wernicke's encephalopathy
    d. Rasmussen's encephalitis
67. Following tumors are known to occur with VHL disease except:
    a. Endolymphatic sac tumors
    b. Pheochromocytomas
    c. Mandibular osteomas
    d. Islet cell tumors
68. A 16-year-old girl with complex partial seizures and mild mental retardation has an area of deep red discoloration (port-wine nevus) extending over her forehead and left upper eyelid. A CT scan of her brain would be likely to reveal:
    a. Hemangioblastoma

b. Charcot-bouchard aneurysm
c. Arteriovenous malformation
d. Leptomeningeal angioma

69. Tests for suspected cases of cerebrovascular syncope include the following except:
    a. Carotid Doppler
    b. MRI brain
    c. EEG
    d. MRA

70. The 'Light-bulb' sign on DWMRI?
    a. Agarwal's disease
    b. Hyperacute stroke
    c. Vanishing bone disease
    d. Marchiafava-Bignami disease

71. High-signal, oblong, elliptical lesions at the callososeptal interface and subependymal periventricular white matter oriented perpendicular to the ventricular surface on FLAIR and T2W MR images are diagnostic of:
    a. Multiple sclerosis
    b. Moya Moya disease
    c. Periventricular leukomalacia
    d. Posterior reversible encephalopathy syndrome

72. The "salt-and-pepper" appearance on T1MRI is hallmark of paragangliomas. The 'salt' and 'pepper' of which represent respectively.
    a. Zallbens and multiple flow voids
    b. Zallbens and discrete calcific foci
    c. Subacute hemorrhages and calcific foci
    d. Subacute hemorrhages and flow voids

73. A 33-year-old woman has the acute onset of right orbital pain. On examination, she has a mild right ptosis and anisocoria. The right pupil is 2 mm smaller than the left, but both react normally to direct light stimulation. Visual acuity, visual fields, and eye movements are normal. Magnetic resonance imaging (MRI) in this patient would be expected to show which of the following?
    a. Increased t2 signal in a periventricular distribution
    b. Contrast enhancement along the tentorial margin
    c. Increased t1 signal in the wall of the right carotid artery
    d. Enlarged optic nerve in the orbit

74. A 75-year-old man with a history of recent memory impairment is admitted with headache, confusion, and a left homonymous hemianopsia. He has recently had two episodes of brief unresponsiveness. There is no history of hypertension. CT scan shows a right occipital lobe hemorrhage with some subarachnoid extension of the blood. An MRI scan with gradient echo sequences reveals foci of hemosiderin in the right temporal and left frontal cortex. The likely diagnosis is:
    a. Gliomatosis cerebri
    b. Multi-infarct dementia
    c. Mycotic aneurysms
    d. Amyloid angiopathy

75. Transfemoral angiogram is most useful in diagnosis of:
    a. Cerebral aneurysms
    b. Gliomas
    c. Multiinfarct dementia
    d. Venous sinus thrombosis

76. A 73-year-old man with a history of hypertension complains of a transient 10-min episode of left-sided weakness and slurred speech. On further questioning, he relates three brief episodes in the last month of sudden impairment of vision affecting the right eye. His examination now is normal. Which of the following would be the most appropriate next diagnostic test?
    a. Holter monitoring
    b. Spect scan
    c. Carotid Doppler study
    d. Cerebral angiography

77. "Eye of tiger" sign on brain MRI is characteristic of:
    a. Krabbe's disease
    b. Joubert syndrome
    c. Lhermit duclos disease
    d. Hallervorden-Spatz disease
78. The most definitive test for identifying intracranial aneurysms is:
    a. MRI scanning
    b. CT scanning
    c. Positron emission tomography
    d. Cerebral angiography
79. Corpus callosum lesions are characteristically seen in the following conditions:
    a. SSPE
    b. Krabbe's disease
    c. Phytanic acid deficiency
    d. Butterfly glioma
80. The location of the cerebellar tonsil in the MRI scan is helpful in diagnosis of:
    a. Arnold-Chiari type 1 malformation
    b. Neurofibromatosis type 2
    c. Giant cisterna magna
    d. Dandy-walker syndrome
81. The tentorium cerebelli which separates the superior cerebellum from the cerebrum is a common site of origin for:
    a. Meningiomas
    b. Ependymomas
    c. Hemangioblastomas
    d. Medulloblastomas
82. Radiological findings in meningioma include all of the following except:
    a. Calcification
    b. Vascular markings
    c. Hyperostosis
    d. Absent dural-tail sign
83. Which one of the following brain tumors is highly vascular in nature?
    a. Glioblastoma
    b. Meningiomas
    c. CP angle epidermoid
    d. Pituitary denomas
84. A 43-year-old man experiences dizziness and tinnitus. CT shows enlarged internal acoustic meatus. What is the diagnosis?
    a. Vestibular schwannoma
    b. Arachnoid cyst
    c. Pituitary adenoma
    d. Medulloblastoma
85. "Ice-cream cone" sign on MRI brain is seen in:
    a. Pilocytic astocytoma
    b. Acoustic neuroma
    c. Glomus jugulare
    d. Meningioma
86. In skull X-ray commonest cause of intracerebral calcified shadow is:
    a. Pituitary adenoma
    b. Oligodendroglioma
    c. Astrocytoma
    d. Glioma
87. Which of the following variety of craniopharyngioma characteristically occurs in childhood?
    a. Cellular   b. Melanotic
    c. Tanycytic
    d. Admantinomatous
88. Premature closure of coronal, sagittal, and lambdoid sutures results in:
    a. Dolichocephaly
    b. Turricephaly
    c. Plagiocephaly
    d. Trigonocephaly
89. In the diffuse axonal injury, the typical location of lesions in the brain include:
    a. Parasagittal region
    b. Cerebral cortex
    c. Ventricles
    d. White matter of cerebral hemispheres, corpus callosum and the upper brain stem

90. 'Tear-drop' appearance on PNS X-ray is seen in:
    a. Fracture of medial wall of the orbit
    b. Fracture of maxillary sinus
    c. Fracture of ethmoidal sinus
    d. Fracture floor of the orbit

91. "Hair on end" appearance in skull X-ray is characteristic of:
    a. Sickle cell anemia
    b. Thalassemia
    c. Megaloblastic anemia
    d. Hemochromatosis

92. Imaging tool of choice for cjd:
    a. DW MRI with ADC mapping
    b. HMPAO spect scan
    c. MR spectroscopy
    d. PET scan

93. A patient with 2 months history of trauma to eye. Now he presents with ocular damage & multiple cranial nerves involvement. What is the best investigation?
    a. MRI   b. CT
    c. DSA   d. MRA

94. Investigation of choice for meningeal carcinomatosis:
    a. Non-contrast CT
    b. Contrast MRI
    c. SPECT   d. PET

95. A 21-year-old woman presents with right arm loss of sensation that has been progressive over a few days. Her physician is concerned that this might be some type of demyelinating disorder. A relatively small plaque of demyelination, should be evident on which of the following?
    a. T1-weighted MRI
    b. T2-weighted MRI
    c. Precontrast CT
    d. Diffusion-weighted MRI

96. Calcification around foramen of monro with raise ICT; periventricular calcification with mass below 3rd ventricle:
    a. Ependymoma
    b. Subependymal-astrocytoma
    c. Medulloblastoma
    d. DNET

97. Frontal Sinus can be best visualized by:
    a. Caldwell's view
    b. Water's view
    c. Towne's view
    d. Schüller's view

98. Which of the following feature of thyroid nodule on Ultrasonogram is not suggestive of malignancy?
    a. Hyperechogenicity
    b. Hypoechogenicity
    c. Nonhomogeneous
    d. Microcalcification

99. Empty delta sign is seen in:
    a. Dissecting aortic aneurysm
    b. Jugular venous thrombosis
    c. Superior sagittal sinus thrombosis
    d. Deep venous thrombosis

100. First sign of hydrocephalus in children is:
    a. Post clinoid erosion
    b. Large head
    c. Sutural diastasis
    d. Thinned out vault

101. Punched out lesions and floating teeth are seen in:
    a. Metastasis
    b. Osteitis fibrosa
    c. Histiocytosis
    d. Asbestosis

102. Hyperintense corticospinal tract on T2W/MRI is/are seen in:
    a. Astrocytoma
    b. Amyotrophic lateral sclerosis
    c. Hemochromatosis
    d. Wilson disease

103. Prevertebral space thickness in adult is:
    a. 7 mm   b. 14 mm
    c. 22 mm   d. 30 mm

104. 'Thumb print' sign seen in:
    a. Candida
    b. Aspergillus
    c. Thermomyces
    d. Epiglottitis

105. Dawson finger in brain seen in which condition?
    a. Cortical vein thrombosis
    b. Multiple sclerosis
    c. Lacunar infarcts
    d. Alzheimer's disease

106. Water's view is used for
    a. Maxillary sinus
    b. Frontal Sinus
    c. Sphenoid sinus
    d. Mastoid air cells

107. In which stage of neurocysticercosis edema is not seen?
    a. Vesicular stage
    b. Colloid -vesicular
    c. Granulo-nodular
    d. Calcified

108. A 12-year-old boy has left body weakness. An MRI scan reveals a well-demarcated cystic lesion in right parietal lobe. There is no perilesional edema or calcification. The lesion is showing no enhancement on contrast scan. The mass effect is negligible. The likely cause of the lesion is?
    a. Taenia solium
    b. Schistosoma haematobium
    c. Taenia echinococcus
    d. Diphyllobothrium latum

109. Which of the following fractures is most commonly associated with CSF rhinorrhea?
    a. Le Fort I
    b. Le Fort II
    c. Le Fort III
    d. Pyramidal fracture

Multiple Correct Questions

110. Normal brain calcifications are present in:
    a. Pineal gland
    b. Choroid plexus
    c. Thalamus
    d. Dura mater
    e. Hypothalamus

111. Bare orbit sign seen in:
    a. Metastasis
    b. Neuroblastoma
    c. Optic nerve glioma
    d. Osteomyelitis
    e. Pseudotumor cerebri

112. J-shaped sella is/are seen in:
    a. Mucopolysaccharidoses
    b. Achondroplasia
    c. Opticchiasmglioma
    d. Neurofibromatosis
    e. Hydrocephalus

113. Physiological calcification of skull in X-ray is seen in:
    a. Pineal gland
    b. Choroid plexus
    c. Red nucleus
    d. Basal ganglion
    e. Habenular

114. Which one of the following tumors shows calcification on CT scan?
    a. Ependymoma
    b. Medulloblastoma
    c. Meningioma
    d. CNS lymphoma

115. Ring enhancing lesion in brain is/are seen in:
    a. Brain abscess
    b. Resolving hematoma
    c. Primary CNS lymphoma
    d. Encephalopathy
    e. Infarction

116. Caldwell view (occipito-frontal) can visualize:
    a. Spenoid sinus
    b. Nasal bone
    c. Maxillary sinus
    d. Ethmoid sinus
    e. Frontal sinus

Recently Asked Questions

117. Empty thecal sac sign on MRI is seen in:
    a. Arachnoiditis
    b. Discitis
    c. Vertebral osteomyelitis
    d. Tethered cord syndrome

118. A 45-year-old female complains of progressive weakness and spasticity of the lower limb with urinary hesitancy MRI shows a mid-dorsal intradural enhancing lesion. What is the most probable diagnosis?
    a. Meningioma
    b. Neuroeptithelial cysl
    c. Intradural lipoma
    d. Dermoid cyst

119. Growing fractures' are seen in:
    a. Skull
    b. Epiphysis of long bones.
    c. Cancellous bones.
    d. Ribs.

ANSWERS

1. **Ans. c.** Corpus callosum lipoma
2. **Ans. c.** Moyamoya disease

   Moyamoya is a rare idiopathic vaso-occlusive disease characterized by progressive irreversible occlusion of main blood vessels to the brain as they enter into the skull. The occlusive process stimulates the development of an extensive network of enlarged basal, transcortical and transdural collateral vessels. In Japanese, Moyamoya means hazy. The disease derives its peculiar name from the angiographic appearance of cerebral vessels in the disease that resembles "puff of smoke".

3. **Ans. b.** Germinoma

   Intracranial germinomas, also known as dysgerminomas or extra-gonadal seminomas, are a type of germ cell tumor and are predominantly seen in pediatric populations. They tend to occur in the midline, either at the pineal region (majority) or along the floor of the third ventricle/suprasellar region. On MRI, these lesions are usually homogenously isointense on T1 and T2-weighted images with marked homogenous contrast enhancement.

4. **Ans. b.** Restricted diffusion
5. **Ans. c.** Gadolinium enhanced MRI
6. **Ans. c.** Meningioma
7. **Ans. d.** Reticulated popcorn-like configuration
8. **Ans. a.** NCCT Head
9. **Ans. b.** Neurofibromatosis
10. **Ans. b.** Basal ganglia
11. **Ans. b.** Myelomalacia
12. **Ans. b.** Schizencephaly
13. **Ans. b.** Amyotrophic lateral sclerosis

    ALS, also known as motor neuron disease, is a neurodegenerative disorder characterized by a progressive muscular paralysis reflecting degeneration of motor neurons in the primary motor cortex, brainstem, and spinal cord. In patients with ALS, signal-intensity changes on conventional MR imaging (i.e, T2-weighted, PD-weighted, and FLAIR sequences) can be observed along the Cortico-Spinal Tract. Typically, Cortico-Spinal Tract changes, which are best followed on coronal scans, appear as areas of bilateral increased signal intensity from the centrum semiovale to the brainstem. Routine anatomic imaging of the brain and/or the spinal cord is helpful in ruling out diseases that mimic ALS with varying degrees of UMN and LMN signs. The revised criteria of the World Federation of Neurology Research Group on Motor Neuron Diseases state that conventional MR imaging studies are not required in those cases that have a clinically definite disease with a bulbar or a pseudobulbar onset. On the other hand, in patients with clinically probable or possible ALS, MR imaging can be useful in excluding several ALS-mimic syndromes, including cerebral lesions (e.g. multiple sclerosis and cerebrovascular disease), skull base lesions, cervical spondylotic myelopathy, other myelopathy (e.g. foramen magnum lesions, intrinsic and extrinsic tumors, and syringomyelia), conus lesions, and thoracolumbar sacral radiculopathy.

14. **Ans. c.** T1 WI are most diagnostic for acute plaques

    Ref: Dahnert Wolfgang 7/e p3131.

15. **Ans. a.** White matter

    Ref. Dahnert Wolfgang 7/e p313.

16. **Ans. a.** Absent oligoclonal band

    Natural history studies have shown that a younger age at disease onset is associated with a higher risk of conversion to clinically definite multiple sclerosis (CDMS) and that male gender is associated with a greater accumulation of disability according to the Kurtzke Expanded Disability Status Scale (EDSS) (Kurtzke, 1983; Weinshenker et al., 1989a, b; Confavreux et al., 2003; Confavreux and Vukusic, 2006a, b; Tremlett et al., 2006; Leray et al., 2010; Scalfari et al., 2010). Regarding the clinical characteristics, patients with CIS presenting with optic neuritis exhibit a lower risk of developing both multiple sclerosis and disability accumulation compared with CIS patients displaying other topographic characteristics (Weinshenker et al., 1989a; Runmarker and Andersen, 1993; Confavreux et al., 2003). Regarding biological factors, a recent meta-analysis showed that the presence of IgG oligoclonal bands increases both the risk of experiencing a second attack and the risk of disability accumulation (Dobsonet et al., 2013). To date, brain MRI remains the most reliable tool to predict future conversion to multiple sclerosis or the accumulation of disability. In this context, it has been demonstrated that a larger number of brain T2 lesions or Barkhof criteria based on a baseline MRI correlates with an increased risk of developing multiple sclerosis and disability in the mid- to long-term

17. **Ans. b.** Krabbe's disease
18. **Ans. c.** Blurring of grey and white matter junction of ipsilateral temporal lobe
19. **Ans. d.** Vein of Galen malformation

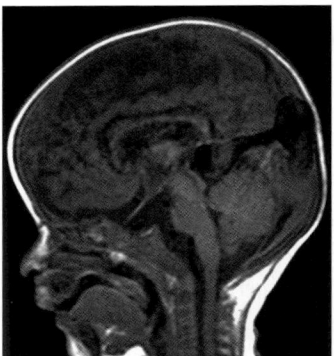

Vein of Galen malformations (VOGMs) are rare anomalies of intracranial circulation that constitute 1% of all intracranial vascular malformations. However, they represent 30% of vascular malformations presenting in the pediatric age group. It is thought to result from the development of an arteriovenous connection between primitive choroidal vessels and the median prosencephalic vein of Markowski. They can cause severe morbidity and mortality, particularly in neonates but also in infants and older children. Most of these malformations present in early childhood, often causing congestive heart failure in the neonate.

20. **Ans. b.** Ballooning of sella
21. **Ans. b.** Diffuse axonal injury
22. **Ans. d.** Video EEG with Ictal 99m Tc-HMPAO Brain SPECT
23. **Ans. a.** Tuberculous meningitis
24. **Ans. a.** Toxoplasmosis
25. **Ans. b.** Craniopharyngioma
26. **Ans. b.** Craniopharyngioma
27. **Ans. b.** Craniopharyngioma
28. **Ans. b.** Medulloblastoma
29. **Ans. c.** Astrocytoma (Pilocystic)
30. **Ans. b.** Hemangioblastoma
31. **Ans. a.** Hemangioblastoma
32. **Ans. c.** Tumors of Schwann cells are common

33. **Ans. a.** Subependymal giant cell astrocytoma (SGCA)
34. **Ans. a.** CT
35. **Ans. a.** Neurofibromatosis type 1
36. **Ans. a.** Solid dural masses
37. **Ans. d.** Wyburn-Mason syndrome

    Sturge-Weber syndrome or encephalotrigeminal angiomatosis a cutaneous, facial angioma in the distribution of the trigeminal nerve, and an ipsilateral, parietal/parietal–occipital vascular malformation.

    Rendu-Osler-Weber syndrome (hereditary hemorrhagic telangiectasia) is an autosomal-dominant dominant syndrome of multiple visceral, mucosal and cerebral vascular malformations.

    Wyburn-Mason (Bonnet-Blanc- Dechaume syndrome) or mesencephalo-oculofacial angiomatosis corresponds to facial angiomatosis, unilateral retinal angiomatosis and a cutaneous hemangioma in an ipsilateral trigeminal distribution with an AVM located in the midbrain

38. **Ans. a.** Sturge-Weber syndrome
39. **Ans. d.** Vertebral hemangiomas
40. **Ans. a.** Erosion of dorsum sella
41. **Ans. c.** Craniopharyngioma
42. **Ans. b.** Wilson's disease
43. **Ans. c.** Sutural diastasis
44. **Ans. c.** Erosions
45. **Ans. d.** Intra-axial tumor
46. **Ans. c.** Cavernous sinus hemangioma
47. **Ans. b.** CMV infection
48. **Ans. c.** Injury to cortical bridging veins
49. **Ans. c.** Crescent-shaped hyperdense lesion
50. **Ans. c.** Extradural hematoma
51. **Ans. c.** Intramedullary
52. **Ans. a.** Non-contrast computed tomography
53. **Ans. a.** Gadolinium enhanced MRI
54. **Ans. b.** MRI
55. **Ans. a.** MRl
56. **Ans. a.** NIRS (Near infra red spectroscopy)

    Continuous real-time monitoring of the adequacy of cerebral perfusion can provide important therapeutic information in a variety of clinical settings. The current clinical availability of several non-invasive near-infrared spectroscopy (NIRS)-based cerebral oximetry devices represents a potentially important development for the detection of cerebral ischaemia. NIR light can be used to measure regional cerebral tissue oxygen saturation (rSO_2). This technique uses principles of optical spectrophotometry that make use of the fact that biological material, including the skull, is relatively transparent in the NIR range. However, because of the poor signal-to-noise ratio as a result of the low intensity of transmitted light, most commercially available devices use reflectance-mode NIRS in which receiving optodes are placed ipsilateral to the transmitter and exploit the fact that photons transmitted through a sphere will traverse an elliptical path in which the mean depth of penetration is proportional to the transmitter and receiver optode separation. Fundamental challenges posed in utilizing transcranial reflectance NIRS to measure cerebral tissue oxygen saturation include the potential requirement for knowledge of the photon path length, the presence of non-heme chromophores, and variable light absorption by overlying extracerebral tissue.

57. **Ans. b.** Lumbar puncture
58. **Ans. b.** Intracerebral calcification
59. **Ans. c.** Lateral view
60. **Ans. b.** Non-contrast CT of the nose and para-nasal sinuses
61. **Ans. c.** Sphenoid sinus

Skull-SMV (Submentovertex) (also called Basal)

Area Covered: This view looks at the base of the skull, including structures such as the foramen ovale, foramen spinosum, and sphenoid sinuses

62. **Ans. a.** Bilateral subdural hematoma in CT
63. **Ans. c.** Agenesis of corpus callosum
64. **Ans. a.** Wilson's disease
65. **Ans. d.** Hallervorden-Spatz disease
66. **Ans. b.** Japanese encephalitis
67. **Ans. c.** Mandibular osteomas
68. **Ans. d.** Leptomeningeal angioma
69. **Ans. c.** EEG
70. **Ans. b.** Hyperacute stroke
71. **Ans. a.** Multiple sclerosis
72. **Ans. d.** Subacute hemorrhages and flow voids
73. **Ans. c.** Increased t1 signal in the wall of the right carotid artery
    Internal carotid artery dissection is a result of blood entering the media through a tear in the intima. The classical presentation includes local pain, headache, ipsilateral Horner syndrome, ischemic stroke and retinal ischemia

    ON MRI, the common features include:
    - High signal **crescent sign** within the wall of the vessel
    - Absent **flow-void**
    - Abnormal vessel contour on MRA
    - Evidence of cerebral ischemia
74. **Ans. d.** Amyloid angiopathy
75. **Ans. a.** Cerebral aneurysms
76. **Ans. c.** Carotid Doppler study
77. **Ans. d.** Hallervorden-Spatz disease
78. **Ans. d.** Cerebral angiography
79. **Ans. d.** Butterfly glioma
80. **Ans. a.** Arnold-Chiari type 1 malformation
81. **Ans. a.** Meningiomas
82. **Ans. d.** Absent dural-tail sign
83. **Ans. b.** Meningiomas
84. **Ans. a.** Vestibular schwannoma
85. **Ans. b.** Acoustic neuroma
86. **Ans. b.** Oligodendroglioma
    - *Most common intra axial brain tumor to show calcification is oligodendroglioma*
    - *90% of Oligodendroglioma show calcification when only 20% of astrocytoma shows calcification*
    - *Most common brain tumor to show calcification is Craniopharyngioma however, it is extra axial*
87. **Ans. d.** Admantinomatous
    - *Adamantinomatous (paediatric) ~90%*
    - *Papillary (adult) ~10%*
    - *Mixed: ~15%, but share imaging and prognosis similar to adamantinomatous*
88. **Ans. b.** Turricephaly
89. **Ans. d.** White matter of cerebral hemispheres, corpus callosum and the upper brain stem
90. **Ans. d.** Fracture floor of the orbit
91. **Ans. b.** Thalassemia
92. **Ans. a.** DWMRI with ADC mapping
93. **Ans. a.** MRI
94. **Ans. b.** Contrast MRI
95. **Ans. b.** T2-weighted MRI
96. **Ans. b.** Subependydomal-astrocytoma (SEGA of TS)
97. **Ans. a.** Caldwell's view
98. **Ans. a.** Hyperechogenicity
99. **Ans. c.** Superior sagittal sinus thrombosis
100. **Ans. c.** Sutural diastasis

101. **Ans. c.** Histiocytosis
102. **Ans. b.** Amyotrophic lateral sclerosis
103. **Ans. b.** 14 mm
104. **Ans. d.** Epiglottitis
105. **Ans. b.** Multiple sclerosis
106. **Ans. a.** Maxillary sinus
107. **Ans. a.** Vesicular stage
108. **Ans. c.** Taenia echinococcus
109. **Ans. c.** Le Fort III

Multiple Correct Answers

110. **Ans. a.** Pineal gland, **b.** Choroid splexus
111. **Ans. a.** Metastasis, **b.** Neuroblastoma
112. **Ans. a.** Mucopolysaccharidoses, **b.** Achondroplasia, **c.** Opticchiasmglioma, **d.** Neurofibromatosis, **e.** Hydrocephalus
113. **Ans. a.** Pineal gland, **b.** Choroid plexus, **d.** Basal ganglion, **e.** Habenular
114. **Ans. a.** Ependymoma, **c.** Meningioma
115. **Ans. a.** Brain abscess, **b.** Resolving hematoma, **c.** Primary CNS lymphoma
116. **Ans. b.** Nasal bone, **d.** Ethmoid sinus, **e.** Frontal sinus

Answers of Recently Asked Questions

117. **Ans. a.** Arachnoiditis
118. **Ans. a.** Meningioma
119. **Ans. a.** Skull

CHAPTER 3

Cardiothoracic Radiology

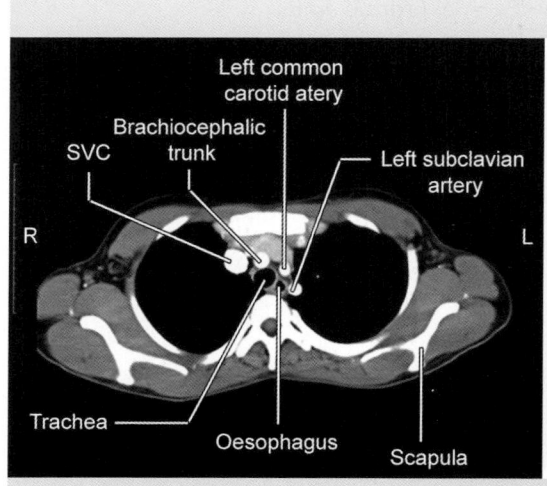
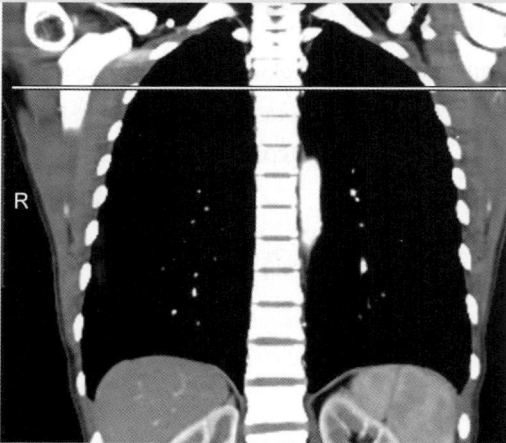
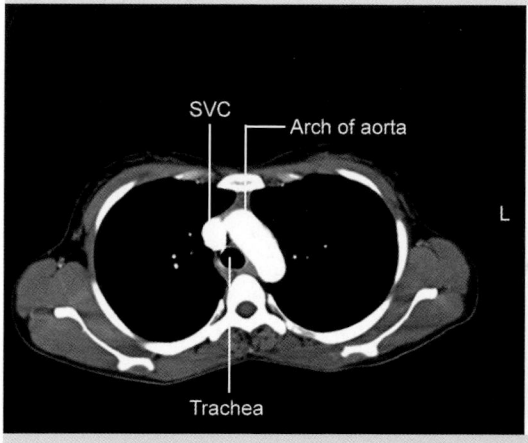
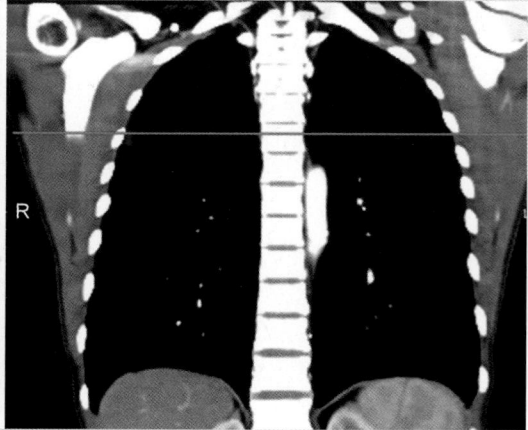

Cardiothoracic Radiology

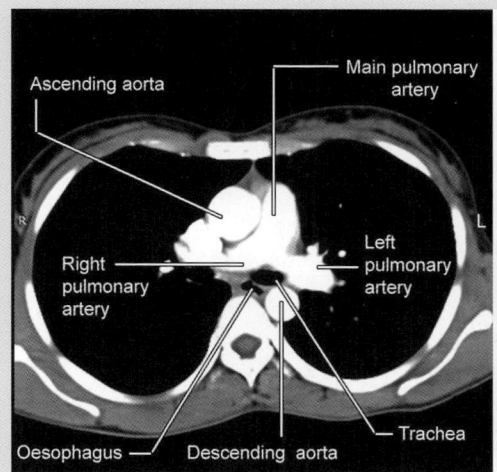
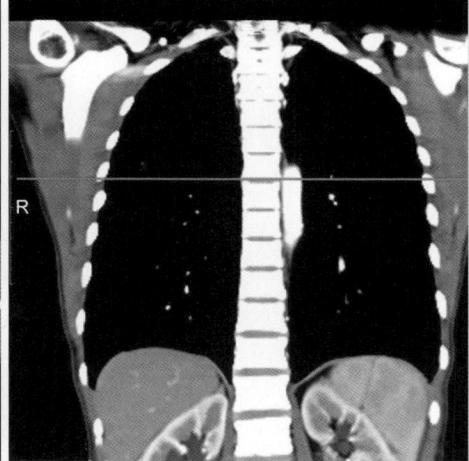
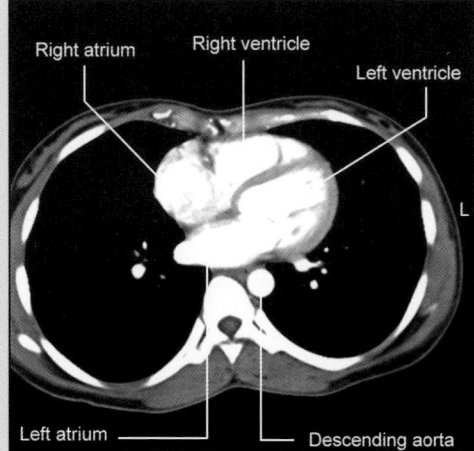
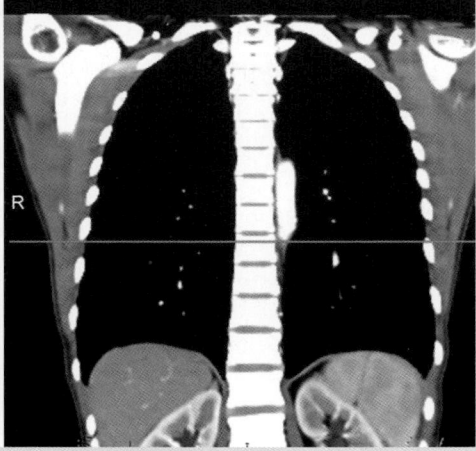
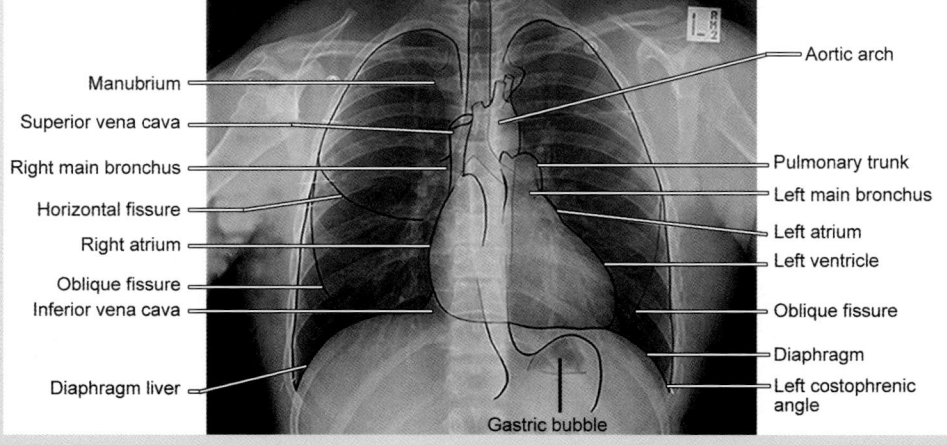

Normal chest X-ray

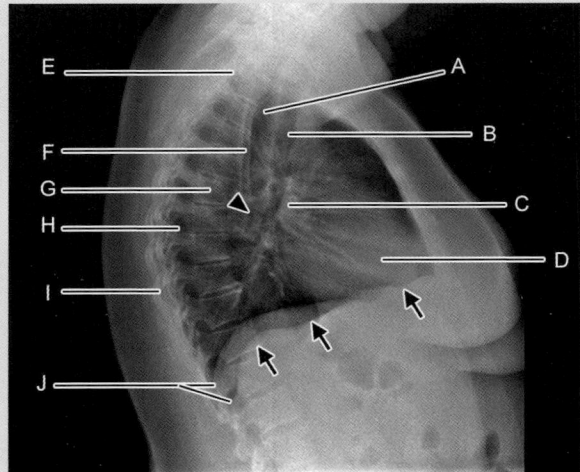

Lateral chest X-ray: Esophagus. (A), Trachea (B), Lung hili (C), Heart silhouette (D), Lung apices (E), Scapulae (F), Thoracic vertebra (G), Thoracic intervertebral foramen (H), Superimposed posterior ribs (I), Costophrenic angles (J), and diaphragm (Black arrows).

RADIOLOGICAL APPROACH

Chest

Investigations

Chest X-ray	–	Initial/first investigation to be done for common symptoms like cough, pain, dyspnea
CT	–	IOC for most chest and mediastinal pathologies
HRCT	–	IOC for ILD/bronchiectasis/Miliary nodules
USG	–	Very sensitive to detect noninvasively a small (pregnant/child) pleural effusion
MRI	–	IOC for pancoast tumor/neurenteric cyst
PET	–	IOC for nodal metastasis/myocardial viability
Angiography	–	Gold standard for pulmonary embolism

Additional views

Lateral decubitus view
- Recommended by American Thoracic Society guidelines for all patients presenting with community-acquired pneumonia (if thickness of effusion < 1 cm, it does not require intervention)
- To check movement of fluid

Expiratory film
- To demonstrate small pneumothorax and obstruction of airflow in FB inhalation

CT Reformat Techniques

Multiplanar and curved multiplanar reconstruction	– Airway and PE
MIP (max intensity projection)	– Vascular and micronodular disease
Min IP	– Air trapping/emphysema
Shaded surface display	– Airway abnormalities
Volume rendering	– Angiographic examination/large airway abnormalities
Virtual bronchoscopy	– For endoluminal pathology

USG

- Guided Aspiration in ICU
- Real time diaphragmatic paralysis
- Absence of sliding pleura sign in pneumothorax
- Absence of echogenic line when infiltrated by tumor
- Transesophageal EUS-for staging of mediastinal node.

MRI

- Heart and Great Vessels
- PE if radiation and contrast to be avoided
- Cystic nature of mediastinal lesions (non-serus fluid solid on CT).

PET

- False (–ve)
  - < 1 cm lesion
  - Carcinoid
  - Bronchoalveolar carcinoma (BAC)

Normal Chest X-ray

> **important**
> FFD is 180 cm in CXR to reduce magnification of heart shadow.

- Film focus distance is 100 cm for all X-rays except **chest X-ray** → 180 cm/6 feet
- **PA view** → 40% of lungs are covered by ribs and soft tissue
- Exposure made by centering at T5, full inspiration and breasts compressed to avoid obscuration of lungs.

Signs of AP X-ray

> **important**
> Hilar point—where superior pulmonary veins cross the descending lower lobe artery. (Left at a bit higher level than right).

- Scapulae overlie the lungs
- Ribs more horizontally
- Stomach bubble usually absent
- Clavicles project over the apices.

    High KVP—Preferred to reduce visibility of bony rib cage (120–170 KVP) → Penetrate even mediastinum/heart to see retrocardiac areas.

> **important**
> Transverse diameter of lower lobe arteries before their segmental division is 9–16 mm on PA view.

    Low KVP → To see miliary nodules and calcifications

Best views:
Right lung → Left anterior oblique
Left lung → Right anterior oblique.

Contributors of Normal Hilum

> **important**
> On right side, the pulmonary artery and vein can give density as if mass while on Left, there is bronchus in between the two.

- **Upper lobe veins and pulmonary arteries (major contribution)**

- Lower lobe veins do not contribute
- Left hilum is higher as left pulmonary artery pass above bronchus
- Lymphatics and lymph nodes do not contribute in normal hilar shadow

Thymus

- By the age of 40 years, replaced by fat except for a few streaks/nodules of residual thymus
- **Sail sign** → Triangular shape of thymus.
- **Wave sign of Mulvey** → indentations on thymus by ribs
- **Notch sign** → Indentation due to heart
    - Shape of thymus change with respiration and position.

> *important*
> If thickening or fat in lower part of oblique fissure/inferior pulmonary ligament-juxtaphrenic peak sign.

Facts

- Calcifications common in benign lesion
- Midline nodes considered ipsilateral in malignant spread
- Blunting of CP angle can be Normal in athletes
- In few, the Left hemidiaphragm can be higher up to 1.0 cm normally (due to gaseous abdomen) but to call it abnormal, it should be > 3.0 cm higher.

> *important*
> - Right hemidiaphragm is higher than left due to slight depression of left by heart
> - In dextrocardia; hence, right hemidiaphragm is lower

Multicystic Air-Filled/Radiopaque (Intrathoracic Lesions)

A. **Respiratory distress with Contralateral mediastinal shift**
   - *Congenital lobar emphysema (CLE)*
     - Most commonly found in infants and presents with progressive respiratory distress + progressive cyanosis within first 6 months of life.
     - Associated with VSD, TOF, PDA
     - Left upper lobe > Right middle lobe > Right upper lobe whole lung usually not involved
     - CxR → Initially radiopaque → then air-trapping and hyperlucent expanded lobe (after clearing of fluid)
   - *Congenital cystic adenomatoid malformation (CCAM)*

- Communicating with bronchi and Normal pulmonary vascular supply (unlike sequestration)
- CXR: Contralateral mediastinal shift by radiopaque/cystic mass
– *Congenital diaphragmatic hernia*
  - Bochdalek
  - Morgagni
  - Eventration of diaphragm

B. **No Respiratory Distress and No Mediastinal Shift**
   – *Esophageal duplication cyst*
   – *Bronchogenic (lung) cyst (do not communicate with tracheobronchial tree-most common intrathoracic foregut cyst)*
   – *Bronchopulmonary sequestration*
   – *Pneumatocele formation*

Unilateral Translucent/Opaque Hemithorax

Unilateral Translucent/Radiolucent Hemithorax	
Due to ↑ air	• Pneumothorax • Emphysema • Pneumatocele • Bullae • Macleod's syndrome (Swayer James syndrome)
Due to ↓ soft tissue/↓ blood	• Mastectomy • Poland's syndrome (absent pectoralis major) • Polio (atrophy of muscles) • Pulmonary embolism (Westermark's sign) (due to reduced flow) (Focal oligemia)
Due to tilted patient	• Scoliosis • Positional • (most common-Rotation)

Unilateral Radiopaque Hemithorax	
No Mediastinal Shift	• Consolidation • Small effusion • Mesotheliomas
Contralateral Shift	• Massive pleural effusion (Figure) • Diaphragmatic hernia • Massive tumor
Ipsilateral shift (↓ air)	• Collapse • Pulmonary agenesis • Pneumonectomy • Lymphangitis carcinomatosa • Fibrothorax

important
Translucency is proportional to air and inversely to soft tissue and blood flow.
Opacity is inversely proportional to air and proportional to soft tissue, consolidation, effusion, blood flow.

important
Poland's syndrome → Absence/hypoplasia of pectoralis major + i/l hand and arm anomalies (syndactyly) ± p. Minor/± rib anomalies ± hypoplasia of breast and nipple.

Diaphragmatic Hernias

Bochdalek hernia	Morgagni hernia
• Congenital/childhood	• Adults
• Posterior aspect on left	• Anterior at Right cardiophrenic angle
• Defect through pleuroperitoneal canal	• Omentum and gut
• Retroperitoneal fat, spleen, kidney	• May be through esophageal hiatus
• BPL (Bochdalek's → Posterior and left)	• MAR (Morgagani → anterior and right)

HEART

Normal Heart Borders
- **Right**
  - SVC
  - Right lateral aspect of ascending aorta (old age) sometimes Right brachiocephalic trunk
  - Right atrium
  - IVC.
- **Left**
  - Aortic knuckle/knob ± Left subclavian vein
  - Pulmonary conus (MPA)
  - Left atrial appendage
  - Left ventricle

important
Left atrium and right ventricles do not contribute in formation of heart borders.

Signs of Left Atrial Enlargement (Mitral Stenosis)

- Posteriorly–Indentation on anterior wall of esophagus (earliest) but seen only on barium/CT
- Superiorly–Elevation of Left main bronchus (earliest to be seen on radiograph)
- Splaying of carina (n ≈ 60–70°) (X-ray)
- Laterally:
  - Right–double contour/double right heart border/ double atrial shadow
  - Left–prominent left atrial appendage below pulmonary conus- causes straightening of left heart border.

important
LA forms the base of Heart, opposite to apex.

important
Lateral displacement/indentation on descending thoracic aorta toward left by enlarged LA-**Bedford Sign.**

important
In some of the medicine books, straightening of left heart border is given as the earliest sign which is not described in radiology.

Right Atrial Enlargement

- Convex Right margin >3 cm from Right lateral vertebral border

- Enlargement of SVC
- ↑ **Height of Right atrium (Most Reliable)**
  [Top of Aortic arch to SVC/RA junction distance is < height of RA (Normally vice-versa)]

Left Ventricle Enlargement
- Prominent Left heart border with rounding
- **Inferolateral shift of apex.**

Right Ventricle Enlargement
- Elevation of cardiac apex
- Less prominence of aortic knuckle.

Pleural Effusion
Minimum amount required to be detected on
- Lateral view – 75 mL
- PA view – 100–200 mL
- Lateral decubitus – < 10 mL

(best view to detect minimal effusion)
- USG – ≈ 1 mL (best Inv/IOC to detect minimum pleural effusion)
- When posterior and lateral CP angles are blunted —200–500 mL

***Subpulmonic effusion**
- Fluid b/w base of lung and diaphragm
- IOC → CT/USG
- On X-ray → High hemidiaphragm with lateral shift of peak contour.

***Lamellar effusion**
- Effusion between visceral pleura and lung

***Vanishing/pseudotomor**
- Loculated effusion in fissure

Lordotic View—for
- Interlobar effusion (Reverse Lordotic view)
- Middle lobe pathologies.

Bilateral Exudative Pleural Effusion
- Pulmonary embolism
- Lymphoma
- Metastasis
- RA, SLE
- Postcardiac injury syndrome
- Myxoedema

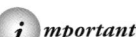
Massive p. Effusion cause → c/l mediastinal shift and depression of diaphragm.
If no shift–rule out associated obstructive collapse of lung/pleuralmalignancy/mesothelioma/metastatic disease.

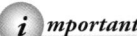
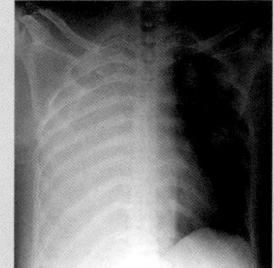
Pleural effusion without mediastinal shift s/o obstructive lesion.

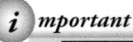
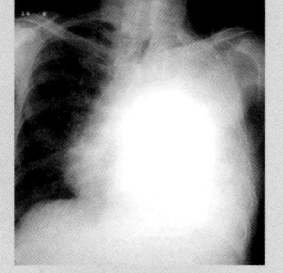
Left sided massive pleural effusion right mediastinal shift.

Right-sided Pleural Effusion
- Liver abscess
- Ascites
- Heart failure

Left-sided Pleural Effusion
- Pancreatitis
- Pericarditis
- Aortic dissection
- Esophageal rupture
If pleural efffusion shows air fluid level-Hydropneumothorax (Figure)
On supine X-ray → veil like haziness with preserved vascular markings
USG:
- Transudate-echo free
- Exudative-echoes (change shape with breathing) septae. Solid lesion does not change shape)

MRI:
- Limited role-Triple echo pulse sequence can differentiate exudative from transudative
Chylous effusion → high signal on T1W (normally fluid low on T1W)

Pneumothorax
- Best X-ray PA–Expiratory
- Best investigation–NCCT
- **USG** →
  - **Sea shore** sign on **M mode** USG suggests motion b/w visceral and parietal pleura. **Absent in Pneumothorax. (Stratosphere sign)**
  - (sliding pleura sign on 'B' mode normally) Absent in pneumothorax.

Pneumothorax-Signs on X-ray
- **Visceral pleura sign with lung laterally devoid of vascular markings**
- Ipsilateral transradiancy
- Deep finger-like costophrenic sulcus (deep sulcus sign)
- Visible anterior costophrenic recess/**double diaphragm sign**
- **Visualization of undersurface of heart-continuous diaphragm sign** → seen in pneumo-mediastinum
- Diaphragm depression.

 mportant
Vanishing/pseudotumor–loculated effusion in fissure (CHF).
Lamellar effusion–effusion b/w visceral pleura and lung (not between visceral and parietal pleura).

 mportant
Infective effusions/empyema shows enhancing visceral and parietal pleura giving **split pleura sign.**

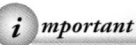 *mportant*

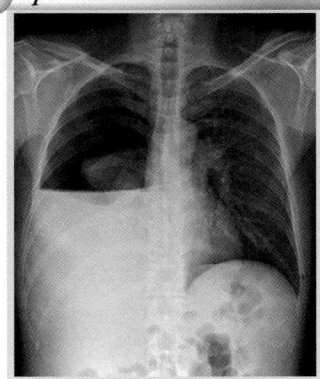
(R) Hydropneumothorax

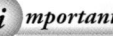 *mportant*

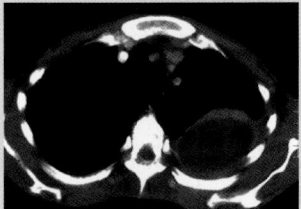
Split pleura sign (empyema)

> **important**

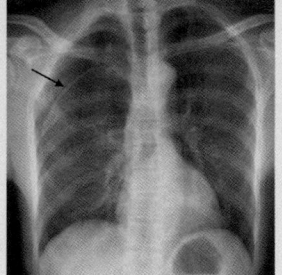

Pneumothorax with visceral pleura sign

> **important**
> Immediate chest tube drainage required for tension pneumothorax, which can cause **Reexpansion edema**, which progresses for 1–2 days and clears within a week.

> **important**

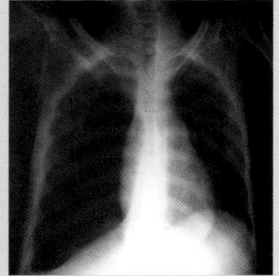

Depressed (R) hemidiaphragm due to tension pneumothorax

> **important**
> *MRI is better than CT for malignant mesothelioma, if extension into diaphragm and chest wall suspected.

> **important**
> *Most common benign tumor of sternum – chondrosarcoma
> *Pleural metastasis – most common pleural neoplasm.

Tension Pneumothorax

Life-threatening condition as it causes adverse effects on gas exchange (intrapleural pressure +ve relative to atmosphere).

Signs on X-ray

- Contralateral mediastinal shift
- Depressed diaphragm (more reliable sign) (Figure on next page).

Pneumo-mediastinum-Signs on X-ray

- Undue clarity of mediastinal border
- Air outlining **thymus (Spinnaker sail sign)**
- Air around pulmonary **artery (ring sign)**
- **Air around bronchi (double bronchial wall sign)**
- **V sign of Naclerio**.
- Over Diaphragmatic surface (continuous diaphragmatic sign)

Pneumopericardium

- Gas does not go beyond pericardial reflections superiorly (aortic knuckle) and changes position with position of patient.

Pleural Thickening

- USG–Unreliable until >1 cm (CT more sensitive)
- Fibrous pleural thickening and pancoast tumors can be indistinguishable (CT/MRI can differentiate)
- **Fibrothorax/diffuse pleural thickening**–smooth uninterrupted pleural thickening which extends over at least one quarter of chest wall or > 8.0 cm in craniocaudal direction on CT, 5.0 cm laterally and thickness > 3 mm.

Calcified Pleural Thickening

- **Asbestosis (parietal and diaphragmatic pleura classical)**
- Empyema (TB)
- Sequelae of Hemothorax (visceral pleura).

Malignant Pleural Thickening

- Mesothelioma-CT–circumferential, nodularity, parietal thickening of more than 1 cm and involvement of mediastinal pleura.

Funnel chest/Pectus excavatum → (lower ½ of sternum)

- Isolated

- Marfan's
- Heart disease (ASD)
  CXR
    - Left shift of heart
    - Straightening of Left heart border
    - Prominence of main pulmonary artery segment
    - Loss of descending aortic interface
    - Increased opacity of Right cardiophrenic angle
    - Loss of clarity of Right heart border–mimicking Right middle lobe disease
    - Steep inferior slope of anterior ribs
    - Undue clarity of the lower dorsal spine seen through the heart.

Pigeon Chest (Pectus Carinatum)

MEDIASTINUM

Division of Mediastinum

- Anterior (anterior to 1st line)
- Middle (b/w 1st and 2nd line)
- Posterior (posterior to 2nd line)

On Lateral X-ray 1st line passing from anterior wall of trachea and then posterior surface of heart.

2nd line–Line passing 1 cm behind the anterior margin of vertebral bodies.

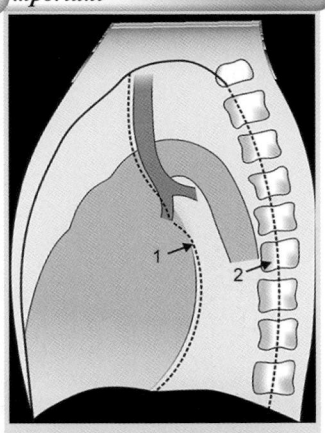

Division of mediastinum

Anterior Mediastinal Masses

(4Ts)-Terrible tetrad
- **Thyroid**
- **Thymic:** thymomas (most common)
- **Germ cell tumors/teratomas**
- **Lymphadenopathy/Terrible lymphoma**

Middle Mediastinal Masses

(ABCDE)
- Vascular masses aneurysm (MC)
- Bronchogenic cyst (2nd most common)
- Carcinoma bronchus
- Distant metastasis/lymph nodes (MC)
- Enteric cyst

Posterior Mediastinal Tumors

Neurogenic (most common)

Mediastinal Masses

- Neurogenic (most common overall)

> *important*
> *Uni/biplanar fluoroscopy– 1st imaging technique to guide percutaneous pleural interventions.

> *important*
> - Remote pleural metastasis from transpleural spread-invasive thymoma.

> *important*
> CT more useful than radionuclide studies for intrathoracic thyroid masses.

- Thymic (most common tumor of anterior mediastinum–thymoma which is most common tumor of thymus in adults)
- Nodal

Pediatric
- **Neuroblastoma/ganglioneuroma (Most common)**
- Foregut cysts
- Germ cell tumors

MDCT → IOC for most mediastinal pathologies

MRI → IOC for
- For suspected neurogenic tumors with intraspinal extension
- Distinguishing solid mass and vessel
- Relationship with pericardium and vessels/diaphragmatic invasion

USG → ECHO/endoscopic
- **Solid vs cystic diff (Most important indication)**
- Cardiac vs paracardiac mass diff
- **Guided mediastinal biopsy**

PET-CT-better for
- Lymph node metastasis
- Neuroendocrine tumors

> *important*
> Foamy appearance of LN in PCP in AIDS patients and metastasis from mucinous tumors.

Thymomas
- Most common tumors of thymus in adults
- CT most sensitive to detect thymoma

Features on CT
- Cyst
- Round/oval
- Punctate/curvilinear calcification
- Enhancement

Rebound thymic hyperplasia
- Poststress/Poststeroid/antineoplastic drug
- Difficult to differentiate from tumor recurrence

Germ Cell Tumor
- Mediastinum is MC extragonadal site of germ cell tumors. Usually anterior to thymus
- Seminoma most common-malignant GCT

> *important*
> **Egg Shell Calcification**
> - TB
> - Lymphoma after RT
> - **Sarcoidosis**
> - **Silicosis (most common)**
> - Coccidioidomycosis
> - Histoplasmosis
> - Pneumoconiosis

- Mature Teratomas are MC Mediastinal GCT-Most are Cystic
- Usually stable but hemorrhage and infection — rapid increase in size
- Fat and Ca^{++} are present

Nodal Ca^{++}

- TB
- Fungal
- Sarcoidosis
- Amyloidosis
- Metastasis from Pri. calcifying tumors:
    - Osteosarcoma
    - Chondrosarcoma
    - Mucinous colorectal
    - Ovarian tumor

LN calcification is rare in metastatic neoplasm otherwise.

Fat in Nodes

- Fatty replacement of inflammatory nodes
- Whipple's disease

Strikingly Enhancing Nodes

- Highly Vascular Tumor Metastasis
    - Melanoma
    - Carcinoid
    - Leiomyoma/sarcoma
    - Renal
    - Thyroid
- Rarely–Castleman's disease

Investigation of choice for nodes-CECT

> **important**
> IOC for nodes- CECT

> **important**
> Most common tumor of posterior mediastinum is neurogenic tumor MRI-IOC

Foregut Duplication Cyst

- **Bronchogenic**
    - **Thin respiratory lining and cartilage** (Ca^{++} - rare/displace carina anteriorly and esophagus posteriorly-**like thyroid and aberrant Left p. artery-pulmonary sling**
- Enteric (Esophageal Duplication Cyst)
    - Can have hemorrhage/thicker walls
    - Barium: extrinsic/intramural compression
    - More intimate contact with esophagus

> **important**
> Posterior mediastinum is most common location of extra-abdominal neuroblastoma.

- Neurenteric cyst
  - Usually have a fibrous connection to intraspinal contents
  - Wall: both gastrointestinal and neural elements
  - Nearly always associated with vertebral body defects.
  - IOC-MRI

Mediastinal pseudocyst
- Post. mediastinal-CECT-IOC
- Continuity with pancreas/any peripancreatic collection

Peripheral neurogenic tumor (neurofibroma)
- In intercostal/paraspinal space with scalloping of adjacent bones
- Punctate foci of calcification
- **Target sign on T2W images**
- **Dumb bell shape**
- Differential diagnosis- lateral meningocele

Ganglioneuroma/ganglioneuroblasma
- Elliptical orientation vertical in paravertebral location anterolateral to 3–5 vertebral bodies.
- Homogenous intermediate signal on both T1 and T2

Paragangliomas →
- Chemodectomas-most common–close to arch of aorta
- Pheochromocytomas (functional)-Post. mediastinum (Close to Left atrium or interatrial septum)
- Imaging features
  - **Rounded-very vascular**
  - Enhance intensely
  - **MRI–high signal on T2 (light bulb sign) (IOC for adrenal paraganglioma)**
  - MIBG/somatostatin receptor scintigraphy-IOC for extraadrenal pheochromocytoma (DOPA-PET, if given in the option is the best answer)

Extramedullary Hematopoiesis
- Expansion of marrow/bone–**lace like trabeculae**
- Masses in paravertebral gutter of lower thorax usually. Bilateral, symmetrical, smooth.

Fibrosing Mediastinitis
- Infiltrative soft tissue with calcification
- IOC-CT > MRI

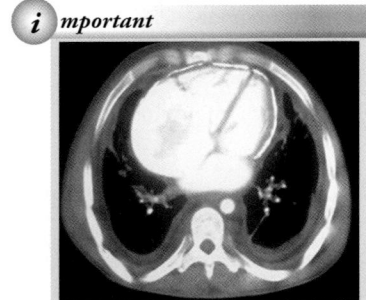

important
Chronic calcific pericarditis- TB

important
Substernal fluid collections and dots of air are (n) in 1st 20 days following sternotomy.

- MRI cannot pick calcifications (required to differentiate from lymphoma and metastasis which usually do not have Ca^{++})

PERICARDIUM

USG-most common investigation for initial assessment of pericardium
    Best – CT
    Flask or water bottle configuration → pericardial effusion

> **important**
> Mach effect → abrupt change in the density b/w the lung and adjacent heart and mediastinum-pnemomediastinum.

Constrictive Pericarditis

- Predominantly anterior to RV
- ≥ 4 mm → MRI ≈ CT but CT is better for calcific pericarditis. (ECHO – most sensitive)
- ECHO and clinical details: IOC for diagnosis of cardiac tamponade
- CT and MRI: IOC for the diagnosis of cause of cardiac tamponade

Malignant mesothelioma is most common primary pericardial neoplasm.
Metastatic melanoma to pericardium neoplasm, Hyper on T1 and hypo on T2W.
Echo–initial IOC
MRI → IOC

> **important**
> Finding a (N) pericardium excludes a diagnosis of constrictive pericarditis. However, finding of thickened pericardium does not necessarily imply presence of constriction.

Hypertrophic Cardiomyopathy (HOCM)

Echocardiography
- Asymmetric septal hypertrophy
- Banana-like left ventricular cavity
- Abnormal systolic anterior motion (SAM) of mitral valve

Causes of Massive Cardiomegaly

- Multiple valvular disease
- Dilated cardiomyopathy
- Pericardial effusion
- Ebstein's anomaly
- ASD

Small Heart

- Normal
- Emphysema
- Addison's disease
- Malnutrition (PEM)
- Constrictive pericarditis

Cardiothoracic Ratio

- Largest transverse diameter of heart/widest internal diameter of thorax

Cardiomegaly if

- Ratio >50% (adults)
- >60% (infants)

LUNG PARENCHYMAL PATHOLOGIES

Consolidation

Air space/alveoli opacification with obliteration of vascular markings
- **Depending upon contents consolidations can be**
  - *Infective exudates* → Pneumonia
  - Fluid-pulmonary edema
  - Blood → contusion
  - Tumor cells → malignancy
  - Pus cells → abscess

Ground Glass Opacification

If air space opacifies, without obliteration of vessels (Active and reversible stage of disease- alveolitis)
- Initial stages of
  - Pneumonia
  - ILDs
  - PCP

TUBERCULOSIS

Primary TB

- Homogenous opacity mimics community acquired
- (Multifocal involvement and cavitation) → rare in pneumonia
- Lymphadenopathy is hallmark with or without pnumonia (Ipsilateral hilar and mediastinal) (also in TB with AIDS)
- Nodal pressure and erosion can cause segmental collapse (ante. Seg. of RUL and middle lobe)
- Bronchial perforation → Endobronchial spread → Tree in bud (like broncho-pneumonia)
- Hematogenous spread – miliary TB (uncommon in primary TB)

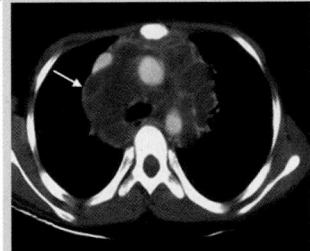

Multiple conglomerate necrotic rim enhancing mediastinal lymph nodes

*Pleural effusion is also common in children
*Peripherally enhancing conglomerate-Necrotic lymph nodes on CT

Primary TB-Focus → Ghon focus/lesion (commonly subpleural perifissural)

Usually resolves completely but 1/3rd cases may have well-defined rounded or irregular/linear with or without calcification (Ghon focus).

Postprimary TB (PPT)

Either due to previous infection or due to BCG vaccination hypersensitivity to tubercular proteins

Greater inflammatory reaction and caseous necrosis most common sites → **Apicoposterior** of upper and superior segments of lower lobes. (Poorly marginated nodular and linear opacities).

Features

- Cavitation: Rasmussen aneurysm-Rare life-threatening complication of cavitary tuberculosis caused by granulomatous weakening of **pulmonary arterial wall**
- **Endobronchial spread** → Tree in bud (Figure)
  Tree in bud also seen in
  - Bronchiolitis
  - PCP (AIDS)
  - **TB (most common)**
  - Pseudomonas aeruginosa
- P. effusion → more likely empyema
- **Miliary pattern**-Hematogenous spread (more common than Pri)
- **Healing by fibrosis** → Nodular linear fibrosis, volume less, bronchiectasis, cyst, bullae, lung distortion.

*Hemoptysis → First vessel to be studied however in bronchial artery

Miliary shadows

- More typical of progressive primary in older
- Multiple small (2 to 5 mm) discrete nodules scattered randomly and evenly throughout both the lungs
- Usually do not reach beyond 5 mm size
- Usually seen in
  - TB,
  - Sarcoidosis,
  - Pneumoconiosis,
  - Silicosis,

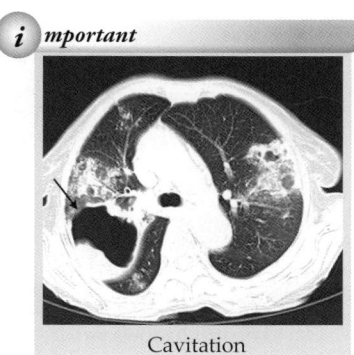

Cavitation

important
(Ghon focus) + calcified nodes (I/L) ± draining lymphatic = Reinke's complex (s/o prior-pri. TB)

important
*Isolated involvement of anterior segment (except in contiguous spread) excludes the diagnosis of tuberculosis.

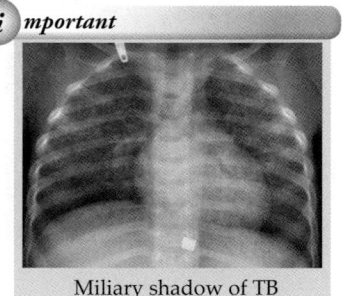

Miliary shadow of TB

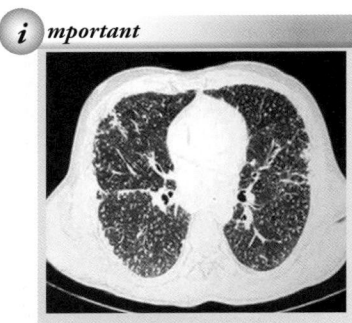
Miliary shadows on CT

- Metastasis,
- Chickenpox (Ca^{++}),
- Histoplasmosis,
- Hemosiderosis (MS),
- Oil embolism,
- Alveolar microlithtisis (sand-like calculi in alveoli–familial).

Tuberculomas (Pri/post pri)

- Localized parenchymal disease that alternatively activates and heals show → satellite lesions and **calcifications (features of benign disease)**
- IOC–CECT for both Pri and Post Pri

Activity/Features

- Ill-defined coalescing nodules
- Poorly marginated linear opacities
- Cavitary disease.

D/d of Cavitary Lesion on Chest X-Ray

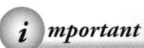
Tree in bud appearance after bone marrow transplant
Early (< 1 month)
- Aerobic bact
- Candida
- HSV

Middle (1–4 months)
- CMV
- RSV

Late (> 6 months)
PCP

- Wegener's granulomatosis
- Septic emboli
- Infections-TB, anerobes, pneumocystis/staph. (pneumatoceles)
- RA
- LCH
- LAM
- Sarcoid
- Metastatic/malignant
- Developmental (sequestration)

Nontubercular mycobacteria-M. kansasii → like post. pri.
Mycobacterium avium complex → Multiple nodules with bronchiectasis in lingula and middle lobes Right

*P. effusion and nodes are (Rare)

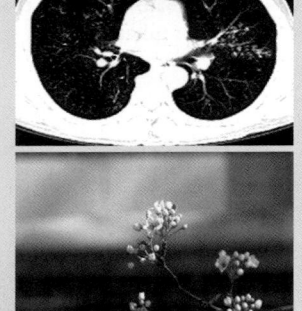
Endobronchial spread-tree in bud

OTHER INFECTIONS

Alveolar (lobar) or Interstitial (bronchopneumonia) pattern
- **Lobar pneumonia**
  - Unifocal, distal air space near visceral pleura,
  - Spread via col-lateral air drift (homogenous)
  - As airways are patent → (air-bronchogram) → Little to no volume loss

- **Bronchopneumonia**
  - Causes multifocal, distal airway,
  - e.g. atypical pneumonia/viral → Reticular/reticulonodular (mycoplasma pneumonia)

Other Causes of Air Bronchogram (arrow in Figure)
- Pneumonic consolidation
- Contusion
- Pulmonary edema
- Hyaline membrane disease (HMD)
- ARDS
- Bronchioalveolar carcinoma
- Round pneumonia (in children due to collateral spread via canals of Lambert)

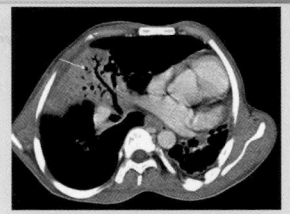

Air bronchogram on CT

Bulging Fissure Sign
- **Klebsiella pneumonia (due to very exudative response)**
- Lung abscess and **tumor (due to direct mass effect)**

Lobar Collapse

Causes increased opacity of lung and features of volume loss.

Direct Signs of Collapse
- Displacement of interlobar fissure, P. vessels and bronchi (Most Reliable)
- Hilar elevation upper lobe collapse
- Depression → Lower lobe collapse

Indirect Signs
- Compensatory shift-hyperinflation of other lobes
- Crowding of ribs
- Mediastinal shift

Other Indirect Signs
- Shifting granuloma sign
- **Luftsichel sign (air crescent)** → overinflation of superior segment of Ipsilateral lower lobe with paramediastinal translucency
- Displacement of anterior junctional line
- Divergent or parallel pattern of vessels in upper lobe collapse
- Tracheal shift
- Diaphragm shift

> *important*
> **Golden 'S' sign** → central mass compressing bronchus with collapse distal lung with Inferior bulge of medial horizontal fissure due to mass and superior bulge/convexity of lateral part of horizontal fissure due to collapse.

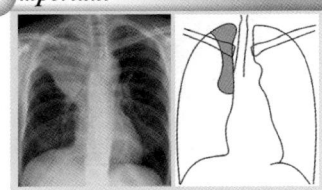

Golden 's' sign

> *important*
> CECT is IOC for both collapse and consolidation.

> *important*
> Collapse shows relative homogenous enhancement unlike pneumonia (due to crowding of vessels and obliteration of airspace).

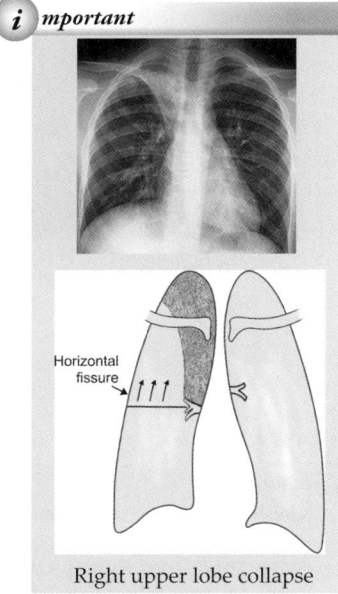

Right upper lobe collapse

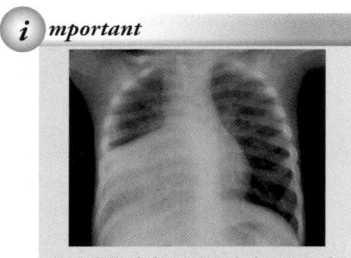

Middle lobe consolidation silhoutting the right heart border

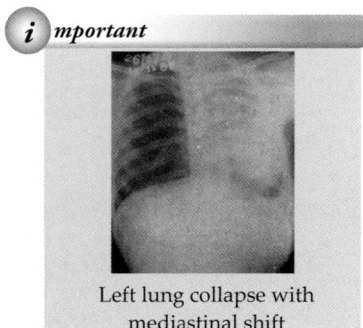

Left lung collapse with mediastinal shift

*Least mediastinal shift with → Middle lobe collapse
*Maximum mediastinal shift with → Lower lobe collapse

Silhouette Sign

- Given by Felson
- When there is density/collapse/consolidation **in lung, it obliterates that part of SVC/aorta/heart/diaphragm, which is in direct anatomical contact.**
  For example, Middle lobe → Right heart border, lingular Left heart border basal lung → diaphragm.

Silhouette structure	Contact with lung
Upper right heart border/ascending aorta	Anterior segment of RUL
Right heart border	RML (medial)
Left heart border	Lingula (anterior)
Aortic knob	Apical portion of LUL (posterior)
Anterior hemidiaphragms	Lower lobes (anterior)

Middle lobe syndrome → Collapsed Right middle lobe with bronchiectasis due to focal bronchostenosis secondary to pulmonary TB.

Superior triangular sign → Triangular density to Right of mediastinum in Right lower lobe collapse due to displacement of junctional line.

Flat waist sign → Extensive collapse of Left lower lobe (flattening of aortic and pulmonary knuckle due to rotation of heart and shift).

Anaerobic Infections

- Due to aspiration in ventilated patients
- **Apicoposterior of upper lobe**
- **Superior/posterior basal of lower lobes.**

Histoplasmosis

- Nodule with central calcification → **Target lesion (specific)**

Coccidioidomycosis

- Miliary nodules.

Staph

→ Pneumatocele (Figure) and septic emboli in drug addicts

PCP

→ Pneumatocele/tree in bud in AIDS/GGO/no lymphadenopathy or effusion perihilar opacification

Pseudomonas A

→ Tree in bud/GGO

North American Blastomycosis

- Mimics-Progressive pri TB → fibrocavitary

Aspergillus

Aspergilloma → air crescent around a freely mobile ball in a cavity (most common-old TB cavities) (Figure)

D/d of Air Crescent

- Aspergilloma/fungal ball
- Inspissated pus in a cavity
- Tumor in a cavity
- Hematoma in old cavity due to bleed
- Hydatid cyst

Allergic Bronchopulmonary Aspergillosis (ABPA)

- Branching thick tubular opacities
- Bronchiectasis (central)
- Finger in glove (due to mucous impaction)
- Type-III immune reaction

Chronic Necrotizing (semi-invasive) → Like TB Invasive (Immunocompromised)

- One or more poorly marginated homogenous areas
- Cavities
- Wedge-shaped infarct
- Miliary nodules
  IOC-CECT-Ground glass halo around nodules (hemorrhage)
  HRCT → angioinvasive nature with occluded vessels (Halo sign due to haemorrhage)

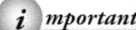

CT mucous bronchogram sign → obstructing lesion causing lobar collapse
Mucus-filled bronchi in enhancing collapsed lung.

If incomplete fissure → The lung might not collapse completely due to collateral drift of air.

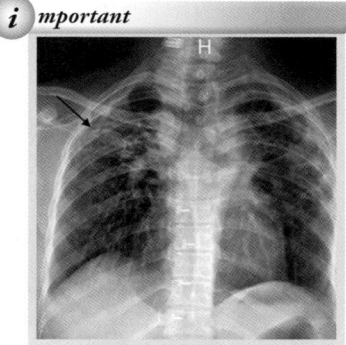

Air crescent sign

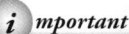

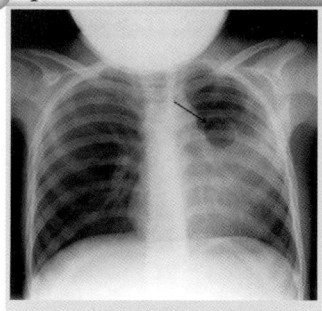

Pneumatocele in staph infection

Atoll/Reverse halo sign → Cryptogenic organizing pneumonia.
(Ring shadow of consolidation around GGO)

Hydatid Cyst of Lung

CXR

- Homogenous Roughly Spherical/Oval
- Sharply demarcated
- No/Rarely calcify (as no stable nidus due to breathing)
- Air crescent [(If pericyst Ruptures-Due to fibrous host Reaction (Not a true membrane)]
- Complex Rupture (Rupture of cyst walls endo/ectocyst)

CT- IOC

- Air fluid level (floating membranes/water lilly/camalote sign (Figure)
- Double wall
- Dry cyst with crumpled membranes (Rising sun sign)
- Empty cyst (If contents expectorated out if communication with bronchus)
- Air bubble sign (perforated hydatid)

> **important**
> If collapse of both (R) middle and lower lobe S/o → obstruction of bronchus intermedius.

> **important**
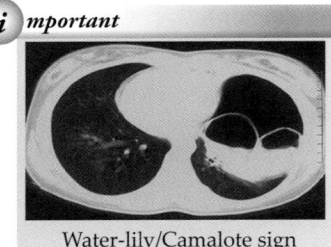
> Water-lily/Camalote sign

Pulmonary Complications of HIV and AIDS Infections

- PCP
- TB
- Cryptococcus
- Kaposi sarcoma
- LIP (lymphocytic interstitial pneumonia)
- CMV

Pneumocystis Jirovecii Pneumonia

CXR

- Bilateral Reticular opacities and GGOs
- Miliary
- Cavitary nodules
- **P. Eff./L.N. rare**
- **Pneumatoceles/Pneumothorax**
- Bronchopleural fistulas

> **important**
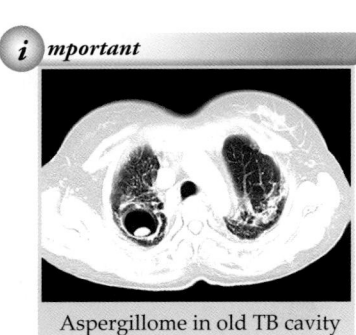
> Aspergillome in old TB cavity

*Pentamidine aerosol causing increased frequency in upper lobes

IOC-CT → Unilateral/Bilateral-GGO or homogenous opacities in geographical distribution

Cryptococcus Neoformans

- Diffuse reticular opacities
- **P. Effusion**
- **Lymphadenopathy** } Contrary to PCP
- Cavitation

Kaposi Sarcoma

- Coarse linear opacities in perihilar region, pleural/pericardial effusion, mediastinal lymphadenopathy (most common AIDS associated malignancy).

CMV

- Most common cause of pneumonia in renal transplant
- **Most common cause of chorioretinitis in AIDS.**

AIRWAY

Post-tracheostomy Stenosis

- Typically begins at 1–1.5 cm distal to the inferior margin of tracheostomy stoma.

Relapsing Polychondritis

- Posterior wall of trachea in early stage but involved in later stages.
- Flaccid which collapses on expiration.

Tracheobronchopathia Osteochondroplastica

- Multiple cartilaginous nodules and bony submucosal nodules on inner surface of trachea.

Sabre Sheath Trachea (Reduced coronal diameter)

- Diffuse narrowing (COPD)
- Intrathoracic trachea narrowing with abrupt normal caliber at thoracic inlet

Tracheobronchomegaly (Mounier-Kuhn disease)

- Marked dilatation of trachea and main branch
- Tracheal diverticulosis

> *important*
> ABPA → most common acute changes → transient consolidation mucoid impaction and atelectasis
> Permanent → bronchiectasis

> **important**
> Bilateral Upper Lobe → cystic fibrosis and ABPA severity
> → cystic > varicoid > cylindrical
> Unilateral-UL → TB
> Lower lobes → viral infections (childhood)

Tracheobronchomalacia (Weakened cartilage)

- Radiographs → with almost 300% reduction **in AP diam on exp.** on CT- narrowing of > 50% on exp.
- Coronal diameter '↑' → lunate configuration-lunate/crescentic → due to bowing of postmembranous trachea.

Bronchiectasis

CXR–thickened bronchial walls
- Parallel → tramlines or tramtract
- End on → signet ring/oval opacity
- Cystic bronchiectasis → multiple thin-walls ring shadows → bunch of grapes [Figure]

HRCT Findings of Bronchiectasis
- Dilatation of bronchi
- With or without bronchial wall thickening
- Lack of tapering of bronchial lumen (cardinal sign)
- Internal diameter greater than adjacent p. artery (signet ring sign)
- Visualization of bronchus within 1 cm of costal pleura
- Abutting mediastinal pleura
- Mucus filled dilated bronchi

Varicose bronchiectasis → beaded appearance → (string of beads)
- Mucus-filled lobulate 'V' or 'Y'-shaped densities → glove finger
- End on-homogenous nodular opacities adjacent to vessels
- Infectious bronchiolitis → **tree in bud** (linear branching)

> ***IOC → MDCT with thin collimations > HRCT misses within interval of slices

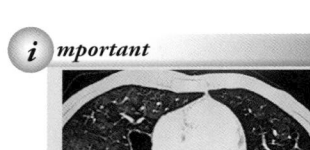

Cystic-Bronchiectasis

> **important**

Broncholithiasis CXR
- Disappearance of previously identified calcified nidus.
- Change in position of a calcified nidus.
  CT and fiberoptic bronchoscopy–evidence of airway obstruction, atelectasis, mucoid impaction, obstructive pneumonitis.

Emphysema
- **Barrel-shaped kyphotic chest**

- Increased intercostal space
- Tubular Heart-
- **Imaging feature**
  - **Overinflation (best predictors of severity)**
  - **Height of Right lung > 29.9 cm**
  - Location of Right hemidiaphragm at or below 7th rib anteriorly
  - Flattening of diaphragm **(Terrace pattern)**
  - Enlargement of retrosternal space
  - Widening of sternodiaphragmatic angle
  - **Narrowing of transverse cardiac diameter**
  - Reduced vessels in affected lung.
- Large progressive upper lobe bullae occupy significant vol. of hemithorax
- CT-IOC
- Four types
  - Paraseptal
  - Centrilobular
  - Panacinar/panlobular
  - Irregular/paracicatricial

Assessment of Air-Trapping by

- **Expiratory MDCT/HRCT** → in obliterative bronchitis
- Texture analysis technique
- CT densitometer by calculating Pixel Index (objective)

Lung Malignancy (WHO)

- Sq. cell ca
- Adenocarcinoma
- Small cell ca
- Large cell ca

Benign

- Uniform cavitation
- Smooth margin/sharply defined
- **Central/lamellated Ca^{++}**
- **Popcorn Ca^{++} hamartoma (fat)**
- **Very long doubling time**
- No enhancement in soft tissue nodule
- Pleural tail

> *important*
> Giant bullous emphysema/vanishing lung syndrome/pri. bullous disease.

> *important*
> Central (sq cc/small cc) peripheral (adenocarcinoma).

> *important*
> Bulky mediastinal adenopathy and fastest rate of growth-Small cell carcinoma.

> *important*
> Squamous cell carcinoma → More likely to cavitate.

> *important*
> Bullae > 1 cm thin but perceptible wall
> cyst → imperceptible wall.

> *important*
> - Density mask technique by CT → for emphysema
> - **Expiratory HRCT is superior to inspiratory**
> - Increased lung markings → 'dirty chest' → bronchitis (loss of clarity of lung vessels).

> **important**
> Diagnosis of chest wall extension is unreliable on CT even, if mild-thickened pleura:
> - Local chest wall pain remains the single-most specific indicator of whether or not the tumor has spread to the parietal pleura or chest wall
> - On CT → only if bone destruction or large soft tissue.

> **important**
>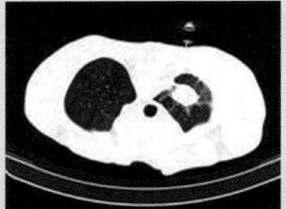
> Malignant nodules showing corona Radiata appearance

> **important**
> Cavitating metastasis
> - Sq cc Head and Neck
> - Ca cervix
> - Osteosarcoma
> - TCC
> - RCC (rare)

> **important**
> Solitary metastasis
> - Colon
> - Kidney
> - Breast
> - Testicular tumors
> - Bone sarcomas
> - Malignant melanoma

> **important**
> Black bronchus sign (seen in GGO)–more black air in bronchus than lobule which is usually more in secondary lobule.

Malignant Nodules

- Doubling time 1–18 months
- Amorphous cloud like dystrophic/eccentric/stippled calcification (metastasis from cartilage or bone forming tumors)
- Umbilicated border
- Thick irregular inner wall of cavity (SCC-most common)
- Lobulated spiculated margins
- Sub solid nodules- GGO nodules/partly solid and GGO
- Corona radiate-highly suggestive but nonspecific (fibrotic nodules) (Figure)

CECT-IOC
PET:
- Indeterminate nodule/staging
- **False negative in**
  - <1 cm
  - Carcinoid
  - Low-grade adenocarcinoma.

PET-CT → now investigation of choice for distant spread (but outside the CNS)

INTERSTITIAL LUNG DISEASE

ILD Interstitial shadows
Fine inter-/intralobular septal thickening/GGO
Coarse → Reticular
- IPF → mediastinal lymphadenopathy
- **Sarcoidosis → Hilar and mediastinal nodes** > skin > peripheral nodes > eyes > spleen > central nervous system > parotid > **bones (least)**

Stage-I → only L.N. (lambda sign/ panda sign)
II → L.N. + lung parenchyma
III → only lung parenchyma
IV → pulmonary fibrotic nodules-irreversible

Bilateral symmetrical → as evenly distributed throughout mediastinal and hilar

Nodular sarcoidosis → **galaxy sign**→ **confluent nodules**

If very small nodules below resolution of HRCT → GGO (alveolar sarcoidosis)

Parenchymal consolidation and GGO → Reversible

while reticulation and architectural distortion → nonreversible

- RA→ Intrathoracic manifestations
  - **Pleural effusion (most common)**
  - **UIP-pattern ILD**
  - Constrictive obliterative bronchiolitis
  - Bronchiectasis
  - Organizing pneumonia
  - Follicular bronchiolitis
  - **Necrobiotic nodules (uncommon)**
    - May cause pneumothorax
    - **FDG-uptake**
- SLE
  - Pleuritis → with pain → P. effusion (most common)
  - Diaphragmatic dysfunction (shrinking lung syndrome)-↓ Lung vol
  - Restricted diaphragmatic movement → band atelectasis
- SJS
  - Most common lung manifestation is NSIP
- **Asbestosis (Predilection for lower lobes)**
  - Parietal pleural plaque (most common) (does not cause significant impairment of lung function)
  - Diaphragmatic
  - Paravertebral (most common to get miss on CxR)
  - Spares → apices, CP angles and visceral pleura
  - Pleural calcification – Round atelectasis (Pseudotumor)
  - Round-Atelectasis/**Crow's feet sign/Vacuum cleaner sign**/Swiss cheese air bronchogram/ Folded Lung/**comet tail sign**: crowding of bronchi and blood vessels that extend from border of mass till hilum) Strong and homogenous enhancement after i/v inj of contrast (indicative of atelectasis rather than neoplasm)

ACUTE THORACIC CONDITIONS

Pulmonary Embolism

CXR- Normal in 30% →

- Westermark's sign (area of focal peripheral oligemia) (most specific)

> *important*
> **Comet tail sign**
> CT Chest – Round atelectasis
> USG Abdomen–Adenomyomatosis of GB

> *important*
>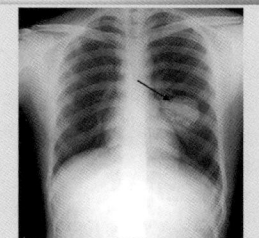
> Popcorn calcification in a nodule- pulmonary hamartoma

> *important*
> *Pneumothorax → seen with metastasis from osteosarcoma

> *important*
> **Upper Lobe Involvement (BREAST)**
> - Beryllium (Barytosis)
> - Radiation
> - Extrinsic allergic alveolitis
> - AS
> - Silicosis/Sarcoidosis
> - TB

> *important*
>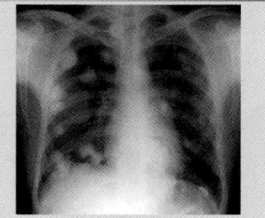
> Cannon Ball nodules- metastasis

> **important**
> **Lower Lobe Involvement (Fail)**
> - Fibrosing alveolitis
> - Asbestosis
> - Idiopathic pulmonary fibrosis
> - Lymphangiomyomatosis

> **important**
> **CTPA-Signs of RV Strain**
> - Dilatation of RV
> - Left shift of septum
> - Reflux in IVC
> - Enlarged central P. artery.

> **important**
> TB → only draining nodes involved → asymmetrical

> **important**
> Nodal enlargement does not appear after parenchymal opacities have developed in sarcoid. While in lymphoma-both prog-ress in unison.

> **important**
> **Honeycombing**
> Histiocytosis
> Sarcoidosis
> Scleroderma
> Pneumoconiosis
> RA
> UIP
> Fibrosing alveolitis

> **important**
> Upper lobe venous diversion (MS/Pulmonary venous hypertension) → **Stag-antler's sign** Reverse moustache sign Cephalization of pulmonary veins

> **important**
> T/t → Pulmonary edema in 1st 3 days of treatment resolution with diuretic (leads to worsening of C × R in 1st 3 days).

- **Knuckle sign/Palla's sign** → enlarged Right descending pulmonary artery
- **Hampton's hump**-peripheral wedge-shaped opacity with convexity toward hilum
- **Melting sign** → infarcts show rapid clearing contrary to pneumonic consolidation
- **Fleischner's lines** → long curvilinear densities reaching pleural surface
  Fleischner's sign → elevated hemidiaphragm
  Felson's sign-pleural effusion L > R
  - Initial Screening-D-Dimers
  - IOC → CECT > V/Q scanning
  - Gold standard → Pulmonary angiography/arteriogram (most specific) However, CT pulmonary angiography has virtually replaced the invasive angiography-hence IOC

Ventilation Agents
- Xe-133
- Kr-81
- Technegoce

Perfusion
- Tc99MAA (macroaggregates of albumin)
  V/P mismatch - sign of emboli
  Reverse mismatch → COPD (abnormal ventilation)
  V/Q scanning (IInd line) when one cannot tolerate i/v contrast
- **CEMRI-Excellent for diagnosis of DVT (MR venography)**
- Can detect large proximal PE but unreliable for smaller segmental PE
- **D-dimer → High negative predictive value to exclude PTE**

Pulmonary Edema: (Excess of extravascular lung water)
- **Cardiogenic-(due to ↑ hydrostatic pressure LVF, MS, atrial myxoma)**
- **Noncardiogenic (↑ vascular permeability)**
  - Volume overload due to renal failure
  - Increased capillary permeability

Stages

*Earliest is equalization of vessels (13–15 mm Hg)

- 16–19 mm Hg → upper lobe diversion of blood (cephalization)/reverse moustache sign
- 20–24 mm Hg → interstitial peribronchial cuffing edema/pleural effusion/kerly lines
- > 25 mm Hg (acute) alveolar edema → perihilar fluffy opacities (Bat wing on X-ray or white out)
- > 30–35 (in chronic phase) (due to thickening of lymphatics/connective tissue)

    Kerley A → Thickened deep interlobular septae (2–6 cm long) from hilum (nonbranching)

    Kerley B → Nonbranching transverse (1–3 cm) perpendicular to pleura

    Thick interlobular septae Kerly C→ Spider web appearance

Causes

- LVF
- MS
- Pneumoconiosis
- Lymphagitic carcinomatosis
- Interstitial fibrosis, sarcoidosis, alveolar cell carcinoma, lymphoma, lymphatic obstruction, lymphangiectasia, lymphangiomyomatosis

Causes of ARDS

- Trauma, septicemia, shock, fat embolism, burns, pancreatitis near drowning, Mendelson's syndrome, oxygen toxicity.

Cardiogenic (LVF)	Noncardiogenic (ARDS)
• Central	• Peripheral
• Upper lobe veins prominent	• Nearly symmetrical
• Cardiomegaly	• Heart usually Normal
• Enlarged mediastinal nodes	
• ↑ attenuation of mediastinal fat	

Pulmonary Arterial Hypertension (PAH)

Mean pulmonary arterial pressure
- > 30 mm Hg during exercise
- > 25 mm Hg at rest in systole

> **important**
> - P edema: Very rapid change in opacity (clearing) (fastest) (in a matter of hours)
> - IInd fastest to get clear → P. hemorrhage (few days).

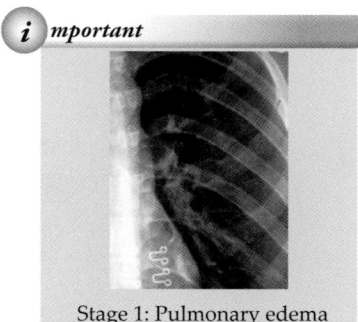

Stage 1: Pulmonary edema Cephalization

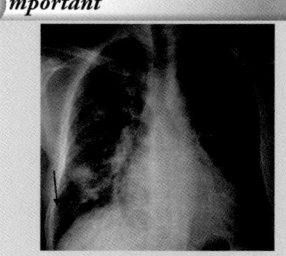

Peribronchial cuffing and subpleural Kerley B lines stage 2

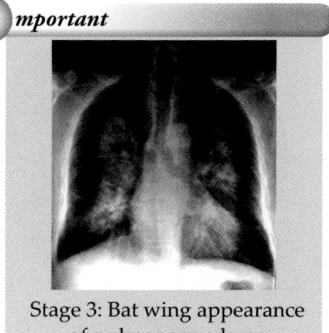

Stage 3: Bat wing appearance of pulmonary edema

Vascular Signs

- Enlargement of central and segmental pulmonary arteries and tapering of peripheral arteries (**peripheral pruning**)
- Diameter ratio of MPA/ascending aorta > 1
- Max. diameter of descending branch of pulmonary artery (1 cm medial and 1 cm lateral to hilar point) > 16 mm (M), > 15 (F)
- **Disproportionately small peripheral arteries**
- Subplural pulmonary infarct
- Calcified plaques of central p. arteries (**pathognomonic**)

Mediastinal and Cardinal Signs

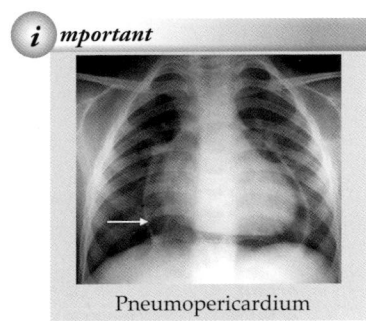

Pneumopericardium

- Cardiac enlargement right sided with hypertrophy
- Dilatation of IVC, SVC, and coronary sinus
- Mosaic perfusion without dilatation of bronchi

Pulmonary Venous Hypertension (PVH)

- LVF, MS, Left atrial myxoma
- **Long-standing PVH** → Fine miliary calcification or fine nodular pattern scattered throughout lung (**pulmonary hemosiderosis**)
- **Severe long-standing PVH → (pulmonary ossicles)**
- Opacification pattern
  - Perihilar bat-wing
  - Right upper zone alveolar edema in severe MR.

Trauma

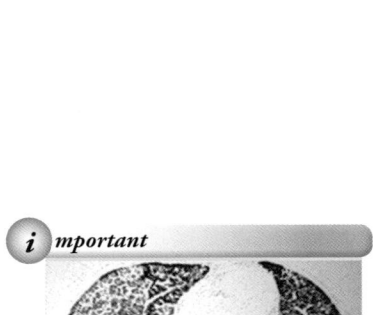

Pulmonary alveolar proteinosis

FAST → focussed assessment with sonography for trauma.

Stable-fast helical MDCT is the most useful imaging investigation.

Two-phase intravenous contrast-enhanced single CT data acquisition-from skull base to mid-femur-dilute contrast in portovenous phase and then high concentration contrast agent injected later, providing arteriographic image in the same examination.

For metallic beam-hardening artefacts

- High Kv CT

- Alternating the angle of acquisition (either by gantry or position of patient)

Majority of acute traumatic aortic injury (ATAI)
- At aortic isthmus (2.0 cm distal to origin of Left SCA)
- Aortic root (5%)
- **Osseous Pinch** → Thoracic spine and sternoclavicular junction
- **Water hammer effect** → Increased intravascular pressure within aorta

Mediastinal Hematoma

- Mediastinal widening (> 25% of chest width)
- Blurring of margins of the aortic arch
- Loss of definition of aortopulmonary window

Indirect

- Deviation of trachea and NG tube
- Widening of paratracheal stripe

Direct

- Intimal Flap
- Pseudoaneurysm
- Pseudocoarctation (sudden change in caliber)
- Contained ruptures

> **Important**
> Photographic negative of pulmonary edema.
> Patchy opacities are peripheral and seen parallel to chest wall in chronic **eosinophilic pneumonia**.

Tracheobronchial Injury →

- Pneumothorax persistent to treatment by chest drain
- **Fallen lung sign** (parenchyma in dependent part)

Esophagus → Mostly Iatrogenic Injury

- **Pneumothorax on supine film**
  - **Deep costophrenic sulcus**
  - Hyperlucency over the hemidiaphragm
  - Well-defined mediastinal or cardiac border
- **Sucking chest wound**
  - Wound with flutter valve
  - Unilateral air flow
  - Pneumothorax resistant to treatment

> **Important**
>
> | | N | Pneumothorax |
> |---|---|---|
> | B Scan | Sliding pleura sign | Loss of Sliding Peura sign |
> | M Node | Seashore sign | Stratosphere sign |

Lung injury

- Most common-parenchymal injury is → contusion

- Delay of 6 hours for it to be visible on X-ray → immediate on CT
- Blast lung (survivors of near proximity explosive)
  - Bilateral diffuse pulmonary infiltrates in butterfly pattern on CxR
- Multiple fractures in '3' contiguous ribs–flail chest
- Injury to upper '3' ribs-most dangerous due to involvement of
  - Brachial plexus
  - Sub clavian vessel
  - Trachea
  - Spine

Diaphragmatic Injury

- Hour glass/collar sign → on CT in case of diaphragmatic rupture
- Dependent viscera sign → due to lack of support from torn diaphragm

Foreign Body Inhalation

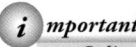

important
Solitary nodule on X-ray
↓
CT scan (Next investigation)
↓
Image-guided biopsy (Best)

- Enter commonly in Right bronchus (wide and vertical orientation)
- **Peanuts - (most common)**
- **Expiratory – CXR - best**
  - Hyperinflation due to air-trapping (most common) (50%)
  - Atelectasis (collapse) → Radiopaque
  - Recurrent pneumonia (5%)

Congenital Heart Diseases

Indications of MDCT

- **Vascular rings-as assessment of airways is necessary**
- **MAPCAS-major aorto pulmonary collateral arteries**
- **Abnormal pulmonary venous return**
- **Vascular stents**
- **Coronary artery disease assessment**
- **Contraindication to MRI**

Causes of increased pulmonary flow-plethora (L to R shunt)	Reduced pulmonary flow oligemia
ASD (most common detected in adults) VSD PDA TGA TAPVC Vein of galen malformation Truncus arteriosus	Ebstein's anomaly Triscupid atresia Tetrology of Fallot TGA with stenosis of pulmonary artery

Acynotic Heart Diseases

Septal Defects

- Normal left atrium-ASD (dilated RA and RV)
- Dilated left atrium-VSD, PDA

Coarctation of Aorta

- Inferior rib notching of bilateral 3rd to 9th ribs due to dilated intercostals collateral vascular channels.
- Inferior rib notching of right 3rd to 9th rib- if pre isthmic coarctation (before origin of left SCA)
- Inferior rib notching of left 3rd to 9th rib – if aberrant origin of right SCA from post isthmic area
- Reverse '3' sign on X-ray due to impression by left SCA and post-stenotic dilatation

Cyanotic Heart Diseases

Increased Pulmonary Vascularity

- Total anomalous pulmonary venous return (**TAPVR**) (types I and II)
- Transposition of the great arteries (**TGA**)
- Truncus arteriosus (**TA**)

Decreased Pulmonary Vascularity

- **Tetralogy of Fallot (normal heart size)**
- **Double outlet right ventricle (DORV) with pulmonary stenosis**
- **Ebstein anomaly with atrial septal defect**

Tetrology of Fallot (Most Common Cyanotic Congenital Heart Disease)

- **Infundibular pulmonary stenosis**
- **Hypertrophy of right ventricle**
- **VSD**
- Overriding of aorta over right ventricle

Pentalogy of Fallot
- Ventricular septal defect (VSD)
- Right ventricular outlfow tract narrowing or complete obstruction
- Right ventricular hypertrophy
- Over riding aorta
- **Atrial septal defect (ASD) or patent ductus arteriosus (PDA)**

Ebstein's Anomaly
- Apically shifted septal and mural valves
- Atrilization of ventricle
- Gross enlargement of the heart (Box shaped heart)
- Functional pulmonary stenosis
- Right to left shunt

Pentalogy of Cantrell
- Omphalocoele
- Ectopia cordis (abnormal location of heart)
- Diaphragmatic defect
- Pericardial defect or sternal cleft
- Cardiovascular malformations

Radiological Appearance of Heart in Various Diseases

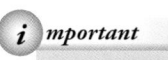

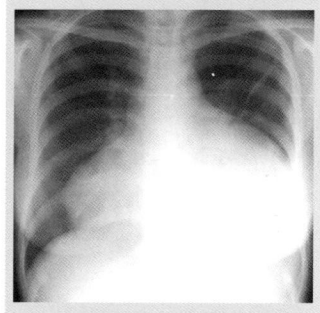

Money bag/flask shaped heart-pericardial effusion

*Fallot's Tetralogy: Boot shaped heart
*Tricuspid Atresia: Box shaped heart
*TAPVC (total anomalus pulmonary venous connection): Snow man appearance, 8 shaped heart, cottage loaf appearance.
*Constrictive pericarditis: Egg in cup
*Pericardial effusion: Water bottle, pear shaped.
*Pulmonary hypertension: Jug handle
*Transposition of vessels: Egg shell cracking/egg on side
*Hilar dance on fluoroscopy is seen in cases of ASD and Bronchiectasis

Coronary Calcium Score-Agatston Scoring
- Calcifications as densities ≥ 130 HU

Score	>	<
1	130	199
2	200	299
3	300	399
4	400	

Total score by summing scores from all the slices →
Indicate risk of cardiovascular events
Total score: 10 → no risk, 1–10 Symbol minimal, 11–100 – mild, 101–400 = moderate, > 400 = severe

*Presence of large amount of calcification does not indicate the presence of significant stenosis.

CARDIAC MRI

MRI is a well-established modality for evaluating congenital and acquired cardiac diseases. The high soft-tissue contrast, availability of a large FOV, multiplanar acquisition capability, and lack of ionizing radiation are particularly appealing features of cardiac MRI. However, the main limitation of cardiac MRI compared with CT is the evaluation of coronary calcifications. There are certain technical challenges unique to cardiac MRI. Most notably is the rapid and complex motion of the heart and pulsatility of the great vessels due to normal contractility. In addition, the effects of respiratory motion and systolic ventricular blood velocities up to 200 cm/s further complicate cardiac imaging. Nevertheless, these issues are generally mitigated by implementation of ECG (cardiac) gating; navigator echo respiratory gating; breath-hold techniques; rapid, high-performance gradients; improved field homogeneity; and advanced pulse sequences.

Enhancement Patterns on Post Contrast MRI

IV injection of Gadolinium is taken up into both normal and injured myocardium. In normal myocardium there will be early wash out of contrast where as in injured myocardium the wash out is very slow resulting in delayed enhancement after 10 - 15 minutes when compared to the normal myocardium.

When a coronary artery is occluded the infarction always starts subendocardially and progresses towards the epicardium depending on the duration of the occlusion.

Both acute and chronic infarctions enhance.

In acute infarctions the contrast enters the damaged myocardial cells due to myocyte membrane disruption.

In chronic infarctions the late enhancement is a result of retention of contrast material in the large interstitial space between the collagen fibers in the fibrotic tissue

important
Infarcted myocardium is bright on delayed images.

Stunned and Hibernating Myocardium

Stunning is defined as post ischemic myocardial dysfunction that persists despite restoration of normal blood flow. Over time there can be a gradual return of contractile function depending on the transmurality of the ischemia. If the degree of transmurality as seen on the delayed enhancement images is less than 50%, the myocardial function is likely to recover.

Hibernation is a state in which some segments of the myocardium exhibit abnormalities of contractile function at rest. This phenomenon is highly significant clinically because it usually manifests itself in the setting of chronic ischemia, that is potentially reversible by revascularization. The reduced coronary blood flow causes the myocytes to enter a low-energy 'sleep mode' to conserve energy. There is an inverse relationship between the transmural extent of hyperenhancement, and the likelihood of wall motion recovery following revascularization. If the transmural extent of late enhancement is less than 50% the function is likely to improve after revascularization

> *important*
> Cine imaging in combination with delayed-enhancement MR allows identification of:
> - Myocardial stunning following acute myocardial infarction and
> - Hibernating myocardium in the setting of chronic ischemic heart disease.

Hypertrophic Cardiomyopathy

Hypertrophic cardiomyopathy (HCM) is characterized by a hypertrophied left ventricle, defined as diastolic wall thickness 15 mm or more, without any identifiable cause such as hypertension or valvular disease. (Normal ventricular septal measurement is 8-12 mm).

Usually there is asymmetric thickening of the wall most prominently involving the ventricular septum without abnormal enlargement of the ventricular cavities.

In about 25% of patients there is obstruction of the left ventricular outflow tract (LVOT) due to hypertrophy of the basal septum and a systolic anterior motion of the mitral valve (SAM).

Constrictive Cardiomyopathy

The most important differential diagnosis of restrictive cardiomyopathy is constrictive cardiomyopathy. MRI can differentiate between those two diagnoses:
- Pericardium is usually thickened in constrictive cardiomyopathy
- Diastolic septal bounce is seen in constrictive, but not in restrictive cardiomyopathy

Dilated Cardiomyopathy

- Dilated cardiomyopathy is defined as dilatation with an end diastolic diameter greater than 55 mm measured on the left ventricular outflow image and an ejection fraction < 40%.
- Patients with idiopathic dilated cardiomyopathy show either no enhancement or linear midmyocardial enhancement.
- This enhancement is explained by the presence of fibrosis.
- This indicates a poorer prognosis.
- Patients with midmyocardial enhancement are at higher risk of sudden cardiac death and arrhythmias

Arrhythmogenic Right Ventricular Cardiomyopathy (ARVC)

- It is an inherited cardiomyopathy whose hallmark is fibrofatty replacement of the RV myocardium.
- The left ventricle is also involved in at least 15% of patients.
- The patients develop progressive RV failure and present with ventricular arrhythmias which can cause sudden cardiac death especially in young people.
- Morphologically the right ventricle can have regional wall thinning, hypertrophy, dilatation and microaneurysms. Functionally cine images are evaluated for RV dysfunction, microaneurysm formation, and focal areas of RV dyskinesia. MR scans may be overinterpreted since the RV has substantial normal variations including variable trabeculation and small outward bulges near the insertion of the moderator band.

Myocarditis

- Myocarditis is often caused by a viral infection.
- Acute myocarditis can be a cause of sudden cardiac death.
- Most patients spontaneously recover, however 5-10% of the patients will develop a dilated cardiomyopathy [30].
- Acute myocarditis may clinically mimic an acute myocardial infarction with chest pain.
- Abnormal laboratory findings and ECG changes may also suggest an acute coronary syndrome.
- The MRI findings however are discriminatory between those two diagnoses. The late enhancement

images are key, as the late enhancement in myocarditis is subepicardially or midmyocardially located, and does not originate from the subendocardium

Takotsubo Cardiomyopathy

- Takotsubo cardiomyopathy or apical ballooning syndrome is a transient cardiomyopathy affecting postmenopausal women after physical or emotional stress.
- Patients present with symptoms mimicking an acute myocardial infarction.
- The ECG changes and abnormal laboratory findings may also mimic an infarction.
- However, coronary angiography is usually normal, but if a left ventricle angiogram is performed, marked hypokinesia of the apical cardiac segments is noted
- The Japanese word takotsubo means octopus pot.
- This pot was used to capture octopus and resembles the shape of the left ventricle during systole in these patients.

QUESTIONS

1. Radiological features of left ventricular heart failure are all, except:
   a. Kerley B lines
   b. Cardiomegaly
   c. Oligemic lung fields
   d. Increased flow in upper lobe veins

2. A patient presents with cough and fever. On X-ray examination, a homogenous opacity silhouetting the right heart border with ill-defined lateral margins is seen. What would be the most probable diagnosis?
   a. Pneumonia affecting medial zone of right middle lobe
   b. Pneumonia affecting superior zone of right lower lobe
   c. Loculated pleural effusion
   d. Pneumonia of anterior zone of right middle lobe

3. Patient with h/o tachyarrhythmias is on implantable cardioverter defibrillator. He develops shock. Best method to know the position and integrity of ICD is to do:
   a. Contrast CT
   b. MRI
   c. USG
   d. Plain radiograph

4. Best noninvasive investigation to check for viability of myocardium is:
   a. Echocardiogram
   b. FDG-18 PET CT
   c. MIBI scintigraphy
   d. Thallium scintigraphy

5. Water lily sign is seen in:
   a. Hydatid cyst of lung
   b. Aspergilloma lung
   c. TB
   d. Silicosis

6. Left border of heart on chest X-ray is formed by:
   a. Left pulmonary artery
   b. Right atrium
   c. Left ventricle
   d. Right ventricle

7. Ground glass appearance is not seen in:
   a. Hyaline membrane disease
   b. Left to right shunts
   c. Pneumonia
   d. Obstructive TAPVC

8. All of the following are true about loculated pleural effusion except:
   a. It makes an obtuse angle with the chest wall
   b. The margins are diffuse when viewed end on
   c. Not confined to any bronchopulmonary segment
   d. Air bronchograms are seen within the opacity

9. A patient presented with minimal Rt. sided pleural effusion. The best method to detect this would be:
   a. Right lateral
   b. Left lateral
   c. Left lateral decubitus
   d. Right lateral decubitus

10. Extensive pleural thickening and calcification especially involving the diaphragmatic pleura are classical features of:
    a. Coal worker's pneumoconiosis
    b. Asbestosis
    c. Silicosis
    d. Siderosis

11. The most likely diagnosis in a newborn who had a radiopaque shadow with an air fluid level in the chest

along with hemivertebrae of the 6th thoracic vertebra on plain X-ray is:
   a. Congenital diaphragmatic hernia
   b. Oesophageal duplication cyst
   c. Bronchogenic cyst
   d. Staphylococcal pneumonia

12. Pappu 3-year-old boy presents in the causality with H/O sudden onset of respiratory difficulty and stridor on auscultation, decreased breath sound and wheeze on the RT side. The X-ray shows right opaque hemothorax what will be the diagnosis:
   a. Pneumothorax
   b. Acute epiglottitis
   c. Massive pleural effusion
   d. Foreign body aspiration

13. A child with acute respiratory distress and hyperinflation of unilateral lung in X-ray is due to:
   a. Staphylococcal bronchopneumonia
   b. Aspiration pneumonia
   c. Congenital lobar emphysema
   d. Foreign body aspiration

14. A neonate presents with respiratory distress, contralateral mediastinal shift and multiple cystic air filled lesion chest. Most likely diagnosis is:
   a. Pneumonia
   b. Congenital lung cyst
   c. Congenital diaphragmatic hernia
   d. Congenital lobar emphysema

15. A 3-year-old female child developed fever, cough respiratory distress. On chest X-ray consolidation is in right lower lobe. She improved with antibiotics but follow up at 8 weeks was again found to have consolidation in right lower lobe. Your next investigation would be:
   a. Bronchoscopy
   b. Bacterial culture of the nasopharynx
   c. CT scan of the chest
   d. Allergen sensitivity test

16. A 55-year-old man who has been on bed rest for the past few days, complains of breathlessness and chest pain. The X-ray is normal. The next step in investigation should be:
   a. Lung ventilation - perfusion scan
   b. Pulmonary arteriography
   c. CT angiography
   d. Echocardiography

17. In pulmonary embolism, findings in perfusion scan is:
   a. Perfusion segmental defect
   b. Perfusion defect with normal lung scan and radiography
   c. Tenting of diaphragm
   d. Normal chest scan

18. Hampton hump is feature of:
   a. Pulmonary tuberculosis
   b. Pulmonary embolism
   c. Pulmonary hemorrhage
   d. Bronchogenic carcinoma

19. A 25-year-old man presented, with fever, cough, expectoration and breathlessness of 2 months duration. Contrast enhanced computed tomography of the chest showed bilateral upper lobe fibrotic lesions and mediastinum had enlarged necrotic nodes with peripheral rim enhancement. Which one of the following is the most probable diagnosis?
   a. Sarcoidosis
   b. Tuberculosis
   c. Lymphoma
   d. Silicosis

20. A patient suffering from AIDS presents with history of dyspnea and non-productive cough X-ray shows bilateral perihilar opacities without pleural effusion and lymphadenopathy. Most probable etiological agent is:

a. Tuberculosis
b. CMV
c. Kaposi's sarcoma
d. Pneumocystis carinii

21. A bone marrow transplant recipient patient, developed chest infection. On CT scan, tree in bud appearance is present. The cause of this is:
    a. Klebsiella   b. Pneumocystis
    c. TB   d. RSV

22. A 35-year-old with a history of asbestos exposure presents with chest pain. X-ray shows a solitary pulmonary nodule in the right lower zone. CECT reveals an enhancing nodule adjoining the right lower costal pleura with comet tail sign and adjacent pleural thickening. The most likely diagnosis is:
    a. Mesothelioma
    b. Round atelectasis
    c. Pulmonary sequestration
    d. Adenocarcinoma

23. Which of the following organs should always be imaged in a suspected case of bronchogenic carcinoma.
    a. Adrenals   b. Spleen
    c. Kidney   d. Pancreas

24. Tumor sensitive to chemotherapy is:
    a. Pancreatic cancer
    b. Renal carcinoma
    c. Small cell ca of lung
    d. Melanoma

25. Which of the following is not a cause of an elevated dome of the diaphragm?
    a. Diaphragmatic paralysis
    b. Pulmonary and lobar collapse
    c. Subphrenic abscess
    d. Large pleural effusion

26. Which among the following is a cause of posterior mediastinal opacity on posterior-anterior (PA) and lateral view of chest radiograph:

a. Tortuous innominate artery
b. Bochdalek's hernia
c. Enlarged pulmonary artery
d. Thymoma

27. For chest X-ray best view is:
    a. PA view
    b. AP view
    c. Lateral view
    d. None

28. Decubitus view is useful in diagnosing:
    a. Pleural effusion
    b. Pleural effusion with dependent hemithorax
    c. Pericardial effusion
    d. Middle lobe consolidation

29. Minimal pleural effusion is best detected by which X-ray view:
    a. AP   b. PA
    c. Lateral decubitus
    d. Oblique

30. What minimal amount of pleural fluid is seen on chest radiograph PA view?
    a. 10 ml   b. 150 ml
    c. 500 ml   d. 800 ml

31. Best view to diagnose pneumothorax:
    a. Lateral oblique
    b. PA view in full expiration
    c. PA view in full inspiration
    d. AP view in full expiration

32. Air bronchogram may be seen in the following except:
    a. Consolidation of lung
    b. Lung collapse
    c. Bronchoalveolar ca
    d. Normal variant

33. Silhouetting of left border of heart (silhouete sign positive) on chest radiograph indicates what pathology:
    a. Upper lobe   b. Hilar
    c. Lingular   d. Lower lobe

34. Base of heart is formed by:
    a. Rt. ventricle
    b. LV
    c. LV + RV
    d. RA + RV
    e. RA + LA

35. Consolidation of which portion of the lung is likely to obliterate the Aortic knuckle on X-ray chest:
    a. Apicoposterior segment of Left upper lobe
    b. Lingula
    c. Right upper lobe
    d. right middle lobe

36. A triangular opacity with clear borders, base towards midline and obliterating right heart border on a chest radiograph suggest that the pathology is likely to be in:
    a. Apical segment of right lower lobe
    b. Medial segment of right lower lobe
    c. Right middle lobe
    d. Any of the above

37. Bulging fissures in lungs in seen in:
    a. Klebsiella pneumonia
    b. Staphylococcal pneumonia
    c. Pulmonary odema
    d. Pneumoconiosis

38. Floating water lily sign is a feature of:
    a. Lung hydatid
    b. Bronchial adenoma
    c. Lung abscess
    d. Aspergilloma

39. Which of the following is a cause of unilateral hyperlucent lung on chest radiography?
    a. Poland syndrome
    b. Asthma
    c. Acute bronchiolitis
    d. Pleural effusion

40. The cause of homogenous opacity on X-ray is all except:
    a. Pleural effusion
    b. Diaphragmatic Hernia
    c. Massive consolidation
    d. Emphysema

41. Solitary nodule in lung cannot be:
    a. Tuberculoma
    b. Neurofibroma
    c. Bronchogenic carcinoma
    d. Lymphoma

42. Which of the following signs suggest benign nature in the evaluation of solitary pulmonary nodule on CT scan?
    a. Air-bronchogram in nodule
    b. Presence of amorphous calcification
    c. Fat density within the lesion
    d. Spiculated outline

43. A patient presents with a solitary pulmonary nodule (SPN) on X-ray. The best investigation to come to a diagnosis would be:
    a. MRI
    b. CT scan
    c. USG
    d. Image-guided biopsy

44. Popcorn calcification is characteristically seen in:
    a. TB
    b. Metastasis
    c. Pulmonary hamartoma
    d. Fungal invagination

45. Characteristics of BENIGN tumour of lung in X-ray:
    a. Size > 5 cm diameter
    b. Cavitation
    c. Peripheral location
    d. Concentric dense calcification

46. Features of pneumothorax are all except:
    a. Devoid of lung markings
    b. Hypertranslucency
    c. Shift of mediastinum to same side
    d. Collapse of ipsilateral lung

47. All of the following are indirect radiological signs of collapse of lung except:
    a. Mediastinal displacement
    b. Hilar displacement
    c. Compensatory hyperinflation
    d. Loss of aeration

48. In patient with high clinical suspicion of pulmonary thromboembolism, best investigation would be:
    a. D-dimer
    b. CT angiography
    c. Ventilation perfusion scan
    d. Color Doppler

49. Gold standard for diagnosing pulmonary embolism is:
    a. X-ray chest
    b. Ventilation perfusion scan
    c. Blood gas analysis
    d. Pulmonary catheter angiography

50. A 40 years old man presents with a recurrent hemoptysis. X-ray was found to be normal. The next investigation done to aid in diagnosis is:
    a. MRI   b. Bronchoscopy
    c. HRCT
    d. CT-guided biopsy

51. The following is not the differential diagnosis of an anterior mediastinal mass:
    a. Teratoma
    b. Neurogenic tumor
    c. Thymoma   d. Lymphoma

52. Commonest mass in the middle mediastinum is:
    a. Lipoma
    b. Aneurysm
    c. Lymph node mass
    d. Congenital cysts

53. In all of the following increased cardiac silhouette size is seen except:
    a. Tetralogy of Fallot
    b. Pericardial effusion
    c. Aortic regurgitation
    d. Ebstein anomaly

54. Sequestrated lung is most commonly supplied by:
    a. Bronchial artery
    b. Subclavian artery
    c. Pulmonary artery
    d. Aorta

55. Which among the following is not a chest radiographic feature of left atrial enlargement?
    a. Double left heart border
    b. Elevated left main bronchus
    c. Splaying of carina
    d. Enlargement of left atrial appendage

56. Earliest sign of left atrial enlargement is:
    a. Posterior displacement of esophagus
    b. Widening of carinal angle
    c. Elevation of left bronchus
    d. Double shadow of right heart border

57. High resolution computed tomography of the chest is the ideal modality for evaluating:
    a. Pleural effusion
    b. Interstitial lung disease
    c. Lung mass
    d. Mediastinal adenopathy

58. Best method to diagnose Bronchiectasis is:
    a. X-ray
    b. Bronchography
    c. MRI
    d. HRCT

59. All are radiological features of Mitral stenosis except:
    a. Straight left border of heart
    b. Oligemia of upper lung fields
    c. Pulmonary hemosiderosis
    d. Lifting of left bronchus

60. Earliest radiological sign of pulmonary venous hypertension in chest X-ray is:
    a. Cephalization of pulmonary vascularity
    b. Pleural effusion
    c. Kerley B lines
    d. Alveolar pulmonary edema

61. Earliest of venous hypertension is:
    a. Upper lobar vessel dilatation
    b. Kerley B lines
    c. Left atrial enlargement
    d. Pleural effusion

62. All are seen in congestive cardiac failure except:
    a. Kerley- B lines
    b. Prominent lower lobe vessel
    c. Pleural effusions
    d. Cardiomegaly

63. Egg-on-side appearance on X-ray chest is seen in:
    a. Tetralogy of Fallot
    b. Uncorrected TGA
    c. Tricuspid atresia
    d. Ebstein's anomaly

64. Prunning of pulmonary arteries is seen in:
    a. Pulmonary hypertension
    b. Chronic bronchitis
    c. Pulmonary infections
    d. Pulmonary transplant

65. In which of the following a 'Coeur en Sabot' shape of the heart is seen?
    a. Tricuspid atresia
    b. Ventricular septal defect
    c. Transposition of great arteries
    d. Tetralogy of Fallot

66. Which is the objective sign of identifying pulmonary plethora in a chest radiograph?
    a. Diameter of the main pulmonary artery >16 mm
    b. Diameter of the left pulmonary artery > 16 mm
    c. Diameter of the descending right pulmonary artery >16 mm
    d. Diameter of the descending left pulmonary artery >16 mm

67. Which of the following is the most common feature of Aortitis on chest X-ray?
    a. Calcification of ascending aorta
    b. Calcification of descending aorta
    c. Calcification of pulmonary artery
    d. Calcification of abdominal aorta

68. Drug used to perform stress ECHO:
    a. Thallium   b. Dobutamine
    c. Adrenaline   d. Adenosine

69. Investigation of choice for Aortic dissection is:
    a. Aortography   b. CT scan
    c. MRI   d. X-ray chest

70. Isotope used in myocardial perfusion scan is:
    a. Technetium
    b. Thallium
    c. Stannous pyrophosphate
    d. Gallium

71. Test of choice for Reversible myocardial Ischemia:
    a. Thallium scan
    b. MUGA scan
    c. Resting ECHO
    d. Coronary arigiography

72. Which of the following is not true regarding myocardium?
    a. Late enhancement on Gd MRI is suggestive of scar

b. Akinetic does benfit by revascularization
c. Low dose dobutamine may be used in hibernating myocardium
d. Rest stress thallium is used to evaluate hibernating myocardium

73. In a Down's syndrome patient posted for surgery, the investigation to be done is:
   a. CT Brain
   b. Echocardiography
   c. Ultrasound abdomen
   d. X-ray cervical spine

74. The most accurate investigation for assessing ventricular function is:
   a. Multislice CT
   b. Echocardiography
   c. Nuclear scan
   d. MRI

75. Most sensitive investigation for air embolism is:
   a. Decreased tidal volume of CO_2
   b. Decreased tidal volume of NO_2
   c. Doppler ultrasound
   d. Central venous pressure

76. Which one of the following investigations is considered to be "Gold standard" technique for diagnosis of arterial occlusive disease?
   a. Doppler ultrasound blood flow detection
   b. Duplex imaging
   c. Treadmill
   d. Digital substraction angiography (DSA)

77. Inferior rib notching is seen in:
   a. Coarctation of aorta
   b. Rickets
   c. ASD
   d. Multiple myeloma

78. Bilateral rib notching is seen in:
   a. Coarctation of aorta
   b. PDA
   c. TAPVC
   d. All of the above

79. A child presents with respiratory distress. A vascular ring is suspected. Investigation of choice is:
   a. PET
   b. CT
   c. MRI
   d. Angiography

80. An asymptomatic old patient presents With bruit in the carotid artery. Which of the following is the investigation of choice?
   a. Doppler ultrasonography
   b. Internal carotid angiography
   c. Aortic arch angiography
   d. Spiral CT angiography

81. A young man with pulmonary tuberculosis presents with massive recurrent hemoptysis. For angiographic treatment, which vascular structure should be evaluated first?
   a. Pulmonary artery
   b. Bronchial artery
   c. Pulmonary vein
   d. Superior vena cava

82. A young man with tuberculosis presents with massive recurrent hemoptysis. Most probable cause would be:
   a. Pulmonary artery
   b. Bronchial artery
   c. Pulomary vein
   d. Superior vena cava

83. Increased radiolucency of one sided hemithorax may be caused by all except:
   a. Obstructive emphysema
   b. Pneumothorax
   c. Expiratory film
   d. Patient rotation

84. All are true regarding emphysema finding in X-ray except:
   a. Low flat diaphragm - Tarrace pattern
   b. Tubular heart
   c. Decreased intercostal space
   d. Increased radiolucency

85. All are true about thymus swelling except:
    a. Widening of mediastinum on X-ray
    b. Sharp border with shail like appearance
    c. Steroid administration reduces size of swelling
    d. Shift of trachea on X-ray

86. About diagnosing air embolism with transesophageal echocardiography, which of the following is false:
    a. It can quantify the volume of air embolised
    b. It is a very sensitive investigation
    c. Continuous monitoring is needed to detect venous embolism
    d. Interferes with Doppler when used together

87. Best investigation for cardiac temponade is:
    a. 2D echocardiography
    b. M-Mode Echocardiography
    c. Real time echocardiography
    d. USG

88. Characteristic X-ray finding in ASD is:
    a. Enlarged left ventricle
    b. Enlarged left atria
    c. Pulmonary pletheora
    d. PAH

89. A patient is having Mitral stenosis. His X-ray will show all of the following finding except:
    a. Lifting up of left bronchus
    b. Double atrial shadow
    c. Obliteration of retrosternal shadow on lateral X-rays
    d. Posterior displacement of esophagus on barium swallow

90. Earliest CXR feature of left atrial enlargement is:
    a. Elevation of the left main bronchus
    b. Double cardiac shadow
    c. Widening of carina
    d. Pericardial effusion

91. Plethoric lung fields are seen in all of the following conditions, except:
    a. Atrial septal defect (ASD)
    b. TAPVC (total anomalous pulmonary venous connection)
    c. Ebsteins' anomaly
    d. Ventricular septal defect

92. Investigation of choice for pericardial effusion is:
    a. CT scan
    b. MRI
    c. Echocardiography
    d. X-ray chest

93. Cardiotoxicity caused by radiotherapy and chemotherapy is best detected by:
    a. ECHO
    b. ECG
    c. Radionucletide scan
    d. Endomyocardial biopsy

94. In patient with high clinical suspicion of pulmonary thromboembolism, best investigation would be:
    a. D-dimer
    b. CT angiography
    c. Catheter angiography
    d. Color Doppler

95. Investigation of choice for pulmonary embolism:
    a. CT scan
    b. Contrast CT
    c. Ventilation-perfusion scan
    d. MRI

96. Pulmonary embolism is best diagnosed by:
    a. USG
    b. X-ray chest
    c. Ventilation-perfusion scan
    d. CT Scan

97. Air bronchogram on chest X-ray denotes:
    a. Intrapulmonary lesion
    b. Extrapulmonary lesion
    c. Intrathoracic lesion
    d. Extrathoracic lesion

98. Calcified pulmonary metastasis is seen in which carcinoma
    a. Pancreatic carcinoma
    b. Thyroid carcinoma
    c. Endometrial carcinoma
    d. Osteosarcoma
99. Radiological feature of sarcoidosis:
    a. Hilar lymphadenopathy
    b. Hilar lymphadenopathy with parenchymal lung changes
    c. No hilar lymphadenopathy with parenchymal lung changes
    d. All of the above
100. Water-Lily sign on chest X-ray is seen in:
    a. Primary TB
    b. Aspergillosis
    c. Hydatid cyst
    d. Cryptococcosis
101. Kerley B lines are seen in which part of chest X-ray?
    a. Upper portion
    b. Mid portion
    c. Peripheral lower zone
    d. Upper peripheral zone
102. Water bottle heart is seen in:
    a. PDA
    b. Chronic emphysema
    c. Pericardial effusion
    d. Constrictive pericarditis
103. Thick cavity in lung is caused by all except:
    a. Lung abscess
    b. TB
    c. Emphysematous bulla
    d. Hamartoma
104. Egg on side appearance of heart is seen in the radiograph of:
    a. TAPVC   b. TGA
    c. ASD   d. VSD
105. The following will be most helpful radiological investigation in a patient suspected of left pleural effusion:
    a. Right lateral decubitus
    b. Left lateral decubitus
    c. Left lateral erect
    d. Right lateral erect
106. Gold standard for pulmonary thromboembolism:
    a. CT angiography
    b. USG
    c. Plethysmography
    d. Ventilation perfusion scan
107. Differential diagnosis of solitary pulmonary nodule are all except:
    a. Bronchogenic carcinoma
    b. Mycetoma
    c. Tuberculoma
    d. Hamartoma
108. Which of the following causes rib notching on X-ray?
    a. Coarctation of aorta
    b. SVC occlusion
    c. Modified blalock taussig shunt
    d. All of the above
109. Double shadow behind right atrium and- elevation of left main bronchus indicates:
    a. Right atrium enlargement
    b. Right ventricle enlargement
    c. Left atrium enlargement
    d. Left ventricle enlargement
110. Best view for right pleural effusion in X-ray chest:
    a. Supine
    b. Prone
    c. Right lateral decubitus
    d. Left lateral decubitus
111. Radiological feature(s) of mitral stenosis is/are all except:
    a. Double atrial shadow
    b. Straightening of left heart border
    c. Splaying of bronchi
    d. Prominent aortic knuckle
    e. Kerley B lines

112. Which of the following is not seen in anterior mediastinum?
    a. Thymoma
    b. Ganglioneuroma
    c. Thyroid masses
    d. Lymphoma
113. Which of the following tumour will not show activity on FDG-PET?
    a. Typical Carcinoid
    b. Atypical Carcinoid
    c. Large cell neuroendocrine tumor
    d. Small cell cancer

Multiple Correct Questions

114. Structure forming right border of heart:
    a. SVC
    b. IVC
    c. Rt. atrium
    d. Lt. atrium appendage
    e. Pulmonary vessels
115. Kerley's 'B' lines are found in:
    a. Interstitial edema
    b. Pulmonary venous congestion
    c. Pericardial effusion
    d. Mitral stenosis
    e. Interstitial lung disease
116. "Miliary shadow" on chest X-ray is seen in:
    a. Tuberculosis
    b. Rheumatoid arthritis
    c. Pneumoconiosis
    d. COPD
117. Egg Shell calcification is found in:
    a. Silicosis
    b. Sarcoidosis
    c. Metastatic node
    d. Lymphoma following radiotherapy
    e. Tuberculosis

118. Radiological feature of mitral stenosis is/are:
    a. Double contour of right heart border
    b. Straightening of left heart border
    c. Splaying of carinal angle
    d. Prominent aortic knuckle
119. Features of pulmonary venous hypertension are A/E:
    a. Perihilar haze
    b. Peribronchial cuffing
    c. Upper lobar diversion
    d. Uniformly branching lines parallel to pleura
    e. Pulmonary ossicles and fine nodular pattern
120. Rib notching is found in:
    a. Neurofibromatosis
    b. Lymphangioleio-myomatosis
    c. Aortic aneurysm
    d. Taussig-Bing operation
    e. Aortic obstruction
121. X-ray picture of VSD:
    a. Small Lt. ventricle
    b. Small Rt. Ventricle
    c. Dilated Lt. atrium
    d. Dilated pulmonary veins
    e. Dilated pulmonary arteries

Recently Asked Questions

122. Boot shaped heart is due to:
    a. Left atrial enlargement
    b. Right atrial enlargement
    c. Right ventricular hypertrophy
    d. Biventricular hypertrophy
123. Which heart chamber enlargement can be seen on barium swallow in patient with mitral stenosis?
    a. Left atrium
    b. Right atrium
    c. Left ventricle
    d. Right ventricle

Cardiothoracic Radiology

ANSWERS

1. **Ans. c.** Oligemic lung fields
2. **Ans. a.** Pneumonia affecting medial zone of right middle lobe
3. **Ans. d.** Plain radiograph
4. **Ans. b.** FDG-18 PET CT
5. **Ans. a.** Hydatid cyst of lung
6. **Ans. c.** Left ventricle
7. **Ans. c.** Pneumonia
8. **Ans. d.** Air bronchograms are seen within the opacity
9. **Ans. d.** Right lateral decubitus
10. **Ans. b.** Asbestosis
11. **Ans. b.** Oesophageal duplication cyst
12. **Ans. d.** Foreign body aspiration
13. **Ans. d.** Foreign body aspiration
14. **Ans. c.** Congenital diaphragmatic hernia
15. **Ans. c.** CT scan of the chest

    This is a case of foreign body aspiration and the best step is to do bronchoscopy and remove the foreign body however with modern imaging techniques with low dose CT scanner, A CT scan is usually done for location

16. **Ans. c.** CT angiography
17. **Ans. b.** Perfusion defect with normal lung scan and radiography
18. **Ans. b.** Pulmonary embolism
19. **Ans. b.** Tuberculosis
20. **Ans. d.** Pneumocystis carinii
21. **Ans. d.** RSV

    Though the most common cause of tree in bud opacities is TB. In bone marrow transplant recipient, RSV is a very common infection which give rise to tree in bud pattern

22. **Ans. b.** Round atelectasis
23. **Ans. a.** Adrenals
24. **Ans. c.** Small cell ca of lung
25. **Ans. d.** Large pleural effusion
26. **Ans. b.** Bochdalek's hernia
27. **Ans. a.** PA view
28. **Ans. b.** Pleural effusion with dependent hemithorax
29. **Ans. c.** Lateral decubitus
30. **Ans. b.** 150 ml
31. **Ans. b.** PA view in full expiration
32. **Ans. b.** Lung collapse
33. **Ans. c.** Lingular
34. **Ans. e.** RA + LA

    Base of heart is opposite to apex which is formed by RA + RV

35. **Ans. a.** Apicoposterior segment of Left upper lobe
36. **Ans. c.** Right middle lobe
37. **Ans. a.** Klebsiella pneumonia
38. **Ans. a.** Lung hydatid
39. **Ans. a.** Poland syndrome
40. **Ans. d.** Emphysema
41. **Ans. b.** Neurofibroma

    It is extra parenchymal

42. **Ans. c.** Fat density within the lesion
43. **Ans. d.** Image-guided biopsy
44. **Ans. c.** Pulmonary hamartoma
45. **Ans. d.** Concentric dense calcification
46. **Ans. c.** Shift of mediastinum to same side
47. **Ans. d.** Loss of aeration

    It is a direct sign

48. **Ans. b.** CT angiography
49. **Ans. d.** Pulmonary catheter angiography
50. **Ans. b.** Bronchoscopy

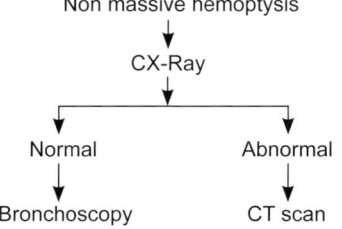

51. **Ans. b.** Neurogenic tumor
52. **Ans. c.** Lymph node mass
53. **Ans. a.** Tetralogy of Fallot
54. **Ans. d.** Aorta
55. **Ans. a.** Double left heart border
56. **Ans. a.** Posterior displacement of esophagus
57. **Ans. b.** Interstitial lung disease
58. **Ans. d.** HRCT
59. **Ans. b.** Oligemia of upper lung fields
60. **Ans. a.** Cephalization of pulmonary vascularity
61. **Ans. a.** Upper lobar vessel dilatation
62. **Ans. b.** Prominent lower lobe vessel
63. **Ans. b.** Uncorrected TGA
64. **Ans. a.** Pulmonary hypertension
65. **Ans. d.** Tetralogy of Fallot
66. **Ans. c.** Diameter of the descending right pulmonary artery >16 mm
67. **Ans. a.** Calcification of ascending aorta
68. **Ans. b.** Dobutamine
69. **Ans. b.** CT scan
70. **Ans. b.** Thallium
71. **Ans. a.** Thallium scan
72. **Ans. b.** Akinetic does benfit by revascularization
73. **Ans. b.** Echocardiography
74. **Ans. d.** MRI
75. **Ans. a.** Decreased tidal volume of CO_2
    - *Most sensitive monitoring device for venous air embolism is TEE (0.02 mL/kg)*
    - *Most sensitive non-invasive technique for venous air embolism is precordial Doppler 0.25 mL of air (0.05 mL/kg)*
    - *Most sensitive gas sensing technique for venous air embolism is ↑ET N_2 (0.5 mL/kg)*
    - *Most convenient and practical for venous air embolism is ↓ET CO_2*

Comparison of method of detection of vascular air embolism				
Method of detection	Sensitivity (mL/kg)	Availability	Invasiveness	Limitation
TEE	High (0.02)	Low	High	Expertise required, expensive, invasive
Precordial Doppler	High (0.05)	Moderate	None	Obese patients
PA catheter	High (0.25)	Moderate	High	Fixed distance, small orifice
TCD	High	Moderate	None	Expertise required
ETN_2	Moderate (0.5)	Low	None	N_2O, hypotension
ETCO_2	Moderate (0.5)	Moderate	None	Pulmonary disease
Oxygen saturation	Low	High	None	Late changes
Direct visualization	Low	High	None	No physiologic data
Esophageal stethoscope	Low (1.5)	High	Low	Late changes
Electrocardiogram	Low (1.25)	High	Low	Late changes

76. **Ans. d.** Digital substraction angiography (DSA)
77. **Ans. a.** Coarctation of aorta
78. **Ans. a.** Coarctation of aorta
79. **Ans. b.** CT

    MRI is very good investigation for assessment of vascular rings however is child with respiration distress, a less time consuming and fast modality should be used. Also the assessment of airways is important for respiratory distress which is better done with CT scan
80. **Ans. a.** Doppler ultrasonography
81. **Ans. b.** Bronchial artery
82. **Ans. b.** Bronchial artery
83. **Ans. c.** Expiratory film
84. **Ans. c.** Decreased intercostal space
85. **Ans. d.** Shift of trachea on X-ray
86. **Ans. d.** Interferes with Doppler when used together
87. **Ans. b.** M-Mode Echocardiography
88. **Ans. c.** Pulmonary pletheora
89. **Ans. c.** Obliteration of retrosternal shadow on lateral X-rays
90. **Ans. a.** Elevation of the left main bronchus
91. **Ans. c.** Ebsteins' anomaly
92. **Ans. c.** Echocardiography
93. **Ans. d.** Endomyocardial biopsy
94. **Ans. c.** Catheter angiography

    Best/gold standard will be Catheter angiography, however is no longer performed due to high sensitivity, easy availability and non-invasive nature of CT angio.
95. **Ans. b.** Contrast CT
96. **Ans. d.** CT scan
97. **Ans. a.** Intrapulmonary lesion
98. **Ans. d.** Osteosarcoma
99. **Ans. d.** All of the above
100. **Ans. c.** Hydatid cyst
101. **Ans. c.** Peripheral lower zone
102. **Ans. c.** Pericardial effusion
103. **Ans. c.** Emphysematous bulla
104. **Ans. b.** TGA
105. **Ans. b.** Left lateral decubitus
106. **Ans. a.** CT angiography
107. **Ans. b.** Mycetoma
108. **Ans. d.** All of the above
109. **Ans. c.** Left atrium enlargement
110. **Ans. c.** Right lateral decubitus
111. **Ans. d.** Prominent aortic knuckle.
112. **Ans. b.** Ganglioneuroma
113. **Ans. a.** Typical carcinoid

Multiple Correct Answers

114. **Ans. a.** SVC, **b.** IVC, **c.** Rt. atrium
115. **Ans. a.** Interstitial edema, **b.** Pulmonary venous congestion, **d.** Mirtal stenosis
116. **Ans. a.** Tuberculosis, **c.** Pneumoconiosis
117. **Ans. a.** Silicosis, **b.** Sarcoidosis, **d.** Lymphoma following radiotherapy, **e.** Tuberculosis
118. **Ans. a.** Double contour of right heart border, **b.** Straightening of left heart border, **c.** Splaying of carinal angle
119. **Ans. d.** Uniformly branching lines parallel to pleura
120. **Ans. a.** Neurofibromatosis, **d.** Taussig-Bing operation, **e.** Aortic obstruction
121. **Ans. c.** Dilated Lt. atrium, **e.** Dilated pulmonary arteries

Answers of Recently Asked Questions

122. **Ans. c.** Right ventricular hypertrophy
123. **Ans. a.** Left atrium

CHAPTER 4

Gastrointestinal and Genitourinary System

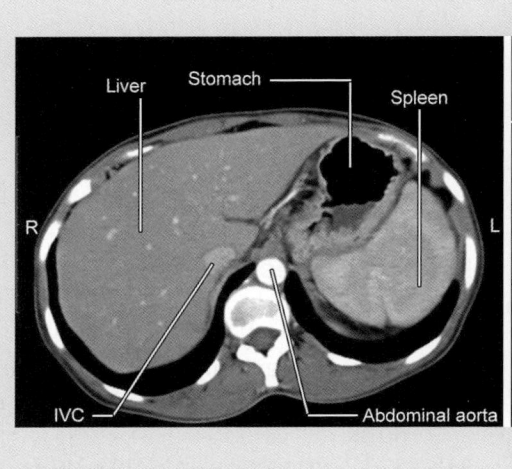
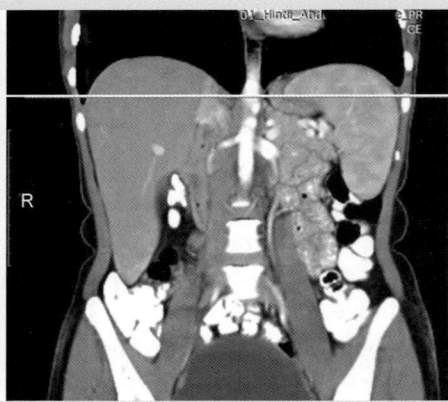
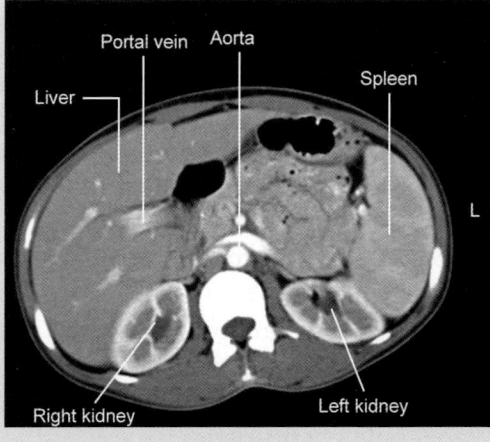
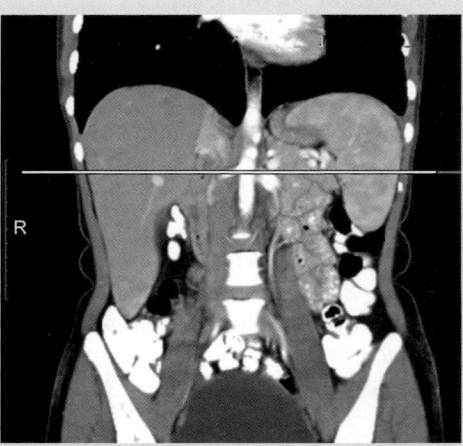

Gastrointestinal and Genitourinary System

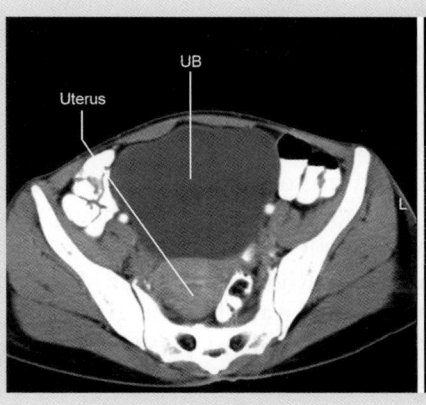
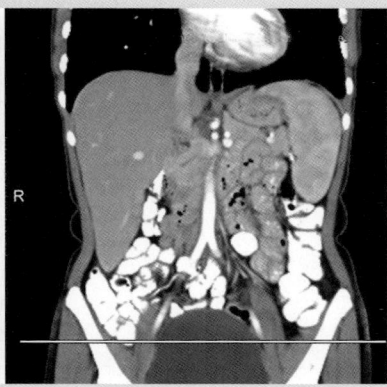

ESOPHAGUS

- Barium studies are **better to diagnose motility disorders** and dysphagia if more for liquids than solids (as seen in achalasia cardia).
- **Gold std** for **motility disorders**^{Q} → **Manometry** like for:
  - Scleroderma
  - Achalasia cardia
  - Diffuse esophageal spasm
- **IOC for intraluminal lesions and complications of esophageal diseases- endoscopy**
- Endoscopic ultrasonography is **investigation of choice** for rest of the esophageal lesions specifically intramural and extraluminal. (Can't be seen on endoscopy)
- EUS: Even can differentiate b/w **T_1 to T_3 lesions for TNM staging-more accurate** [CT/MRI can only d/d b/w (T_1–T_3) and (T4) lesions as these cannot tell exact layer of infiltration in the wall of esophagus] [5-layers]
- EUS even considered IOC for local staging of Ca esophagus over **PETCT But for metastatic workup- PETCT is IOC**

i **mportant**
Barium studies are done under fluoroscopic guidance which is real time X-ray imaging and motility can be assessed unlike other studies where fix images are taken.

i **mportant**

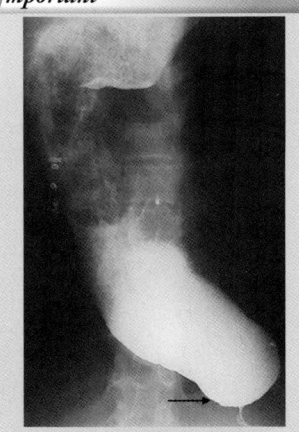

Achalasia Cardia
(Bird's beak sign)

Esophageal Markings on Barium Column
Normal
- Aortic arch and main bronchus
- Impression by LA in front
- At entry into diaphragm

Abnormal
- Right-sided aortic arch indents the esophagus on Right
- Coarctation of aorta → **Reverse '3' sign** (due to pre- and poststenotic dilatations)
- *Aneurysms of aortic arch and descending aorta (dysphagia aortica → dysphagia in old due to unfolding of aorta)
- *Aberrant Right subclavian A → **Indentation on posterior wall (Dysphagia lusoria)**
- LA/LV enlargement (MS) → **Anterior impression on esophagus**

Achalasia Cardia
- **Birds beak at GE junction**^{Q}
- If long duration disease, dilated esophagus with air fluid level can be seen on CXR-PA (Erect)
- If barium retained for > 5 minutes—supportive evidence on barium studies
- Premalignant
- Amyl nitrate and hot water improve while methacholine worsen symptoms.

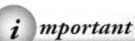
important
Bird's beak has a smooth surface and rat's tail has an irregular surface hence is a feature of carcinoma/secondary achalasia due to Ca.

Diffuse Esophageal Spasm
- Corkscrew on barium, seish kebab, rosary bead

Scleroderma
- Patulous esophagus (GE junction) + lung ILD + mediastinal nodes with GE reflux [Involvement of distal esophagus as scleroderma does not involve voluntary muscles in upper esophagus].

GERD
- 24-h pH monitoring **(Gold std)**^{Q}
- IOC for complications—endoscopy

Ca Esophagus
- If Ca develops in long standing case of achalasia cardia—dilated esophagus can be seen both prox. and distal to lesion on barium.

Features on Barium Study
- Irregular mucosal outline-**Rat tail appearance**^{Q}
- Narrowing
- **Shouldering of ends (arrow in figure)**
  IOC → Endoscopic ultrasound + biopsy

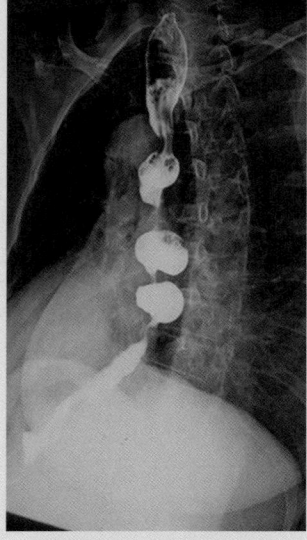
Cork screw appearance in diffuse esophageal spasm

Biopsy for confirmation of malignancy
Endoscopic ultrasound for local staging

Computed Tomography
- Most widely used for distant spread
- Prone position is preferred
- Criteria for Invasion
  - Loss of triangle of fat between esophagus, aorta, and spinal column
  - > 90° contact with Aorta
  - Nodular protrusion into airway

Echo Endoscope/Endoscopic Ultrasonography
- [EUS] (7-12 MHz)-highest spatial resolution.
- **Radial–perpendicular to scope–**for staging.
- **Linear–parallel to axis** → for FNAC/Biopsy.

> **Lower esophageal cancer if epicenter within 5.00 cm from GE junction (AJCC–Guidelines for Ca stomach)
> **Coeliac and perioesophageal cervical nodes are regional rather than metastasis.
> **(N) esophagus < 5 mm thick on CT
> Thickness of wall of esophagus < 5 mm normally on CT

i important

Shouldering in Ca Esophagus

i important
Most malignant nodes do not enlarge and hence nodal enlargement cannot be taken as a criteria for spread of disease. Rounding, loss of central fat and hypoechoic nodes

HERNIA AND DYSPHAGIA

First investigation in patient suspected with dysphagia is barium swallow.

Bochdalek's Hernia
- MC congenital
- Through a defect in posterolateral diaphragm
- Can show 13 pairs of ribs [B-PL]

Post-traumatic
- On barium herniation of bowel loop in thorax through rent → **Love bird sign**

Hiatus Hernia
- GE junction > 2 cm above hiatus [normal in rolling hernia]
- Widened hiatus > 2.5 cm
- > 3 gastric folds above hiatus [under fluoro direct visualization]
- Schatzki's or B-Ring [Sq-columnar junction] > 2 cm above hiatus

i important

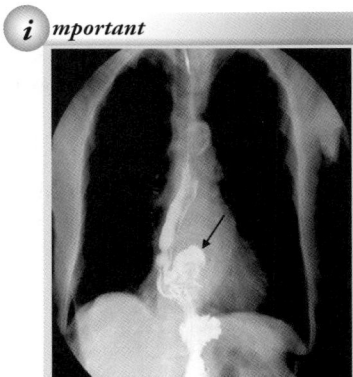

Sliding hiatus hernia on barium swallow study

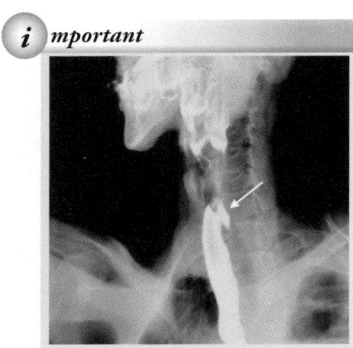
Zenker's diverticulum

> **important**
> - Most common benign sub mucosal lesion of esophgos leiomyoma
> - EUS can show origin from M.mucosa/muscularis propria
> - **Best: biopsy** as GIST and leiomyoma look same on EUS

> **important**
> Acquired hypertrophy of pylorus d/t → peptic ulcer/inflammation → does not show shouldering

High Resolution Manometry is Gold Std for Sliding Hiatus Hernia.

Zenker [Pharyngoesophageal] Diverticulum

- X-ray- can show air fluid level posterior to prox. end of esophagus
- **Barium – IOC** → contrast filled out pouching through killian dehiscence
- Endoscopy is difficult → contraindicated in suspected c/o of Zenker's with potential danger of rupture

Killian-Jamieson Pouch/Diverticula

- Protrusion from anterolateral wall d/t weaknesss in upper cervical esophagus just below the level of cricopharyngeus d/t passage of inferior laryngeal nerve through it.

Dysphagia Lusoria

- Dysphagia due to aberrant vascular loop around esophagus
- MC is aberrant right SCA-**Angiography → gold std**.

Dysphagia Aortica

- In old age due to unfolding of aorta. Loop of aorta causes external compression on lower esophagus

ESOPHAGITIS

Barium Findings

Eosinophilia	– Low caliber esophagus
Barrett's esophagitis	– granular/reticular appearance
Candida	– Large linear mural plaques
Radiation/caustic injury	– Long stricture
HIV/CMV	– Large ovoid/diamond shape.

STOMACH

Hypertrophic Pyloric Stenosis

Hypertrophied muscles lengthens and narrows canal
- **IOC → USG**^{Q}

- **Criterias on USG:** Elongated pylorus with thickened muscle **(most specific)**
  - ≥ 16 mm length
  - ≥ 13 mm transverse diameter
  - ≥ 4 mm circular muscle thickness
- Barium Signs of IHPS
  - String sign [most specific sign] (2)
  - Shouldering (antral) (due to retrograde bulge of muscles) (5)
  - Double track sign/triple track sign/double string sign
  - Beak sign (antral)
  - Pyloric canal is curved upward posteriorly
  - Diamond sign/Twining recess (3)
  - Pyloric teat sign
  - Olive pit sign (4)
  - Caterpillar sign
  - Kirklin mushroom sign → d/t indentation of base of-duodenal bulb (1)
- Treatment of choice is ramstedt pyloromyotomy

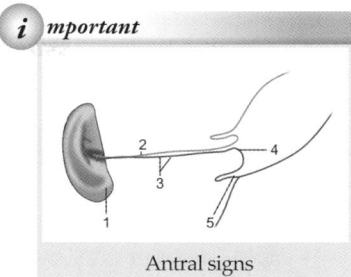

Antral signs

Peptic Ulcer

Benign	Malignant
Margin-Smooth ulcer **mound** d/t mucosal edema [circular filling defect/**ulcer collar**	**Heaped up nodular margins**
Sharpy punched out lesion-dependent position	Overt neoplastic tissue with shaggy and necrotic base
Ring shadow in nondependent ulcer	**Gastric folds do not reach the ulcer crater**
Hampton's line (in fallible sign-pathognomonic) (overhanging mucosa at margin)	**Carman's Meniscus sign**
Penetrating sign if within wall rather than mass with-smooth/clean base of ulcer	Kirkland complex
Radiating folds are smooth symmetric reaching up to edge of ulcer in sponge like manner [spoke wheel patterns] [ulcer crater may extend beyond wall]	Intraluminal crater rather than only in wall

> **important**
> If perforation suspected → use water soluble contrast as barium can lead to granuloma formation/peritoneal fibrosis.

> **important**
> You don't see shouldering in antral narrowing due to gastritis unlike in IHPS.

> **important**
> Breast ca metastasis can also be like linitis plastica i.e. diffuse thickening of stomach wall.

Contd...

> **important**
> - Double bubble sign
>   - Ladd bond/malrotation
>   - Annular pancreas
>   - Duodenal atresia/stenosis
> - Single bubble sign → IHPS
> - **Triple/many multiple bubble** → jejunal/Ileal obstruction
> - **Apple core sign** → Ca colon (mainly → R sided)
> - **Napkin ring** → Ca colon [(L) sided]
> - **Coiled spring sing** → Intussusception
> - **String of Kantor sign** → Crohn's disease
> - **String sign** → IHPS/ICTB
> - **Rams horn shape** → stenotic disease due to scarring and fibrosis causing narrowing of gastric antrum and pylorus into a funnel
> - **Wind sock** appearance → duodenal web/diverticulum.
> - **Hide bound** appearance → scleroderma of intestine

Contd...

Benign	Malignant
Can show area gastricae in ulcer crater	Strong enhancement at the site of ulcer than adjacent wall on CECT
Normal peristalsis	Abnormal peristalsis

**Superficial erosions are till muscularis, mucosa → mound of edema only if complete erosions
Trifoliate duodenum → chronic duodenal ulcer with scarring.
**In barium study it is recommended do both prone and supine views to exclude anterior wall perforation.

Gastritis

- Thick folds > 5 mm (most useful), [For H. Pylori Gastritis]
- Prominent area gastricae [most specific]-for H. Pylori gastritis
- Antral narrowing
- Inflammatory polyps

Gastric Striae

- Transverse folds impressions by gastric mascularis mucosa in c/o antral gastritis.

Emphysematous Gastritis

- It is due to acute gas forming infection

Gastric Emphysema

- Air in wall of stomach, without infection

Phlegmonous Gastritis

- If pan mural inflammation

Linitis Plastica

- Better appreciated on fluoroscopy than endoscopy:
- Causes
  - Adenocarcinoma
  - Diffuse scirrhous carcinoma **[leather bottle appearance]**
  - NHL **[If adenopathy is bulky and also below renal hila and with splenomegaly]**
  - Breast metastasis
  - Kaposi sarcoma

> **important**
> **Presence of gastric varices in absence of esophageal varices is a sign of splenic vein thrombosis [due to pancreatitis/ca pancreas].

> **important**
> **Marked irregular narrowing of antrum and Ist part of duodenum → **Pseudopost Billroth I-appearance** [Crohn's disease].

Bull's Eye Lesions in
Stomach (due to central ulceration)

- Submucosal metastasis [MC-melanoma]
- Lymphoma
- Carcinoma breast, bronchus, pancreas
- Carcinoid
- Leiomyoma
- Kaposi sarcoma
- Ectopic pancreas [central dip due to rudimentary duct]

Rotation/Volvulus

Organoaxial rotation [more common]
- Axis along cardia and pylorus
- If horizontal originally then→Greater curvature up and lesser low (more common)
- If stomach vertically oriented → (R) → (L) shift
- **Mesentericoaxial (mainly traumatic)**
  - Antropylorus at a higher level then fundus and cardia [known as → Upside down stomach]

Radiological Signs of Malabsorption on Barium

- Dilatation
- Rapid transit
- Flocculation of contrast [**Snow flake-like deposits**]
- Segmentation of barium column
- Fold thickening
- Excessive secretion
  - Causing dilution of contrast
  - Reduced mucosal coating

Other Barium Signs

- "Moulage sign"→Tube-like appearance of bowel seen in Crohn's disease
- **Stacked coin appearance** → In HSP due to submucosal hemorrhages
- **Hide bound appearance** → scleroderma
- **Scalloped edges of sigmoid colon**-pneumatosis intestinalis
- **Saw tooth appearance** → Diverticulosis
- **String sing**
  - Crohn's (of Kantor's)
  - TB
  - IHPS

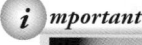
important
Wilkie's SMA compression synd-If compression and dilatation of duodenum (transverse IIIrd part) present even on prone films.

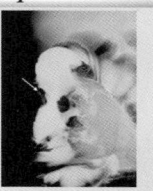
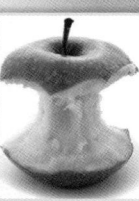
Apple core sign
Ca – ascending color
– apple core sign on barium studies

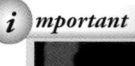
important

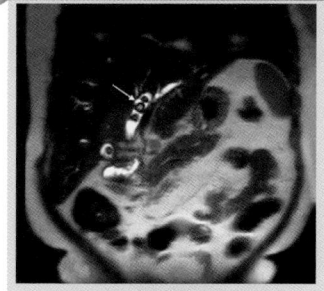
CBD/Gallstone on MRI
Filling defect on T_2W images

Ileocecal Tuberculosis (MC site of intestinal TB)

- Mucosal fold thickening
- Ulcers (transverse/star shaped/circumferential [*Crohn's disease have longitudinal ulcers*]
- Terminal ileum stricture
- Funnelled contracture of cecum
- **Fleischer sign/Inverted umbrella defect** [due to thick, rigid, irregular IC-valve]
- **Sterlein sign** → rapid emptying of narrowed ileum in cecum
- Symmetrical annular napkin ring stenosis and widened ileocecal angle (N) ≤ 90° → it becomes obtuse)
- Amputated cecum → rigid, contracted, cone shaped retracted/pulled up cecum out of ileal fossa.
- **String sign** → on barium d/t narrowing of terminal ileum
- **Goose neck appearance** – ileum hanging from fibrosed, pulled up cecum.
- **Purse string** appearance of cecum

> *important*
> In a case of previous hemicolectomy due to CD, anastomosis is the most common site of recurrence.

> *important*
> *Comb sign, mesenteric edema, layered wall T2 hyperintensity and lymph nodes.
> **Signs of active CD**

Inflammatory Bowel Diseases

- **Crohn's disease** → skip lesions
    - **Aphthoid ulcers (barium sign)** Fissure ulcers, abscess, fistula
    - **Longitudinal ulcer along mesenteric border** → characteristic sign
    - **Cobblestoning** → longitudinal and transverse ulcers separating intact mucosa
    - **Strictures** → Multiple strictures are virtually diagnostic of CD (string sign **of Kantor** if terminal ileum stricture)
    - **Pseudodiverticula** → d/t asymmetrical involvement of intestine [(n) intestine appears as pseudodiverticula in an otherwise sevely involved segment]
    - Inflammatory polyps not frequent in CD (seen as filling defects)
    - **Thickening of wall** → displacement of adjacent barium filed bowel loops [which is also due to fibro fatty proliferation of the peritoneal fat]
    - Stenosis + dilated proximal bowel loops
    - Adhesions
    - Enlarged Ileocecal valve

> *important*
>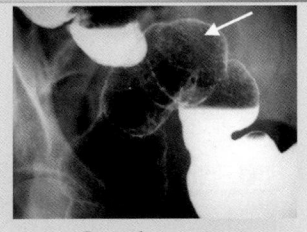
> Granular mucosa

- **CT enteroclysis/CT enterography → IOC**
  - Stratification/target mural thickening of bowel wall unlike malignancy where the wall architecture get loss [active disease]
  - Comb sign – due to ↑ vascularity/Halo sign due to submucosal edema [active disease]
- MRI → better to detect fistula or sinuses.

Ulcerative Colitis

- Granular mucosa **[earliest change]** on barium studies
- **Toxic mega colon** if transverse colon > 5.0 cm [As transverse colon is least dependent in supine position]
- Haustration always absent → if present it should not be because of toxic mega colon
- Collar button ulcers [on barium in profile view]
- Pseudopolyps
- Contiguous-No skip lesion
- Reflex/backwash ileitis
- **Pipe stem colon** [ahaustral]
- ↑ Presacral space [due to proliferation of perirectal fat]
- **Instant Enema** (If active disease → colon is almost always free of fecal matter → no need for bowel preparation before enema in such patients)

Causes of Aphthoid Ulcers (black mound of halo due to edema) on Barium Studies

- CD (not seen in UC)
- Amebiasis
- Tuberculosis
- Behcet's disease
- HIV-related infection

Sacculations

- CD [Pseudodiverticula]
- Ischemic colitis

Accordion sign

- AIDS related ischemic colitis
- Severe edema due to cirrhosis
- Pseudomembranous colitis

Lymphoma

- **Aneurysmal dilatation of bowel loops**

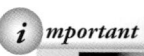 *mportant*
*Free perforation is rare in CD d/t chronic adhesions
*Mural thickening is more in CD than UC

mportant
Crohn's diseases
Aphthoid ulcers [earliest change]
Raspberry-/Rose thorn appearance due to deep ulcers.
**Montreal classification for Crohn's disease

mportant
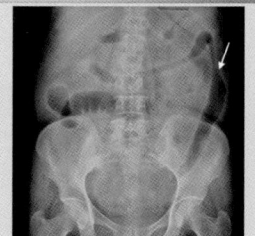
Featureless ahaustral colon- UC

mportant
- Radiation colitis [due to endarteritis] > 4500 rad/45 gray
- *Radiation enteritis* → **Mucosal tacking**

> **important**

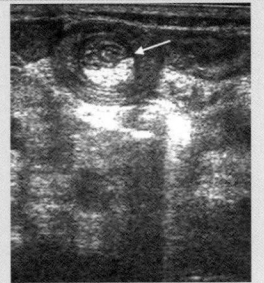

Intussusception target sign

> **important**
> **Hellmer sign** → lucency b/w liver and abdominal wall due to fluid in ascites.

> **important**

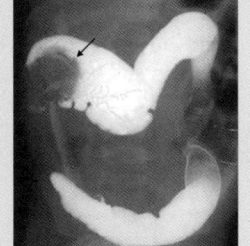

Claw sign of intussusception on barium enema

> **important**
> Soap Bubble appearance is seen in meconium ileus

> **important**
> String of Bead: Three causes
> - Angiography—Fibromuscular dysplasia
> - ERCP—Chronic pancreatitis
> - Plain abdominal radiograph—SBO

- Sandwich-like massive mesenteric lymphadenopathy
- Secondary deposits in RIF → narrowed loops in parallel configuration—**Palisading**

Ascariasis

- **Medusa head** appearance
- Sphagetti appearance
- Bulls eye sign
- Impacted worm sign
- Inner/double tube sign
- Tubular filling defects on BaMFT

Intussusception

- Coiled spring sign-barium
- Target sign–USG (Image) + Hayfork sign–USG
- Claw sign–barium
- Empty right iliac fossa
- Barium enema can be both therapeutic and diagnostic-usually not done
- Preferred T/t is ultrasound guided hydrostatic reduction

Hirschsprung's Disease

- Most common causes of neonatal colonic obstruction
- Characterized by a short segment of colonic aganglionosis
- Smaller calibre affected bowel with dilated normal proximal bowel (6.5 cm) mega rectum
- Most important sign is transition zone with reversal of recto sigmoid ratio (normally rectum is more dilated than sigmoid colon).

CURRENT STATUS

In situation of acute abdomen–supine abdomen and erect chest radiograph (after 10 min of standing are basic standard radiograph)
- **Supine** → with empty bladder, from diaphragm to hernial orifices which in practice means that the obturator foramen should be included.
- **(L) Lateral decubitus**–It can clarify if erect X-ray is confusing for free air **(most sensitive)**
- Erect abdomen is misleading to differentiate acute obstruction with ileus.

- **Valid indications of radiography in (acute abdomen)**
  - Suspected viscus perforation
  - Bowel obstruction
  - Bowel wall pattern [ischemia, colitis]
  - Intraabdominal foreign body.

Signs of Pneumoperitoneum

On supine radiograph
1. **Football sign** (hydropneumoperitoneum)
2. **Right UQ gas**
   - Perihepatic
   - Subhepatic
   - Morison's pouch
   - Fissure for ligamentum teres
   - Triangular air
3. **Rigler's [double wall]**—visualization of both sides of bowel wall (Pathognomonic) (Image)
   - Ligaments
     - Falciform [lig. teres]
     - Medial umbilical lig [inverted 'v' sign]
   - Gas under (R) and (L) hemi diaphragm may join in midline—cupola sign

On standing radiograph
- Gas under diaphragm
- Doge's cap sign

Pseudopneumoperitoneum
- Intestine b/w liver and diaphragm [Chilaiditi synd.] (image) (note the haustra of large bowel arrow)
- Subpulmonary pneumothorax
- Subphrenic abscess
- Curvilinear atelectasis
- Subdiaphragmatic fat
- Cysts in pneumatosis intestinalis
- Diaphragmatic irregularities/multiple humps

BOWEL OBSTRUCTION

- **Acute gastric dilatation**–paralytic–elderly–due to fluid and electrolyte disbalance.
- **Paralytic ileus**—peritonitis, post-op, metabolic, ischemic, renal failure, morphine
  In developed world **MC cause of Small Bowel Obstruction** → adhesions due to previous surgeries.

> **important**
> **Causes of Ca++ in Right Hypochondrium**
> - Gallstone
> - Porcelain GB
> - Calcified (N) costal cartilage
> - Hepatic adenoma, hemangioma, abscess, metastasis, hydatid cyst
> - Calcification in kidney/stone
> - Phlebolith/fecolith

> **important**

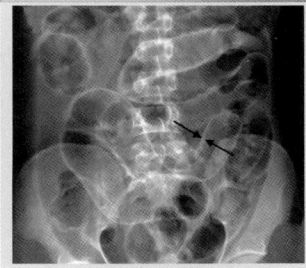

Rigler's sign

> **important**

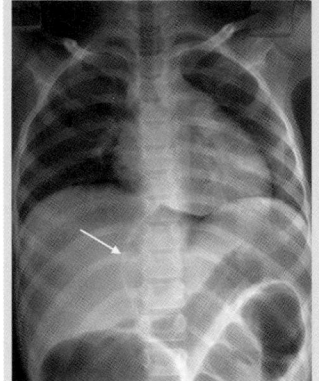

Falciform ligament sign

> **important**
> Gas in soft tissue of (L) thigh–classical site for gas from a diverticular disease/perforation.

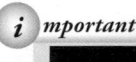
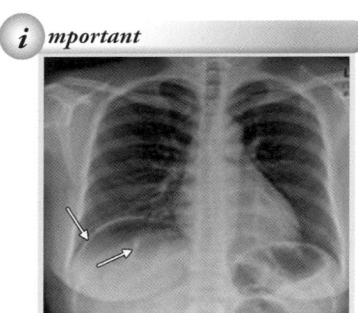
Pseudopneumoperitoneum
[Chilaiditi synd.]

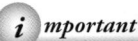
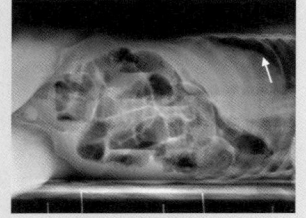
Gas around liver in left lateral decubitus view

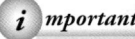
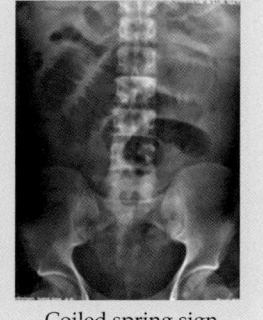
Coiled spring sign

Important
*Best projection to detect pneumoperitoneum is PA Chest X-ray–if patient, cannot get erect then left lateral decubitus view after 10 minutes in that position.

In underdeveloped/developing world is strangulated hernia [3/4th cases].

Radiological Signs of SBO

- Obstruction small bowel → centrally placed bowel loops > 3.0 cm
- **Transition zone** → most reliable CT sign [dilated prox. and collapsed distal]
- **Small bowel feces sign–[pathognomonic** and help in identifying transition zone]
- **String of beads–diagnostic of acute obstruction.** (Small air bubbles along non-dependent wall)

Radiological Signs of Large Bowel Obstruction

- Peripherally Placed bowel loops > 5 cm with Haustra
- **Imminent rupture of cecum > 9 cm diameter**
- **Air in rectum suggests paralytic ileus**

CT Signs of a Closed Loop Obstruction

- Small bowel dilatation
- 'V' shaped or radial fluid-filled loops
- Mesenteric vessels converging toward point of obstruction
- Triangular loop with or without whirl or beak.
- Angulated or tethered loops on CT-adhesions
- Pseudo obstruction—elderly
- US/UK-**Ca colon** MC-for **large bowel obstruction,** diverticulitis—IInd MC cause.
  Underdeveloped → 85% by **volvulus**.

Sigmoid Volvulus

- **Liver overlap sign** → ahaustral sigmoid colon
- Dilated descending colon-**[left flank overlap sign]**
- Left pelvis-**[pelvic overlap sign or inferior convergence]**
- Volvulus apex above T10 on left-side below diaphragm
- Enema-**hooked beak [bird of prey sign]**
- (Screw pattern of mucosal folds at twist)
- **Whirl sign**-due to twisted bowel and mesentery

Cecal Volvulus (30–60 years) Younger Age

- **'x-marks the spot' sign**-two overlapping transition at the site of twist
- Pole of cecum and appendix in (L) upper quadrant (if inversion)
- (L) side of colon is collapsed

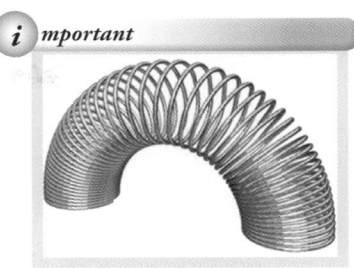

Ischemic Colitis

- **Splenic flexure and adjacent descending colon (MC)**
- Submucosa gets thickened due to edema and hemorrhage
    - **Thumb printing** and functional obstruction with dilated proximal bowel loops

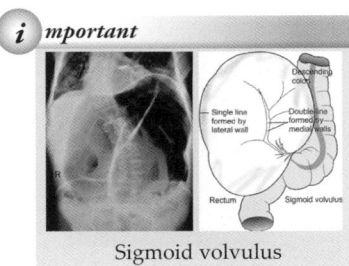

Sigmoid volvulus

Colitis (IBD)

- **Inactive disease if formed feces**.
- **Extensive colitis**-if absence of feces.
    - When haustra disappears → Ulcers have penetrated muscle layer.
    - Daily plain AXR- justified for follow-up
- **Pseudomembranous colitis** →
    - Thumb printing-transverse colon (MC)
    - Accordion sign.

important

String of beads
- FMD on [angiography]
- Chronic pancreatitis (chain of lakes) [MRCP/ERCP]
- Small bowel obstruction [supine X-ray]

important
USG is IOC in pediatric population or pregnant ladies. Cholecystitis – IOC–USG Calculus shows acoustic shadow (an USG artifact)

Appendicitis-IOC-CECT

USG

- Appendix > 7 mm (USG) (> 6 mm) CT [wall to wall diameter]
- Appendicitis can cause generalized ileus
- **On USG-noncompressible, aperistaltic, blind ending tubular structure in RHC arising from cecum**
- Perforated appendix is compressible.
- CT–luminal contrast or air in the cecum pointing toward the obstructed origin of the appendix— **arrowhead sign**.
- Focal cecal thickening due to edema at the origin of the appendix → **cecal bar sign**.
- In pediatric patients, USG is the preferred investigation for acute appendicitis.

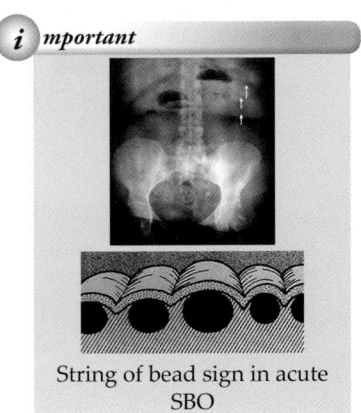

String of bead sign in acute SBO

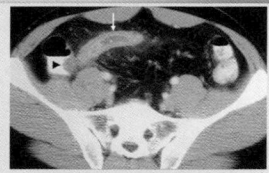

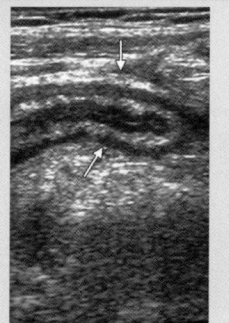

Acute appendicitis- CECT, USG

*i*mportant
*In a c/o chronic intestinal bleeding-demonstration of persistent vitelline artery is a hallmark for angiographic disease of Meckel's diverticulum.

*i*mportant

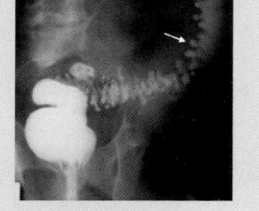

Diverticula on sigmoid colon

*i*mportant
Giant cyst formation in diverticular disease-pseudocyst with no epithelial lining → can mimic duplication cyst.

Ischemia

Arterial

- Acute occlusive **(thrombus)** → Mural thickening, dilatation, **nonenhancement, ascites (66%)**
- Nonocclusive **hypotension** → Mural thickening, mucosal **hyperenhancement** ascites not common.

Venous Thrombosis

- **Mural thickening + mucosal hyperenhancement,** mesenteric stranding + vascular engorgement, **ascites (> 70%)**
- Ischemic colitis → **thumb printing**

Causes of Pneumatosis Intestinalis + Air in Portal/SM Veins

- Ischemia
- Infective/Inflammation
- Asthma
- Neoplastic conditions

Progressive Systemic Sclerosis

- Increased number of mucosal folds
- **Wire spring/hide bound appearance**
- **S**acculations [pseudodiverticula]

Diverticula-Sigmoid Colon MC Site

- **CT-most accurate** in determining the severity of diverticulitis
- Saw tooth appearence on barium enema studies (arrow in image)
- Diverticula filled with diverticulolith [fecal matter]– may appear hyperdense like a polyp.
  - Fistula formation-MC with bladder

Blunt Trauma Abdomen

- **Gold std** → DPL not done now a days
- **IOC** → CECT in stable patient
- **FAST** → It unstable and if time permits (Figure-fluid in Morrison's pouch)
- **Laparotomy** → **If unstable**

Gastrointestinal and Genitourinary System

Gallstones → 90% lucent
- Do not overlap spine on lateral X-ray
- If air in stone → **Mercedes Benz sign**
- IOC-USG → **acoustic shadowing**–also seen in renal stones
- **WES complex** [wall-echo shadow complex] [Fibrosed wall → stone (echo) → shadow] → d/t cholelithiasis and chronic cholecystitis
- Acute cholecystitis → [Tc99 HIDA **best investigation**]
- MRI- GB calculi seen as filling defect on T2W images (Figure)
- CBD stone → MRCP (IOC) → meniscus appearance.

Adenomyomatosis of Gallbladder
Generalized
- Pearl necklace GB (T2WMRI)
- **Comet tail artefact (-USG)** [d/t **reverberation artifact** b/w cholesterol crystals in RA Sinus [pathognomonic]
- **String of beads sign** in thick GB wall (T2WMRI)

Localized–Fundal

Pancreatitis
- Acute pancreatitis diagnosed by clinical and lab parameters
- **IOC for complication of acute pancreatitis** → CECT
  - Necrosis which is most imp. prognostic criteria (Figure).

Diagnosis of Acute Pancreatitis (2-out of 3)
1. Abdominal pain (typical)
2. Three fold or greater ↑↑ in S. amylase or S lipase
3. Confirmatory findings on cross sectional imaging

CECT Findings in Acute Pancreatitis
- Bulky pancreas
- Ill-defined peripancreatic planes with loss of lobulations
- Peripancreatic fluid collections.

Best prognostic scoring by → CTSI (CT severity Index)

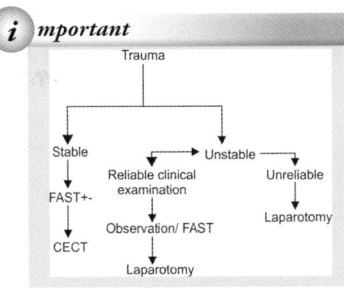

i mportant

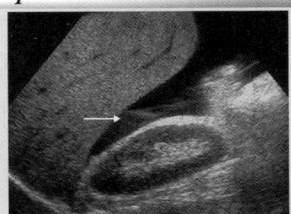

i mportant
Trauma–CECT is IOC
Angiography reserved for embolization of traumatic pseudoaneurysm or A.V. fistula.

i mportant
Comet tail sign is seen on CT in round atelectasis → Asbestosis

i mportant

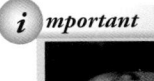

Blunt trauma abdomen
(fluid in Morrison's pouch)

i mportant
Features of Gallstone ileus
- Ectopic calcified gallstone
- Signs of small intestinal obstruction
- Gas in the biliary tree

i mportant

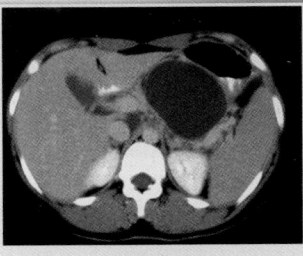

Pseudocyst

X-ray
- Sentinel loop/colon cut-off/duodenal ileus/mottled lucencies/gasless abdomen/Renal halo sign

Causes of Ca⁺⁺ in Pancreas
- Chronic alcoholic pancreatitis
- Hereditary
- Malnutrition
- Parathyroidism

> **Important**
> - IOC for Chronic pancreatitis → EUS > MRCP > ERCP
> - IOC for chronic calcific pancreatitis → NCCT
> - Chain of lakes: in chronic pancreatitis (ERCP/MRCP)

Periampullary Carcinoma
- **Widened 'c' loop of duodenum**
- **Frost berg inverted '3' sign**
- **Double duct sign**
- **Antral pad sign** in c/o ca head of pancreas.

> **Important**
>
> Necrosis in acute necrotic pancreatitis

Acute pancreatitis	- Renal halo sign - Gasless abdomen - Colon cut-off sign - Sentinel loop sign
Chronic pancreatitis	- Beaded/string of pearls/chain of lakes - Rat tail/appearance - Nipping/narrowing of origins of side branches of MPD or CBD ± double duct sign
Calcific pancreatitis	- Double duct - Scrambled egg - Inverted 3 sign - Rose thorning of II part of duodenum

Causes of Air in Biliary Tract
- **Due to fistula with GI tract**
  - Trauma
  - Surgery
  - Malignancy
  - Duodenal ulcer
  - Gallstone ileus
- **Emphysematous cholecystitis**
- **Reflux from duodenum**
  - Passage of stone/ascariasis
  - Sphincterotomy/plasty

> **Important**
>
>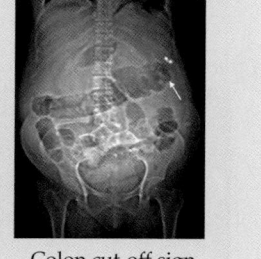
>
> Colon cut-off sign

FOCAL LIVER LESION

- Very commonly encountered lesion on abdominal ultrasound.
- Ultrasound is a very good investigation to differentiate cystic lesion from solid lesion.
- Ultrasound is not very good in characterizing a solid lesion.
- Best investigation for characterization of a liver lesion is triphasic MRI.
- Usually biopsy is not required. It may be done in case of metastatic lesion to look for primary source.

> **_important_**
> **Few important full forms:**
> - HIFU → High frequency ultrasound
> - TACE → Transcatheter arterial chemoembolization
> - FAST → Focused assessment by sonography for trauma
> - ALARA → As low as reasonably achievable
> - BIRADS → Breast imaging reporting and data system
> - FLAIR → Fluid attenuated inversion recovery sequence

Lesions	Classical triphasic CT/MRI findings
Hepatic cyst	Sharply demarcated wall, water density, non enhancing
Hemangioma	Peripheral filling in of contrast over time "Light Bulb Sign" on T2 MRI
Focal nodular hyperplasia (FNH)	Early filling in arterial phase with central filling defect (scar)
Hepatic adenoma	Variable, central changes due to hemorrhage often seen
Metastasis	Mostly multiple low attenuation lesions, rim enhancement without "filling in"
Abscess	Well demarcated hypodense areas with peripheral enhancement, may see gas
Hepatocellular carcinoma (HCC)	Early arterial enhancement, fast washout, delayed fibrous capsule enhancement

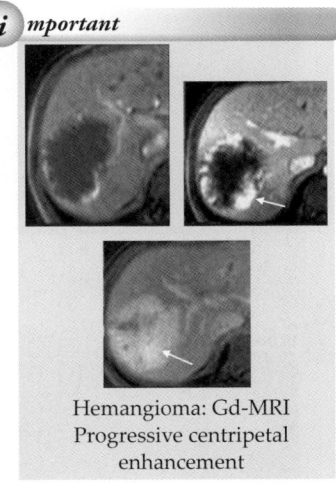

Hemangioma: Gd-MRI Progressive centripetal enhancement

X-ray Signs of Splenic Trauma

- **Obliteration of splenic outline (best)**
- Loss of psoas outline
- Indenting gastric air bubble
- Fracture of lower ribs and elevation of (L) hemidiaphragm

Internal Hernias

(L) Paraduodenal (75%)–through landzert fossa at duodenojejunal junction bowel loops behind stomach and pancreas displacing inferior mesenteric vein anteriorly.

(R) Paraduodenal → [In cases of nonrotated bowel]- Through waldeyer's fossa → behind SMA and inferior to IIIrd part of duodenum
- Encapsulated small bowels in Rt mid-abdomen
- Ante displacement of (R) celiac vein
- Looping of small intestine around SMA

Renal Calculi → 90% Radiopaque

NCCT is investigation of choice
Uric acid and xanthine stones are lucent renal calculi
Ureteric stones overlap spine on lateral X-ray.
Cysteine stones are poorly radiopaque due to sulfur

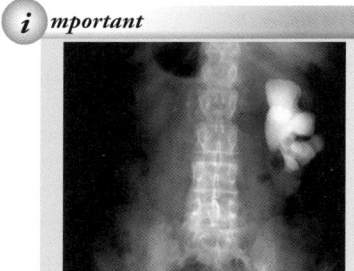

Stag horn calculus

Ureteric Colic/Obstruction

- IOC for ureteric colic → NCCT KUB
- Acutely obstructed kidney → Increasingly dense nephrogram without or delayed contrast in PCS on IVP
- USG → **acoustic shadow/twinkling artifact** on color Doppler
- Chronic obstruction – Hydronephrosis, No persistent nephrogram with poor pyelogram

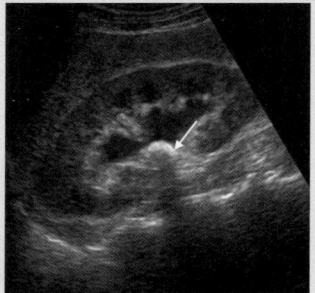

Renal calculus on USG-acoustic shadow

Renal Tuberculosis

- *IOC for early renal TB → IVP/IVU (Feathery outline)
- For Chronic → CT
- MRI: No role
  - Predominantly for evaluation of nonfunctioning kidney.

X-ray

- Lobar distribution of calcification is specific for renal TB (calcification is rare in UB)

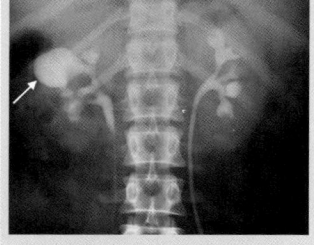

Amputated calyx- TB kidney

IVU

- Early features → loss of definition of minor calyx with **feathery outline**. (Moth eaten calyx)
  - Earlist to be picked by IVP
- Upward pointing renal pelvic calculi due to **hiked up pelvis**
- **Autonephrectomy/putty kidney**
- Strictures with phantom calyx, amputated calyx
- Kinking of pelvis **(Kerr's kink)**
- **Beaded and corkscrew ureter**

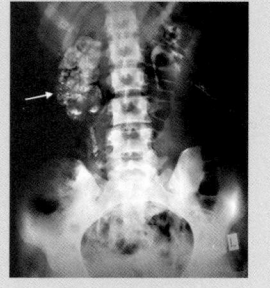

Putty kidney

- Pipe stem ureter
- Caseocavernous type → enlarged sac like poorly functioning kidney
- **Thimble bladder** — contracted (without calcification)
- **Golf hole ureter** on cystoscopy

Cystic Disease of Kidneys

- **Cortical beak sign** on CT → simple cyst → filling defect on IVP
- Swiss cheese/spider leg → IVP → PCKD
- **Sentinel cyst** → tubular obstruction by tumor
- Striated nephrogram → ARPKD → (potter type-I) [ANC USG-bilateral enlarged echogenic kidneys + oligohydramnios]
- **Swiss cheese nephrogram**
  - ADPKD
  - Medullary sponge kidney

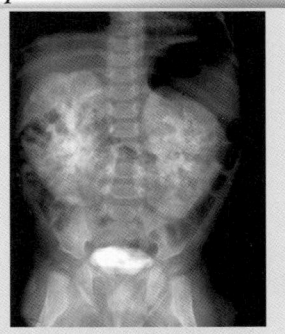

Swiss cheese nephrogram on IVP- medullary sponge kidney

Renal Hydatid

If contrast between ectocyst and pericyst → of Renal hydatid → **Goblet of urine glass or Surraco's sign**.
- Crescent sign

> *important*
> *An extracapsular rim of edema as hyperintensity on T2W MRI and hypoechoic on USG around kidneys in renal failure → **kidney sweat sign**

Horseshoe Kidney

- **Flower vase appearance on** → IVP
- IVP → medially projecting lower pole calyces → **'Hand shaking sign'**
- More prone to → calculi/trauma/Wilm's tumor/obstruction

Ureterocele

- **Adder head/ cobra head** → IVP
- Alternating distending and collapsing anechoic cyst at VUJ on — USG

> *important*
> *Chalice/Bregman's sign → TCC [Distal margin of soft tissue mass extending into the distended part of opacified ureter].
> [Not seen in nonopaque calculus as ureter not distended distal to nonopaque calculi].

Immediate Faint Persistent Nephrogram

- Chronic glomerular disease
- Acute glomerulonephritis
- Renal vein thrombosis
- Chronic severe ischemia

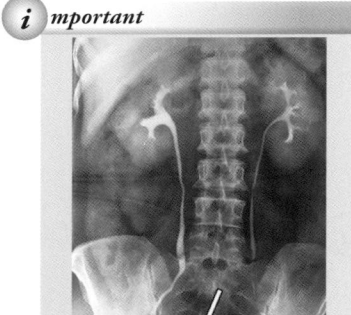
Right ureterocele- adder head appearance

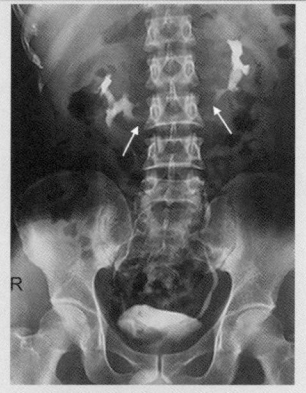
Horseshoe kidney- shaking hand sign

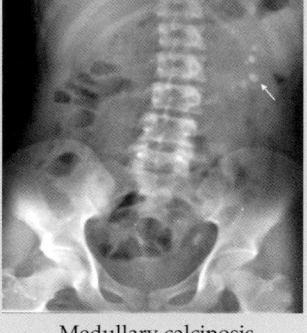
Medullary calcinosis

Unilateral Delayed Nephrogram
- Obstructive uropathy
- ↓Renal blood flow due to Renal artery stenosis/RVT

Increasingly Dense Nephrogram
- Acute renal obstruction
- Hypotension/dehydration
- Acute Papillary necrosis
- Renal ischemia
- MM/Myeloid
- Acute glomerular disease
- Intratubular obstruction
- Acute Renal vein thrombosis

Immediate Dense Persistent Nephrogram
B/L
- Acute tubular necrosis/obstruction
- Severe inflammatory renal disease
- Systemic hypotension

U/L
- Renal artery stenosis
- Renal vein thrombosis
- Urinary tract obstruction

Striated Nephrogram: Prominent nephrons seen extending into the medulla as medullary rays.

U/L
- Obstructive nephrogram (acute)

U/L or B/L
- Pyelonephritis
- Polyarteritis nodosa (PAN)
- Trauma

B/L
- Medullary cystic kidney disease/sponge
- ARPKD

Cortical Rim Sign: Enhancement of only most peripheral rim of renal cortex:

- Acute cortical necrosis
- Renal infarction
- Renal vein thrombosis
- ATN
- Acute arterial obstruction
- Severe hydronephrosis.

Nephrocalcinosis

Cortical	Medullary
Acute cortical neurosis	Distal renal tubular acidosis
Alport's synd.	Hyperparathyroidism
Graft rejection	Sarcoidosis/hypercalcemia
Hemolytic-uremic synd.	Medullary sponge kidney
Chronic glomerulonephritis	Hyperoxaluria

Radionuclide

IOC for GFR	– Tc^{99}DTPA (only glomerular filtration)
IOC for R. function	– MAG 3 (both glomerular and tubular excretion)
IOC for scar/reflux nephropathy	– Tc^{99} DMSA
Screening for renovascular hypertension	– captopril DTPA scanning
IOC for Renal artery stenosis	– MR Angiography
Gold standard	– Renal angiography

Medially Placed Ureters

B/L

- Retroperitoneal fibrosis
- Pelvic lipomatosis
- Abdominoperineal resection
- Ureterolysis

U/L

- Retrocaval ureter

Duplex Pelvicalyceal System

Weigert-Meyer law
- Upper moiety drains lower and more medial than lower moiety in UB.

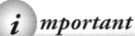
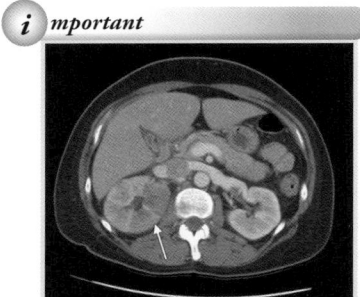
Acute pyelonephritis

- Upper moiety more prone to ureterocele which is usually obstructive
- Lower moiety → VUR

**If ureters—fused distally → yo-yo reflux from one ureter to the other which is draining non-functioning/excreting moiety.

IOC for reflux (VUR)	– MCU (Micturating cystourethrography)
For posterior urethra	– MCU
For anterior urethra	– RGU (retrograde urethrography)
For posterior Urethral Valve	– MCU

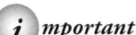
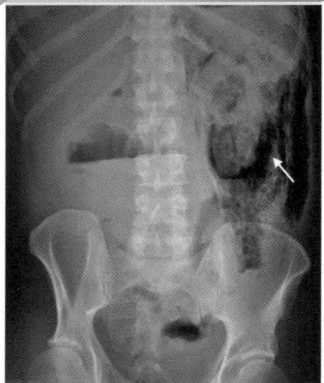
Emphysematous pyelonephritis

Tumors

- **Oncocytoma**
  - Spoke wheel pattern on angiography however not characteristic:
- **Angiomyolipoma**
  - Fat containing lesion [CT attenuation-'– 50' to '– 100' HU]
  - Associated with tuberous sclerosis

Wilms	Neuroblastoma
• Vascular displacement	• Encasement
• Does not cross midline	• Crosses midline
• Calcification rare	• Calcification common
• Pulmonary metastasis	• Usually metastasize to bone
• Necrotic areas	• Usually solid

Renal Artery Stenosis

Signs of significant renal artery stenosis on Doppler
- Percentage of diameter stenosis > 70%
- Collaterals **(most specific-Harrison)**
- Systolic pressure gradient > 20 mm Hg across the lesion
- Poststenotic dilatation of the renal arteries with turbulent and reversed flow.

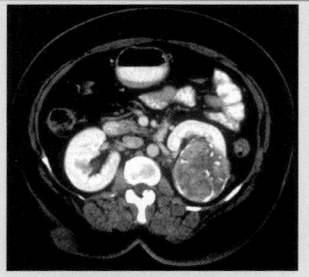
Renal cell carcinoma

Direct Signs

- ↑Peak systolic velocity (> 150 cm/sec)
- Peak renal artery to aorta ratio (RAR) > 3.5
- Absence of blood flow during diastole.

Indirect Signs of Renal Artery-Stenosis

- Tardus parvus wave form in segmental renal arteries.
- Loss of early systolic acceleration
- Acceleration time (AT) delay > 0.05–0.08 sec increased
- **Reduced acceleration index (AI) [single most sensitive screening parameter]**
- Reduced resistive index (RI) and pulsatility index (PI)

Painful Hematuria

- Stone (MC)
    - X-ray—KUB—Ist baseline investigation
    - NCCT – IOC
    - USG – Initial IOC

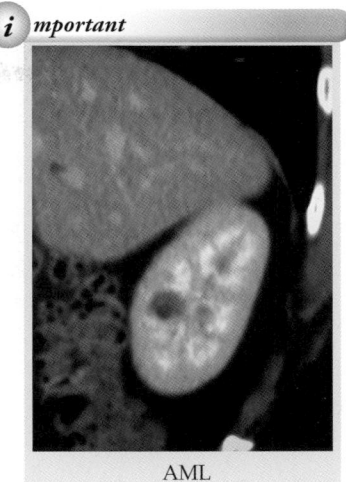
AML

Painless Hematuria

- Malignancy
    - USG–initial baseline Investigation
    - IVU–Ist investigation
    - CECT (CT urography)–IOC

Child with UTI

- IVU and cystourethrography (first investigation)
- VCUG (voiding cystourethrography)-IOC for VUR

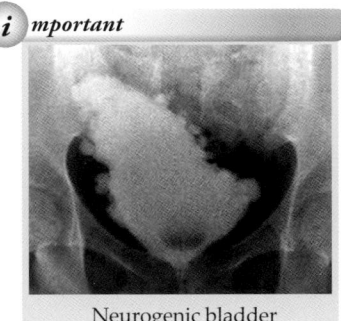
Neurogenic bladder

Obstructive Uropathy in Pregnant and Children

- MR urography is preferred over IVU

    IOC for pretransplant workup → angiography (MDCT > conventional)
Posterior urethral valve → IOC -VCUG (key hole appearance)

Renal Papillary Necrosis

- Analgesic (acute)
- DM, dehydration, diarrhea
- Shock
- Obstruction
- Sickle cell disease
- Alcohol
- Coagulopathy
- Trauma
- TB

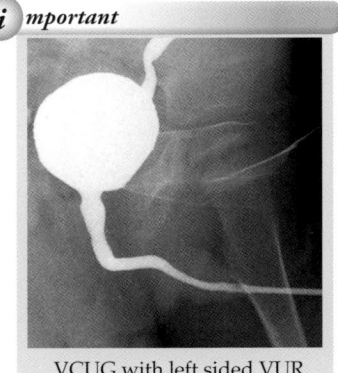
VCUG with left sided VUR

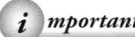

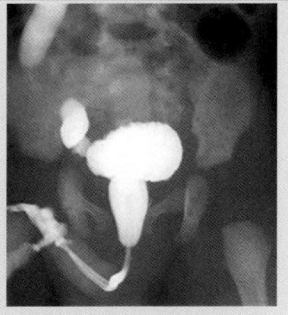

Key hole appearance in PUV

- RVT
- Rejection

Imaging features:
- **Ring-shaped calcification in sloughed papilla (X-ray)**
- IVP (best)
  - **Ball/egg in cup**
  - **Signet ring**
  - **Ring shadow**
  - **Club shaped/saccular calyx**
  - **Lobster claw sign**
  - **Filling defects in PCS**
  - ↓ **Density of contrast material in nephrogram**
  - Amputated calyx and formation of cavities

Acute Pyelonephritis

- Global/focal renal enlargement (IVU)
- Striated nephrogram (CT)
- Sloughed papilla/fungal ball (CT)

USG

- Focal/diffuse enlargement with hypoechogenicity
- Focal areas of hypoperfusion
- Perinephric fluid
- IOC in pregnant/pediatric patients

FEMALE PELVIS

MR imaging has become a valuable modality in the evaluation of the female pelvis. In many cases, it follows the performance of HSG or US. These cases include infertility and pelvic pain.
- Test of choice for local staging of cervical cancer and the evaluation of pain or disability in the pregnant patient.
- In the evaluation of advanced gynecologic cancers, it is usually a secondary choice with CT preferred.

Cervical incompetence

- USG is currently the **investigation of choice** for diagnosing cervical incompetence during pregnancy.
- The cervical length in normal pregnancy should measure more than 3 cm.

- The **width of the cervical canal is by far the most reliable parameter to predict cervical incompetence** and should measure less than 2 cm in the second trimester.
- If bulging of membranes into the cervical canal is seen, the prognosis is unfavorable.
- US criteria for diagnosing cervical incompetence have not been established in the nongravid patient.
- MRI offers the potential to diagnose cervical **incompetence in the nonpregnant as well as the pregnant patient**.

MRI Findings
- Shortening of the endocervical canal (less than 3 cm)
- Widening of the internal cervical os (greater than 4 mm)
- Asymmetric widening of the endocervical canal
- Thinning or absence of the low signal intensity cervical stroma.

Adenomyosis of Uterus

TVS
- Poorly defined hypoechoic myometrium
- Heterogenous myometrial echotexture
- Assymmetrically thickened myometrial wall
- Poor definition of endomyometrial junction
- Scattered small (<5 mm) myometrial cysts.

MRI
- Ill defined poorly marginated low signal intensity area
- Thickened endomyometrial junction >12 mm
- Multiple scattered small T2W hyperintense cysts.

Corpus Luteal Cysts
- Thickened hyperechoic (due to higher fat) crenulated wall showing increased peripheral vascularity on color Doppler.

Hemorrhagic Cyst
- **Fish net appearance of the cysts on USG**
- **Hyperintense signal on both T1W and T2W images of internal contents**

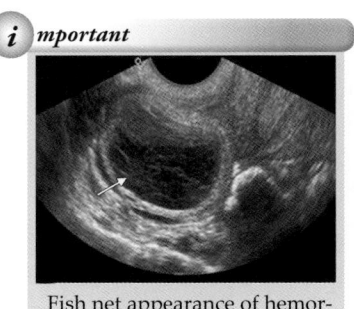

Fish net appearance of hemorrhagic cyst on USG

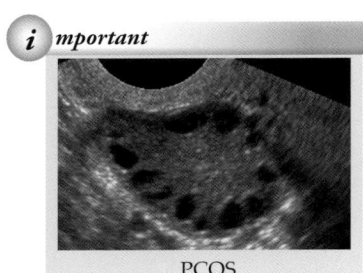

PCOS

Endometrial Cysts
- T1W hyperintense signal which shows shading on T2W images. [d/t old or bleed of various ages]

Polycystic Ovarian Disease
- Bilateral ovarian enlargement with multiple (10 or more) peripherally arranged small cysts (2–8 mm) giving string of pearls appearance on TVS/MRI

Hydrosalpinx
- Dilated tube with incomplete septae
- Cogwheel sign
- Beads on a string sign

Ovarian Torsion
- **USG with Doppler** – initial investigation of choice
- Unilateral ovarian enlargement
- Edematous ovary with multiple small cystic structures at the periphery
- Small amount of fluid in pouch of douglas
- Ovary has a dual blood supply and torsion can lead partial loss of blood flow with absent systolic spike/peak
- Arterial flow may be present in non viable ovaries but absent venous flow may be sensitive of non viability.

ANC
1st trimester scan- for
- Confirmation of pregnancy
- Intra uterine or extrauterine (ectopic)
- No of pregnancies
- Estimation of gestation age
- Adnexal/uterine pathologies
- Viability of fetus

TVS is the method of choice; more accurate and sensitive than transabdominal scan due to use of higher frequency probe.

Crown rump length is the most accurate single parameter for the assessment of gestational age in first trimester.

Earliest congenital anomaly to be detected on ANC USG- Anencephaly (8–10 weeks)- absent ossification of frontal bone.

Exencephaly- brain outside skull (14 weeks)

Routine use of Doppler is avoided although used to assess foetal or maternal complications like ectopic pregnancy and IUGR.

- **Ectopic pregnancy**
  Failure to double the level of –beta HCG in 48 hours and lower levels of B-HCG as compared to gestational age.

important

	TVS	TAS
G. Sac	4 + wks	5 + wks
CA	5 + wks	6 + wks

USG Features of Ectopic Pregnancy

- Heterogenous/complex adnexal mass representing ectopic gestational sac or hematoma separate from the ovary (**Most common finding**)
- Doppler shows a ring of fire due to high velocity, low impedence flow compatible with placental flow
- **Tubal ring- extrauterine G sac with trophoblastic tissue**
- Free fluid in pouch of douglas
- **Doughnut/bagel sign- hyperechoic rim surrounding the gestational sac**
- **Pseudo sac** in the endometrial cavity containing fluid and echogenic areas
- Decidual reaction in the endometrial cavity.

2nd Trimester Scan/Anomaly Scan- 18–20 Weeks

- For gross congenital anomalies and structural/anatomical defects and placental localization
- BPD is most accurate single parameter however multiple parameter assessment is the best and most accurate for dating in 2–3rd trimester.

IUGR (Intrauterine Growth Retardation)

- Doppler is IOC to assess IUGR
- Early diastolic notching is abnormal after 22 weeks of gestation with gradual reduction in diastolic flow with S/D (systolic/diastolic) ration > 3 suggests IUGR [Normal is <2.5]
- Absent diastolic flow is associated with high mortality rate

- Reversal of diastolic flow is associated with worst fetal outcome
- Increased diastolic flow or reduced S/D ratio of cerebral arteries is an indicator of brain sparing IUGR.

Imaging of Male Genital System

Scrotum

Epididymitis- orchitis
- Prehan sign- pain relieved when testes are elevated over pubic symphysis
- USG with Doppler- IOC
- Enlarged hypoechoic epididymis/testis (hyperechoic if hemorrhage)
- Indirect signs of inflammation like- reactive hydrocoele or pyocele, scrotal wall thickening
- Increased number and concentration of identifiable vessels with high flow

Testicular Torsion
- Anomalous suspension of testis by a long stalk of spermatic cord (bell and clapper phenomenon)
- USG- first investigation with Doppler being IOC
- Testicular morphology may be normal if done immediately
- Testicular swelling and decreased echogenecity – most common findings at 4–6 hours duration
- Heterogenous echotexture due to hemorrhage and infarction
- Reduced or absent blood flow on Doppler.
- Presence of color on power Doppler in a patient with clinical manifestations – does not exclude torsion
- Torsion of appendix testis- blue dot sign through overlying skin.
- Reversal of flow in diastole is suggestive of venous infarction.

Carcinoma Prostate
- Location: Peripheral zone 70%, transition zone 20% and central 10%.
- Most important factor affecting **prognosis/choice** of treatment is **presence or absence of extracapsular extension.**
- **TRUS is most widely used imaging modality for local staging.**

- Small prostatic cancer usually appears hypoechoic because of closely packed cells.
- Secondary signs like glandular asymmetry and capsular bulging.
- 3D MR spectroscopy (increased choline and decreased citrate levels) + Endorectal MR imaging increase accuracy in detecting and staging of local and extracapsular extension of prostate carcinoma.
- Pathologically: adults (adenocarcinoma); Children (rhabdomyosarcoma)

Classic Imaging Appearance

- TRUS is most frequently used to assess the primary tumor, but no consistent finding predicts cancer with certainty.
- TRUS is used primarily to direct prostate biopsies.
- Computed tomography (CT) scans lack sensitivity and specificity to detect extraprostatic extension and are inferior to magnetic resonance imaging (MRI) in visualization of lymph nodes.
- **T2WI:** Decrease signal in a normally high signal peripheral zone.

MRI is IOC for Preoperative Staging of Prostatic Cancer

- MRI specificity is improved with an endorectal coil and aids in planning radiation therapy. T1-weighted images demonstrate the periprostatic fat, periprostatic venous plexus, perivesicular tissues, lymph nodes, and bone marrow. T2-weighted images demonstrate the internal architecture of the prostate and seminal vesicles.
- MR spectroscopy is also helpful in identification of malignancy identified by loss of citrate peak [seen in normal gland] and identification of choline peak.
- Radionuclide bone scans are used to evaluate spread to osseous sites.

Spermatic Venography is usefully employed in localisation of undescended testis if this is not identified using cross-sectional imaging. Now for a young man with primary infertility, low volume, fructose negative ejaculate, pathology is most likely to be in seminal vesicles, ejaculatory duct or vas.

Transrectal Ultrasonography (TRUS) is an excellent technique for demonstrating seminal vesicle anatomy and finding ejaculatory duct pathologies.

QUESTIONS

1. Which of the following is not seen on ultrasound in acute pyelonephritis?
   a. Grossly enlarged kidney
   b. Focal area of hypoechogenicity
   c. Perinephric collection (pus in the perinephric space)
   d. Increased vascularity

2. On barium contrast radiography, which among the following is false:
   a. Ileum is featureless
   b. Colon has haustrations
   c. Jejunum is feathery
   d. Distal part of duodenum has a cap

3. Central dot sign is seen in:
   a. Primary sclerosing cholangitis
   b. Liver hamartoma
   c. Caroli's disease
   d. Polycystic liver disease

4. The radiological procedure for studying vesico-ureteric reflux is:
   a. Ascending pyelogram
   b. Cystogram
   c. Intravenous pyelogram
   d. Micturating cystourethrogram

5. Which of the following is true regarding the principle of use of MRCP?
   a. Intraluminal dye is used to create the three-dimensional view of the structures
   b. Dye is instilled percutaneously first, then MRI is used
   c. Use of heavily T2-weighted image without contrast to create the three-dimensional image of the biliary tree using MIP algorithm
   d. Use of systemic gadolinium as a contrast agent to create the three-dimensional image of the biliary tree

6. Micturating cystourethrography is used in the diagnosis of:
   a. Vesicoureteric reflex and posterior urethral valve
   b. Rupture urethra
   c. Stricture urethra
   d. Ca of the bladder

7. Investigation of choice in small renal calculi:
   a. Low dose non-enhanced CT
   b. High dose non-enhanced CT
   c. Low dose enhanced CT
   d. High dose enhanced CT

8. Distribution of functional renal tissue is seen by:
   a. Dimercaptosuccinic acid (DMSA)
   b. Diethylene triamine penta-acetic acid (DTPA)
   c. Mercaptoacetyle triglycine 3 (MAG3) - Tc99
   d. I 123 iodocholesterol

9. On X-ray, small bowel can be differentiated by large bowel by having:
   a. String of beads sign
   b. Haustrations
   c. Peripherally placed concave coil of intestine
   d. Air fluid level
   e. Valvulae conniventes

10. Renal agent used for assessing cortical scarring:
    a. TC-99 m DTPA
    b. TC-99 m DMSA
    c. TC-99 m Glucohepatanate
    d. 1-131- Hippuran

11. For suspected ureteric calculus, the modality of choice is:
    a. Noncontrast CT
    b. Ultrasonography
    c. X-ray KUB
    d. Cystoscopy

12. Which one of the following imaging modalities strive for evaluation of extra-adrenal pheochromocytoma?
    a. Ultrasound
    b. CT
    c. MRI
    d. MIBG scan
13. For renal stone, diagnosis is not done by:
    a. IVP b. MRI
    c. PET-scan d. CT-scan
14. Of the following imaging modality is most sensitive investigation of choice to detect early renal tuberculosis:
    a. Intravenous urography
    b. Ultrasound
    c. Computed tomography
    d. Magnetic resonance imaging
15. Posterior urethra is best visualized by:
    a. Static cystogram
    b. Retrograde urethrogram
    c. Voiding cystogram
    d. Cr cystogram
16. Radiation exposure is least in the following procedure:
    a. Micturating cystourethrogram
    b. IVP
    c. Bilateral nephrostogram
    d. Spiral CT for stones
17. All of the following form radiolucent stones except:
    a. Xanthine
    b. Cysteine
    c. Indinavir associated stones
    d. Allopurinol associated stones
18. Most sensitive and specific investigation for diagnosis of renovascular hypertension:
    a. MRI
    b. Captopril-enhanced radionuclide scan
    c. Spiral CT angiography
    d. Catheter angiography
19. Abdominal ultrasonography in a 3-year-old boy shows a solid circumscribed hypoechoic renal mass. Most likely diagnosis is:
    a. Wilms' tumor
    b. Renal cell carcinoma
    c. Mesoblastic nephroma
    d. Oncocytoma
20. Which of the following is not an appropriate investigation for anterior urethral stricture?
    a. Magnetic resonance imaging
    b. Retrograde urethrogram
    c. Micturating cystourethrogram
    d. High-frequency ultrasound
21. Transrectal ultrasonography in carcinoma prostate is most useful for:
    a. Guided prostatic biopsies
    b. Seminal vesicle involvement
    c. Measurement of prostatic volume
    d. To detect hypoechoic area
22. Papillary necrosis features are all except:
    a. Egg in cup
    b. Hyperdense nephrogram
    c. Calyceal horns
    d. Ring shadows
23. The most important sign of significance of renal artery stenosis on an angiogram is:
    a. A percentage diameter stenosis >70%
    b. Presence of collaterals
    c. Stenosis > 50%
    d. Thrombosed renal artery
24. Dense persistent renogram is obtained by:
    a. Dehydrating the patient
    b. Increasing the dose of contrast media
    c. Rapid (bolus) injection of dye
    d. Using nonionic media

25. Investigation of choice in diffuse esophageal spasm is:
    a. Manometry
    b. Esophagoscopy
    c. Barium examination showing tertiary contractions
    d. CT thorax

26. Double bubble sign with air shadows absent in distal bowel coils on X-ray abdomen is characteristic of:
    a. Duodenal webs
    b. Duodenal atresia
    c. GIPH
    d. Ileal atresia

27. Carman's meniscus sign is diagnostic of:
    a. Peptic ulcer
    b. Cholecystitis
    c. Meconium ileus
    d. Carcinoma of stomach

28. Trifoliate appearance is seen in:
    a. Peptic ulcer
    b. Pyloric stenosis
    c. Carcinomal head of pancreas
    d. Periampullary carcinoma

29. X-ray feature of pyloric stenosis is:
    a. Single bubble appearance
    b. Double bubble appearance
    c. Triple bubble appearance
    d. Multiple air fluid levels

30. String sign is seen in:
    a. Crohn's disease
    b. TB of the ileocaecal region
    c. Idiopathic hypertrophic pyloric stenosis
    d. All of the above

31. "Coffee bean" sign is seen in:
    a. Intussusception
    b. Bowel ischemia
    c. Sigmoid volvulus
    d. Congenital hypertrophic pyloric stenosis

32. Triad of vomiting, abdominal distension and string of beads sign on abdominal X-ray is typically suggestive of:
    a. Duodenal atresia
    b. Small bowel obstruction
    c. Large bowel obstruction
    d. Gastric volvulus

33. String sign of Kantor is seen in:
    a. Crohn's disease
    b. Ulcerative collitis
    c. TB
    d. Carcinoma

34. Ileocecal tuberculosis presents with all except:
    a. Rapid emptying of narrowed terminal ileum
    b. Inverted umbrella sign
    c. Stellate ulcer with elevated margins
    d. Longitudinal ulcers are more common

35. Following are common features of malignant gastric ulcer on barium meal, except:
    a. Location on the greater curvature
    b. Carman's meniscus sign
    c. Radiating folds which do not reach the edge of the ulcer
    d. Lesser curvature ulcer with a nodular rim

36. Findings of pyloric stenosis on USG are all except:
    a. Accuracy 95%
    b. High gastric-residue
    c. Segment length > 16 mm
    d. Thickness of muscle wall > 4 mm

37. A newborn presenting with intestinal obstruction. Abdominal on X-ray multiple air fluid levels are seen. The diagnosis is most likely to be:
    a. Pyloric obstruction
    b. Duodenal atresia
    c. Ileal atresia
    d. Lads's bands

38. The following are radiological features of sigmoid volvulus except:
    a. Inverted U-shaped bowel loop
    b. Liver overlap sign
    c. Bird of prey
    d. Cupola sign
39. Radiological signs of Crohn's disease:
    a. String sign of Kantor
    b. Pipestem colon
    c. Pseudopolyp
    d. Backwash ileitis
40. Lead pipe appearance is seen in:
    a. Crohn's disease
    b. Ulcerative colitis
    c. Schistosomiasis
    d. Carcinoma colon
41. All of the following are diagnostic barium follow-through features of ileocecal tuberculosis except:
    a. Apple-core appearance
    b. Pulled up contracted cecum
    c. Widening of ileocecal angle
    d. Strictures involving terminal ileum
42. Following are features of ischemic colitis except:
    a. Thumb printing
    b. Serrated mucosa
    c. Increased mucosal fold thickness
    d. Dilution of barium
43. The best view to visualize minimum pneumoperitoneum is:
    a. AP view of abdomen
    b. Erect film of abdomen
    c. Rt lateral decubitus with horizontal beam
    d. Lt lateral decubitus with horizontal beam
44. In case of suspected perforation which view is the best:
    a. Erect
    b. Supine
    c. Lateral decubitus
    d. None
45. Radiological feature of ischemic colitis is:
    a. Saw-toothing
    b. Craggy popcorn appearance
    c. Thumb printing
    d. Corkscrew appearance
46. Feathery appearance in jejunum is due to:
    a. Valvulae conniventes
    b. Haustrations
    c. Luminal gas
    d. Vascular network
47. Which among the following is false regarding small bowel appearance on abdominal radiograph?
    a. Valvulae conniventes are present
    b. Peripheral distribution
    c. Radius of curvature is small
    d. Solid faces are absent
48. Small intestine in intestinal obstruction is distinguished radiologically from large intestine by:
    a. Haustration
    b. Valvulae conniventes
    c. Cannot be distinguished
    d. None
49. Soap bubble appearance in X-ray is seen in:
    a. Multiple cystic kidney
    b. Neuroblastoma
    c. Cystic lymphangiectasis
    d. Meconium ileus
50. Which among the following is false regarding need of Supine chest radiograph in the abdominal pathology?
    a. For showing presence of a small pneumoperitoneum
    b. A number of chest conditions can present as acute abdominal condition
    c. Acute abdominal condition may be complicated by the chest pathology
    d. Even when the chest radiograph is normal, it acts as a most valuable baseline.

51. Free gas in abdomen (under the diaphragm) can be best diagnosed by which X-ray?
    a. Standing
    b. Right lateral recumbent view
    c. Left lateral recumbent view
    d. Sitting position
52. Cupola sign:
    a. Radiological finding in supine posture for pneumoperitoneum
    b. Radiological finding in supine posture for pneumothorax
    c. Air in Morrison's pouch
    d. Both walls of bowel is seen
53. Typical "saw-tooth" colon on barium enema is seen with:
    a. Colonic diverticulosis
    b. Colonic volvulus
    c. Colonic carcinoma
    d. Ulcerative colitis
54. Chain-of-lake appearance ERCP is seen in:
    a. Acute pancreatitis
    b. Chronic pancreatitis
    c. Carcinoma pancreas
    d. Ductal adenoma
55. Solitary hypoechoic lesion of the liver without septate or debris is most likely to be:
    a. Hydatid cyst
    b. Caroli's disease
    c. Liver abscess
    d. Simple cyst
56. "Hat sign" on double contrast barium enema is seen in:
    a. Ulcer
    b. Polyp
    c. Carcinoma
    d. Diverticulum
57. Couinaud's segments are used to divide which organ:
    a. Liver   b. Lung
    c. Spleen   d. Kidney
58. A 22-year-old man presents with a solitary 2 cm space-occupying lesion of mixed echogenicity in the right lobe of liver on ultrasound examination. The rest of the liver is normal. Which of the following tests should be done next?
    a. Ultrasound-guided biopsy of the lesion
    b. Hepatic scintigraphy
    c. Hepatic angiography
    d. Contrast-enhanced CT scan of the liver
59. Which one of the following hepatic lesions can be diagnosed with high accuracy by using nuclear imaging?
    a. Hepatocellular carcinoma
    b. Hepatic adenoma
    c. Focal nodular hyperplasia
    d. Cholangiocarcinoma
60. CT findings of acute pancreatitis are all except:
    a. Dilation of pancreatic duct
    b. Fuzzy outline of pancreas
    c. Peripancreatic fluid collection
    d. Edematous pancreas
61. According to Couinaud's classification of functional segments of liver, which of the following is segment IV of liver?
    a. Left lobe   b. Right lobe
    c. Caudate lobe d. Quadrate lobe
62. Radiological signs of acute pancreatitis include the following except:
    a. Colon cut-off sign
    b. Cullen's sign
    c. Renal halo sign
    d. Sentinel loop sign
63. CT findings of acute pancreatitis are:
    a. Fuzzy outline of pancreas
    c. USG has replaced it
    c. Dye used is telepaque
    d. All of the above

64. Colon cut-off sign is seen in:
    a. Acute pancreatitis
    b. Diverticulitis
    c. Appendicitis
    d. Carcinoma colon
65. Widening of the C loop in X-ray is diagnostic of:
    a. Chronic pancreatitis
    b. Carcinoma head of pancreas
    c. Periampullary carcinoma
    d. Calculi in the ampulla of Vater
66. "Spongy appearance" with central sunburst calcification is seen in:
    a. Pancreatic adenocarcinoma
    b. Mucinous cyst adenocarcinomas
    c. Somatostatinoma
    d. Serous cystadenoma
67. Most sensitive investigation for pancreatic carcinoma is:
    a. Angiography b. ERCP
    c. Ultrasound   d. CT scan
68. Investigation of choice for small intestine tumor:
    a. Ba followthrough
    b. Echo
    c. X-ray abdomen
    d. CT scan with contrast
69. Contrast used in barium enema is:
    a. Barium oxide
    b. Barium sulfide
    c. Barium sulfate
    d. Lead sulfate
70. A patient complains of epigastric pain, radiating to back off and on. The investigation of choice is:
    a. MRI
    b. CT scan
    c. USG
    d. Radionucleotide scan
71. Investigation of choice for gallstone:
    a. X-ray
    b. USG
    c. Cholecystography
    d. CT scan
72. The investigation of choice for acute cholecystitis is:
    a. USG   b. HIDA-scan
    c. CT-scan   d. X-ray
73. Which is not required for visualization of gallbladder in oral cholecystography?
    a. Functioning liver
    b. Motor mechanisms of gallbladder
    c. Patency of cystic duct
    d. Ability to absorb water
74. Investigation of choice in obstructive jaundice is:
    a. ERCP   b. USG
    c. Cholecystography
    d. Laparoscopy
75. Minimal ascites can be best detected by:
    a. USG
    b. Plain X-ray abdomen
    c. MRI
    d. CT scan
76. Most common investigation done for obstructive jaundice:
    a. CT scan   b. USG
    c. X-ray   d. ERCP
77. Focal and diffuse thickening of gallbladder wall with high amplitude reflections and 'comet tail' artifacts on USG suggest the diagnosis of:
    a. Xanthogranulomatous cholecystitis
    b. Carcinoma of gallbladder
    c. Adenomyomatosis
    d. Cholesterolosis
78. Which of the following is not a diagnostic feature of gallstone ileus in plain abdominal radiograph?
    a. Ectopic calcified gallstone
    b. Stone < 2.5 cm size in the intestine
    c. Signs of small intestinal obstruction
    d. Gas in the biliary tree

79. Air in biliary tract is seen in all except:
    a. Gallstone ileus
    b. Sclerosing cholangitis
    c. Carcinoma gallbladder
    d. Endoscopic papillotomy

80. Computed tomography (CT scan) is least accurate for diagnosis of:
    a. Aneurysm in the hepatic artery
    b. Lymph node in the para-aortic region
    c. Mass in the tail of pancreas
    d. Gallstones

81. Investigation of choice for recurrent GIST:
    a. MIBG   b. PET CT
    c. MRI   d. CECT

82. Techetium-99 scan is used for diagnosis of:
    a. Meckel's diverticulum
    b. Appendix
    c. Volvulus
    d. Obstruction

83. Best imaging modality for neuroendocrinal tumors:
    a. PET
    b. CECT
    c. Radionucleotide scan
    d. MRI with gadolinium scan

84. Protein-losing enteropathy diagnosis, all used except?
    a. Tc albumin
    b. Tc dextran
    c. In transferrin
    d. Tc seclosumab

85. A dense persistent nephrogram may be seen in all of the following except:
    a. Acute ureteral obstruction
    b. Systemic hypertension
    c. Severe hydronephrosis
    d. Dehydration

86. Calcific hepatic metastases are seen in:
    a. Adenocarcinoma of the colon
    b. Carcinoid tumors
    c. Renal cell carcinoma
    d. Lymphoma

87. For the evaluation of blunt abdominal trauma, which of the following imaging modalities is ideal?
    a. Ultrasonography
    b. Computed tomography
    c. IVP
    d. MRI

88. USG is sensitive in:
    a. Ureteric colic
    b. Gallstone
    c. Appendicitis
    d. Pancreatic pathology

89. Investigation of choice for diagnosis of splenic rupture:
    a. Peritoneal lavage
    b. Ultrasound
    c. CT scan
    d. MRI

90. Which of the following agents is used to measure glomerular filtration rate (GFR)?
    a. Iodohippurate
    b. Tc99m-DTPA
    c. Tc99m-MAG3
    d. Tc99m-DMSA

91. The investigation of choice for Renal Scarring defect in kidney is:
    a. Tc99 DMSA scan
    b. DTPA scan
    c. DEXA scan
    d. MCU

92. A patient presents with acute renal failure and anuria. The USG is normal. Which of the following investigations will give the best information regarding renal function?
    a. Intravenous pyelogram
    b. Retrograde pyelography

c. Antegrade pyelography
d. DTPA scan

93. A patient presented with ARF with complete anuria but a normal ultrasound. Next investigation is:
   a. IVP
   b. Antegrade pyelography
   c. Retrograde pyelography
   d. Radiorenogram

94. A dense renogram is obtained by:
   a. Dehydrating the patient
   b. Increasing the dose of contrast media
   c. Rapid (Bolus) injection of dye
   d. Using nonionic media

95. Nonvisualization of kidney in excretory urogram is seen in:
   a. Duplication
   b. Renal vein thrombosis
   c. Hydronephrosis
   d. Hypoplasia

96. 'Stipple sign' in transitional cell carcinoma of the renal collecting system is best demonstrated by:
   a. Intravenous urography
   b. Retrograde pyeloureterography
   c. Radionuclide scan
   d. Ultrasound scan

97. "Adder-head" appearance on voiding cystourethrogram in bladder is feature of:
   a. Horse-shoe kidney
   b. VUR
   c. Ureterocele
   d. Carcinoma of bladder

98. Cobra head deformity is characteristic of:
   a. Posterior urethral valve
   b. Ureterocele
   c. Bladder tumor
   d. Cystitis

99. IVP is contraindicated in:
   a. Multiple myeloma
   b. Kidney stones
   c. Renal cyst
   d. Transplanted kidney

100. Screening of renovascular hypertension is done by:
   a. MRI
   b. Captopril-enhanced radionuclide scan
   c. Spiral CT scan
   d. Duplex-Doppler flow study

101. The investigation of choice for imaging of urinary tract tuberculosis is:
   a. Plain X-ray
   b. Intravenous urography
   c. Ultrasound
   d. Computed tomography

102. Spider leg appearance is found in:
   a. Polycystic kidney
   b. Pyelonephritis
   c. Hydronephrosis
   d. Renal artery stenosis

103. Tear-drop bladder is seen in:
   a. Pelvic abscess
   b. Pelvic lipomatosis
   c. Bladder rupture
   d. All of the above

104. Renal tuberculosis can be diagnosed earliest by:
   a. CT scan
   b. IVP
   c. Angiography
   d. USG

105. Hypoechoic lesion within prostate in USG is seen in:
   a. Adenocarcinoma
   b. Normal prostate tissue
   c. Infertility
   d. Urethral obstruction
   e. BPH

106. Most accurate assessment of gestational age by USG is done by:
    a. Femur length
    b. Gestational sac size
    c. Menstrual history
    d. Crown rump length

107. Molar pregnancy can be best diagnosed by:
    a. Clinical history and examination
    b. Ultrasound study
    c. Laparoscopy
    d. CT Scan

108. USG can detect gestation sac earliest at:
    a. 5–6 weeks of gestation
    b. 7–8 weeks of gestation
    c. 10 weeks of gestation
    d. 12 weeks of gestation

109. The investigation of choice for an ectopic pregnancy is:
    a. CT scan
    b. Transvaginal USG
    c. Serum hCG levels
    d. Crown rump length

110. Earliest sign of fetal life is best detected by:
    a. X-ray
    b. Fetoscopy
    c. Real time USG
    d. Doppler

111. Parameters used to estimate gestational age in last TM:
    a. CR length
    b. Abdominal circumference suggestive of
    c. BPD
    d. Femur length

112. In second trimester of pregnancy, the diagnosis of IUGR can be best made of by assessing which of the following parameters:
    a. HC   b. AC
    c. CRL   d. BPD

113. Which of the following congenital malformations of the fetus can be diagnosed in first trimester by ultrasound?
    a. Anencephaly
    b. Inencephaly
    c. Microcepha!y
    d. Holoprosencephaly

114. Anencephaly can be diagnosed by USG at:
    a. 10–12 weeks of gestation
    b. 14–18 weeks of gestation
    c. 20–24 weeks of gestation
    d. 24–28 weeks of gestation

115. Ultrasonography of umbilical artery is done to know about:
    a. Heartbeat
    b. Gestational age
    c. Fetal weight
    d. Fetal maturity/growth

116. True about antenatal Doppler analysis is all except:
    a. Reduction in end diastolic flow is associated with poor outcome
    b. Reduction of EDF is associated with IUGR
    c. In normal gestation placental resistance is high
    d. S/D ratio is high in IUGR
    e. Investigation of choice in pregnancy

117. USG done at 18–20 weeks mainly to:
    a. Detect fetal abnormality
    b. Determine sex
    c. Estimate liquo
    d. Determine maturity

118. All are signs/features of ectopic pregnancy on USG except:
    a. Pseudosac
    b. Hyperechoic rim
    c. Adnexal mass
    d. Echogenic mass with multicystic spaces within endometrial cavity

119. Ectopic pregnancy, characteristic finding in USG is:
    a. Absence of gestational sac in uterus
    b. Complex adnexal mass
    c. Resistance in color Doppler
    d. Free fluid in peritoneal cavity

120. USG can diagnose all except:
    a. Anencephaly
    b. Neural tube defect
    c. Placenta previa
    d. Down's syndrome

121. On USG, finding of cystic hygroma in fetus is suggestive of:
    a. Down's syndrome
    b. Marphan's syndrome
    c. Turner's syndrome
    d. Klinefelter's syndrome

122. What is least useful as diagnostic procedure in case of acute hematemesis?
    a. Barium meal
    b. Endoscopy
    c. Gastric content aspiration
    d. Angiography

123. Following are common features of malignant gastric ulcer on Barium meal except:
    a. Location on the greater curvature
    b. Carman's meniscus sign
    c. Radiating folds which do not reach the edge of the ulcer
    d. Lesser curvature ulcer with a nodular rim

124. Gasless abdomen is a feature of:
    a. High obstruction
    b. Acute pancreatitis
    c. Congenital diaphragmatic hernia
    d. All of the above

125. Widening of C loop of duodenum is a feature of:
    a. Pancreatic head growth
    b. Carcinoma stomach
    c. Splenic involvement
    d. Involvement of upper right renal pole

126. X-ray appearance of CBD stone on cholangiography is:
    a. Meniscus appearance
    b. Sudden cut-off
    c. Smooth tapering
    d. Eccentric occlusion

127. A newborn baby has not passed meconium for 48 hours since birth. She has vomiting and distension of abdomen. The most appropriate investigation for evaluation would be:
    a. Anorectal manometry
    b. Rectal biopsy
    c. Lower GI contrast study
    d. Trypsin estimation

128. Papillary necrosis features are all except:
    a. Egg in cup
    b. Hyperdense nephrogram
    c. Calyceal horns
    d. Ring shadows

129. Which of the following regarding antenatal assessments of umbilical arteries by color Doppler study is TRUE?
    a. There is decreased S/D ratio in smoker and nicotine-abusing pregnant females
    b. The reduced diastolic flow at term indicates good prognosis
    c. The flow velocities and the S/D ratio are useful to evaluate high-risk pregnancies
    d. In otherwise normal pregnancies the increased S/D ratio is normal in smoking females

130. Best for unruptured ectopic pregnancy is:
    a. Per abdominal US
    b. BHCG

c. Transvaginal US
d. Amniocentesis

131. Most accurate assessment of gestational age by USG is done by:
    a. Femur length
    b. Gestational sac size
    c. Menstrual history
    d. Crown rump length

132. The method to diagnose misplaced intrauterine device is:
    a. Ultrasound
    b. X-ray abdomen (Erect view)
    c. Uterine sound and hysteroscopy
    d. All of the above

133. Maximum radiopaque shadow in ovary is seen in:
    a. Teratoma
    b. Dysgerminoma
    c. Mucinous cystadenoma
    d. Granulosa cell tumor

134. Missed IUD (IUCD) is recognized by:
    a. X-ray   b. USG
    c. Barium meal   d. CT Scan

135. Radiological investigation of female of reproductive age group is restricted to:
    a. Menstrual period
    b. First 10 days of menstrual cycle
    c. 10–20 days of menstrual cycle
    d. Last 10 days of menstrual cycle

136. Radiological findings of battered baby syndrome is:
    a. Multiple injuries not explained by one cause
    b. Multiple fractures in different stage of healing
    c. Excessive callus formation
    d. All of the above

137. In renal cell carcinoma, investigation of choice to evaluate inferior vena cava and renal vein for thrombus:
    a. IVP
    b. Color Doppler
    c. USG
    d. CT scan

138. Which of the following is the most preferred route to perform cerebral angiography?
    a. Transfemoral route
    b. Transaxillary route
    c. Direct carotid puncture
    d. Transbrachial route

139. Calcification is best detected by:
    a. X-ray   b. USG
    c. CT scan   d. MRI
    e. PET scan

140. Functional analysis of kidney is best done by:
    a. Radionuclide scanning
    b. IVP
    c. Ultrasound
    d. MRI

141. Investigation of choice in obstructive jaundice is:
    a. ERCP
    b. USG
    c. Cholecystography
    d. Laparoscopy

142. Gastro-esophageal reflux is best detected by:
    a. Endoscopy
    b. USG
    c. Barium study
    d. Isotope scan

143. Neural tube defect is best detected by:
    a. USG
    b. Chromosomal analysis
    c. Amniocentesis
    d. Placentography

144. Investigation of choice for Zenker's diverticulum is:
    a. Barium swallow
    b. Endoscopy
    c. Esophageal manometry
    d. CT

145. Which of the following is not a CT feature of Adrenal adenoma?
    a. Low attenuation
    b. Homogenous density and well defined borders
    c. Enhances rapidly, contrast stays in it for a relatively longer time and washes out late
    d. Calcification is rare
146. Fir tree appearance of bladder is seen in:
    a. Schistosomiasis
    b. Tuberculosis
    c. Neurogenic bladder
    d. Pelvic abscess
147. Investigation of choice for posterior urethral valve is:
    a. Micturition cystouretrogram
    b. Retrograde urethrography
    c. Ultrasound
    d. IVP
148. Drooping Lilly sign is seen in:
    a. Duplication of ureters
    b. Renal cyst
    c. Hydatid cyst
    d. Duplication of uterus
149. Earliest finding of renal truberculosis on IVP is:
    a. Cortical scarring
    b. Hydronephrosis
    c. Cavitation
    d. Ill defined calyx
150. Investigation of choice in choledocholithiasis:
    a. CT
    b. PET scan
    c. USG
    d. HIDA scan
151. Invertogram to be done in a new born:
    a. Immediately
    b. After 2 hours
    c. After 4 hours
    d. After 6 hour
152. On CT, Balthazar grading is for:
    a. Acute pancreatitis
    b. Cholecystitis
    c. Pancreatic carcinoma
    d. Chronic pancreatitis
153. Endoscopic USG criteria for chronic pancreatitis, when the diameter of the main pancreatic duct is:
    a. >1 mm
    b. 1.5 mm
    c. >2 mm
    d. >3 mm
154. Corkscrew esophagus on barium swallow is seen in:
    a. Achalasia cardia
    b. Diffuse esophageal spasm
    c. Carcinoma esophagus
    d. Gastroesophageal reflux
155. Colon cut off sign is seen in:
    a. Carcinoma colon
    b. Pancreatitis
    c. Sigmoid volvulus
    d. Diverticulosis
156. Drug administered to increase diagnostic accuracy of HIDA scan in neonatal jaundice is:
    a. Pentagastrin
    b. Phenobarbital
    c. Morphine
    d. Cholecystokinin
157. Apple core appearance is seen in:
    a. Carcinoma esophagus
    b. Carcinoma colon
    c. Sigmoid volumes
    d. Diverticulosis
158. Chain of lakes appearance is seen in:
    a. Chronic pancreatitis
    b. Acute pancreatitis
    c. Gall stone ileus
    d. Subacute intestinal obstruction
159. On DSA, typical 'string of beads' appearance of arteries is seen in:
    a. Takayasu's disease
    b. Atherosclerotic stenosis
    c. Fibromuscular dysplasia
    d. Middle aortic syndrome
160. Pulled up cecum is seen in:
    a. Ileocecal TB
    b. Carcinoma cecum

c. Intussusception
d. Carcinoma

161. Fetal cardiac activity can be detected earliest by USG at which age of intrauterine life:
    a. 1-2 weeks   b. 2-4 weeks
    c. 5-6 weeks   d. 6-8 weeks

162. Gas shadow in heart and great vessels appears in:
    a. IUD
    b. Abortion
    c. Still birth
    d. None of the above

163. Spalding sign is seen in:
    a. Abortion   b. Still birth
    c. IUD   d. infanticide

164. T-sign is seen in:
    a. Genital TB
    b. Membrane in twin pregnancy
    c. Molar pregnancy
    d. Septate uterus

165. What is the most appropriate Ix to be done to confirm a malignant CA head of pancreas.
    a. MRI guided biopsy
    b. EUS guided FNAC
    c. CT guided Biopsy
    d. percutaneous guided Biopsy

166. Asymptomatic abdominal aortic aneurysm is to be operated when more than:
    a. 55 mm
    b. 40 mm
    c. 50 mm
    d. 60 mm

167. Ultrasound is investigation of choice for:
    a. CHPS
    b. H type to fistula
    c. Annular pancreas
    d. Anorectal malformation

168. Which of the following is not true about Xanthogranulomatous pyelonephritis?
    a. Replacement of the renal parenchyma by yellow lipid-containing macrophages
    b. Usually associated with chronic urinary tract infection by Proteus mirabilis
    c. Histologically, cells may resemble hypernephroma clear cells
    d. CT finding of parenchymal destruction or streaky or mottled gas in the parenchyma is diagnostic

Multiple Correct Answers

169. The chemical composition of renal calculi visualized on plain radiographs is:
    a. Calcium oxalate
    b. Uric acid
    c. Magnesium ammonium phosphate
    d. Cysteine

170. Teardrop bladders are seen in:
    a. Pelvic hematoma
    b. Pelvic lipomatosis
    c. TB
    d. Neurogenic bladder
    e. Intraperitoneal bladder rupture

171. Investigations for small intestine include all except:
    a. Enteroclysis.
    b. Radionucleide enteroclysis
    c. MRI enteroclysis
    d. CT enteroclysis
    e. USG enteroclysis

172. True about features of cholecystitis on USG:
    a. Thick fibrosed gallbladder wall
    b. Stone impacted at neck of gallbladder

c. Pericholecystic edema
d. Increased vascularity
e. Comet tail sign

173. **Thickened gallbladder wall in USG is seen in:**
    a. Acute cholecystitis
    b. Mucosal thickening
    c. Cholesterosis
    d. Ascites
    e. AIDS cholangitis

174. **True about MRCP:**
    a. MRI is used to obtain the image
    b. CT is used for the images
    c. It shows the biliary tree
    d. Dye has to be injected endoscopically
    e. It is an invasive procedure

175. **Splenic injury is diagnosed on X-ray by:**
    a. Half stomach shadow
    b. Obliteration of splenic shadow
    c. Rib fracture
    d. Gas under diaphragm

176. **In a CT scan at the level of celiac trunk, following structures will be seen:**
    a. Pancreas
    b. Gallbladder
    c. Inferior vena cava
    d. Duodenum
    e. Portal vein

177. **RHC calcification is seen in:**
    a. Gallstone
    b. Renal stone
    c. Calcification of vessels
    d. Hepatic hemangioma
    e. Calcified costal cartilage

178. **For renal stone, diagnosis is not done by:**
    a. IVP
    b. MRI
    c. PET-scan
    d. USG
    e. CT scan

179. **IVP of polycystic kidney disease shows:**
    a. Cobra head
    b. Dropping lily
    c. Flower base appearance
    d. Spider leg deformity
    e. Fish hook appearance

180. **Diffuse esophageal dilatation on barium swallow is seen in:**
    a. Achalasia
    b. Trypanosomiasis
    c. Etidronate therapy
    d. Scleroderma

181. **Radiological finding in ileal atresia:**
    a. Microcolon on Ba enema
    b. Double bubble sign
    c. Coil spring appearance in Ba-Enema
    d. Obstruction in Ba meal
    e. Napkin ring stenosis

182. **Causes of bladder calcification are:**
    a. Schistosomiasis
    b. Urethral cell carcinoma
    c. TB
    d. Ureterocele
    e. Cystitis

183. **ERCP in pancratitis is done to know about:**
    a. CBD stones
    b. Associated cholangitis
    c. Ascites
    d. Pancreatic divisum
    e. Annular pancreas

Recently Asked Questions

184. **What is true regarding NIPT?**
    a. DNA is extracted from fetal cells circulating in maternal circulation.
    b. It can be used for structural abnormalities in fetus
    c. It is done before 7 weeks
    d. It is a recommended test for fetal sex determination

185. A 3 yrs old child is presented with multiple air-fluid levels on X-ray abdomen erect view. What should be the next step in the management of the patient?
    a. Gastrograffin follow through
    b. USG
    c. CECT abdomen with contrast
    d. Diagnostic laparotomy

186. Where do you find "Gasless abdomen"?
    a. Acute pancreatitis
    b. Intussusception
    c. Necrotizing enterocolitis
    d. Ulcerative colitis

ANSWERS

1. **Ans. d.** Increased vascularity
2. **Ans. d.** Distal part of duodenum has a cap
3. **Ans. c.** Caroli's disease
4. **Ans. d.** Micturating cystourethrogram
5. **Ans. c.** Use of heavily T2-weighted image without contrast to create the three-dimensional image of the biliary tree using MIP algorithm
6. **Ans. a.** Vesicoureteric reflex and posterior urethral valve
7. **Ans. a.** Low-dose non-enhanced CT to reduce penetration and hence ↑ resolution like in mammography
8. **Ans. a.** Dimercaptosuccinic acid (DMSA)
9. **Ans. e.** Valvulae conniventes
10. **Ans. b.** TC-99 m DMSA
11. **Ans. a.** Noncontrast CT
12. **Ans. d.** MIBG scan
13. **Ans. c.** PET-scan
14. **Ans. a.** Intravenous urography
15. **Ans. c.** Voiding cystogram
16. **Ans. c.** Bilateral nephrostogram
17. **Ans. b.** Cysteine
18. **Ans. d.** Catheter angiography
19. **Ans. a.** Wilms' tumor
20. **Ans. a.** Magnetic resonance imaging
21. **Ans. a.** Guided prostatic biopsies
22. **Ans. b.** Hyperdense nephrogram
23. **Ans. b.** Presence of collaterals
24. **Ans. a.** Dehydrating the patient
25. **Ans. c.** Barium examination showing tertiary contractions
26. **Ans. b.** Duodenal atresia
27. **Ans. d.** Carcinoma of stomach
28. **Ans. a.** Peptic ulcer
29. **Ans. a.** Single bubble appearance
30. **Ans. d.** All of the above
31. **Ans. c.** Sigmoid volvulus
32. **Ans. b.** Small bowel obstruction
33. **Ans. a.** Crohn's disease
34. **Ans. d.** Longitudinal ulcers are more common
35. **Ans. d.** Lesser curvature ulcer with a nodular rim
36. **Ans. b.** High gastric-residue
37. **Ans. c.** Ileal atresia
38. **Ans. d.** Cupola sign
39. **Ans. a.** String sign of Kantor
40. **Ans. b.** Ulcerative colitis
41. **Ans. a.** Apple-core appearance
42. **Ans. d.** Dilution of barium
43. **Ans. d.** Lt lateral decubitus with horizontal beam
44. **Ans. c.** Lateral decubitus
45. **Ans. c.** Thumb printing
46. **Ans. a.** Valvulae conniventes
47. **Ans. b.** Peripheral distribution
48. **Ans. b.** Valvulae conniventes
49. **Ans. d.** Meconium ileus
50. **Ans. a.** For showing presence of a small pneumoperitoneum
51. **Ans. c.** Left lateral recumbent view
52. **Ans. a.** Radiological finding in supine posture for pneumoperitoneum
53. **Ans. a.** Colonic diverticulosis
54. **Ans. b.** Chronic pancreatitis
55. **Ans. d.** Simple cyst
56. **Ans. b.** Polyp
57. **Ans. a.** Liver
58. **Ans. d.** Contrast-enhanced CT scan of the liver
59. **Ans. c.** Focal nodular hyperplasia
60. **Ans. a.** Dilation of pancreatic duct
61. **Ans. d.** Quadrate lobe
62. **Ans. b.** Cullen's sign
63. **Ans. a.** Fuzzy outline of pancreas
64. **Ans. a.** Acute pancreatitis
65. **Ans. b.** Carcinoma head of pancreas
66. **Ans. d.** Serous cystadenoma
67. **Ans. d.** CT scan

68. **Ans. d.** CT scan with contrast
69. **Ans. c.** Barium sulfate
70. **Ans. b.** CT scan (IOC for pancreatitis)
71. **Ans. b.** USG
72. **Ans. a.** USG
73. **Ans. b.** Motor mechanisms of gallbladder
74. **Ans. a.** ERCP
75. **Ans. a.** USG
76. **Ans. b.** USG
77. **Ans. c.** Adenomyomatosis
78. **Ans. b.** Stone < 2.5 cm size in the intestine
79. **Ans. b.** Sclerosing cholangitis
80. **Ans. d.** Gallstones
81. **Ans. b.** PET CT
82. **Ans. a.** Meckel's diverticulum
83. **Ans. a.** PET
84. **Ans. b.** Tc dextran
85. **Ans. c.** Severe hydronephrosis
86. **Ans. a.** Adenocarcinoma of the colon
87. **Ans. b.** Computed tomography
88. **Ans. b.** Gallstone
89. **Ans. c.** CT scan
90. **Ans. b.** Tc99m-DTPA
91. **Ans. a.** Tc99 DMSA scan
92. **Ans. d.** DTPA scan
93. **Ans. d.** Radiorenogram
94. **Ans. a.** Dehydrating the patient (c > a)
95. **Ans. d.** Hypoplasia
96. **Ans. a.** Intravenous urography
97. **Ans. c.** Ureterocele
98. **Ans. b.** Ureterocele
99. **Ans. a.** Multiple myeloma
100. **Ans. b.** Captopril-enhanced radionuclide scan
101. **Ans. b.** Intravenous urography
102. **Ans. a.** Polycystic kidney
103. **Ans. d.** All of the above
104. **Ans. b.** IVP
105. **Ans. a.** Adenocarcinoma
106. **Ans. d.** Crown rump length
107. **Ans. b.** Ultrasound study
108. **Ans. a.** 5–6 weeks of gestation
109. **Ans. b.** Transvaginal USG
110. **Ans. c.** Real time USG
111. **Ans. d.** Femur length
112. **Ans. b.** AC
113. **Ans. a.** Anencephaly
114. **Ans. a.** 10–12 weeks of gestation
115. **Ans. d.** Fetal maturity/growth
116. **Ans. c.** In normal gestation (placental resistance is high
117. **Ans. a.** Detect fetal abnormality
118. **Ans. d.** Echogenic mass with (H. mole) multicystic spaces within endometrial cavity
119. **Ans. a.** Absence of gestational sac in uterus
120. **Ans. d.** Down's syndrome
121. **Ans. c.** Turner's syndrome
122. **Ans. c.** Gastric content aspiration
123. **Ans. d.** Lesser curvature ulcer with a nodular rim
124. **Ans. d.** All of the above
125. **Ans. a.** Pancreatic head growth
126. **Ans. a.** Meniscus appearance
127. **Ans. c.** Lower GI contrast study
128. **Ans. b.** Hyperdense nephrogram
129. **Ans. c.** The flow velocities and the S/D ratio are useful to evaluate high-risk pregnancies
130. **Ans. c.** Transvaginal US
131. **Ans. d.** Crown rump length
132. **Ans. d.** All of the above
133. **Ans. a.** Teratoma
134. **Ans. a.** X-ray
135. **Ans. b.** First 10 days of menstrual cycle
136. **Ans. d.** All of the above
137. **Ans. d.** CT scan
138. **Ans. a.** Transfemoral route
139. **Ans. c.** CT scan
140. **Ans. a.** Radionuclide scanning
141. **Ans. a.** ERCP
142. **Ans. c.** Barium study
143. **Ans. a.** USG

144. Ans. a. Barium swallow
145. Ans. c. Enhances rapidly, contrast stays in it for a relatively longer time and washes out late
146. Ans. c. Neurogenic bladder
147. Ans. a. Micturition cystouretrogram
148. Ans. a. Duplication of ureters
149. Ans. d. Ill defined calyx
150. Ans. c. USG
151. Ans. d. After 6 hours
152. Ans. a. Acute pancreatitis
153. Ans. d. >3 mm
154. Ans. b. Diffuse esophageal spasm
155. Ans. b. Pancreatitis
156. Ans. b. Phenobarbital
157. Ans. b. Carcinoma colon
158. Ans. a. Chronic pancreatitis
159. Ans. c. Fibromuscular dysplasia
160. Ans. a. Ileocecal TB
161. Ans. c. 5-6 weeks
162. Ans. a. IUD
163. Ans. c. IUD
164. Ans. b. Membrane in twin pregnancy
165. Ans. b. EUS guided FNAC
166. Ans. a. 55 mm
167. Ans. a. CHPS
168. Ans. d. CT finding of parenchymal destruction or streaky or mottled gas in the parenchyma is diagnostic

Multiple Correct Answers

169. Ans. a. Calcium oxalate, c. Magnesium ammonium phosphate, d. Cysteine
170. Ans. a. Pelvic hematoma, b. Pelvic lipomatosis
171. Ans. b. Radionuclide enteroclysis, e. USG enteroclysis
172. Ans. a. Thick fibrosed gallbladder wall, b. Stone impacted at neck of gallbladder, c. Pericholecystic edema
173. Ans. a. Acute cholecystitis, b. Mucosal thickening, c. Cholesterosis, d. Ascites, e. AIDS cholangitis
174. Ans. a. MRI is used to obtain the image, c. It shows the biliary tree
175. Ans. b. Obliteration of splenic shadow, c. Rib fracture
176. Ans. a. Pancreas, b. Gallbladder, c. Inferior vena cava, e. Portal vein

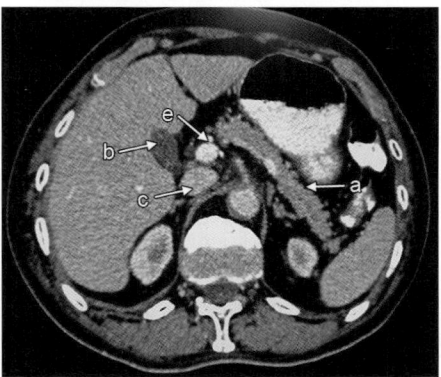

177. Ans. a. Gallstone, b. Renal stone, c. Calcification of vessels, d. Hepatic hemangioma, e. Calcified costal cartilage
178. Ans. b. MRI, c. PET-Scan
179. Ans. d. Spider leg deformity
180. Ans. a. Achlasia, b. Trypanosomiasis, d. Scleroderma
181. Ans. a. Microcolon on Ba enema, d. Obstruction in Ba meal
182. Ans. a. Schistosomiasis, b. Urethral cell carcinoma
183. Ans. a. CBD stones, d. Pancreatic divisum, e. Annular pancreas

Answers of Recently Asked Questions

184. Ans. a. DNA is extracted from fetal cells circulating in maternal circulation.
185. Ans. c. CECT abdomen with contrast
186. Ans. a. Acute pancreatitis

CHAPTER 5

Musculoskeletal Radiology

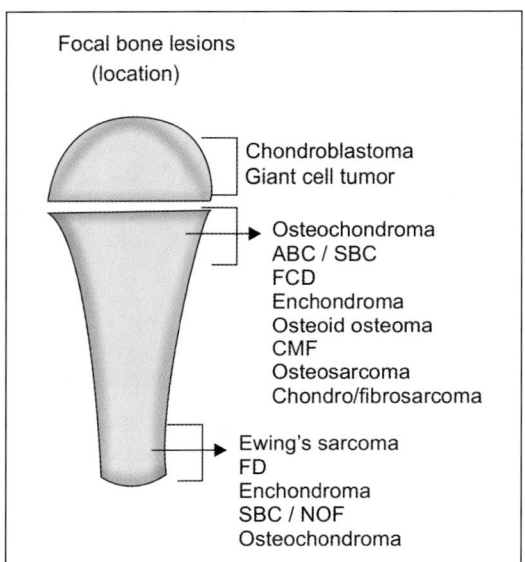

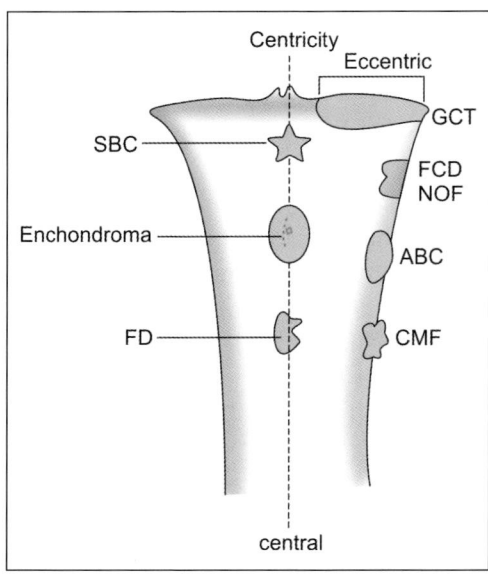

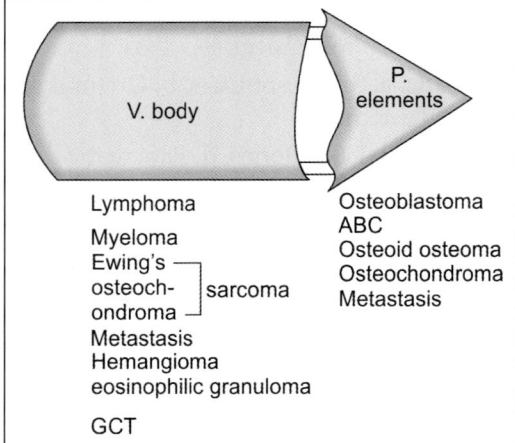

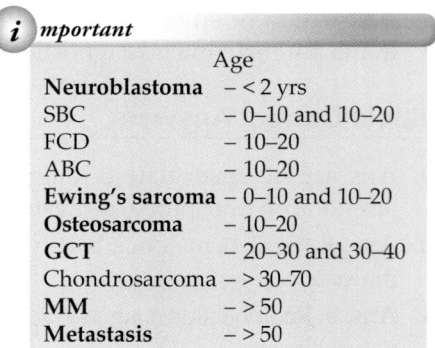

Patterns of Bone Destruction

I. Geographic
- With sclerotic margin—SBC, enchondroma, CMF, FD, Brodie's
- **No marginal sclerosis**—GCT (Figure), also-SBC
- Ill defined margins—osteosarcoma, chondrosarcoma, ABC, osteomyelitis

II. Moth-eaten Bone Destruction–Wide Zone of Transition—Malignant
- Reticulum cell sarcoma, osteosarcoma, chondrosarcoma, fibrosarcoma, round cell tumor (Ewing's), osteomyelitis

III. Permeative Bone Destruction
- Ewing's, reticulum cell sarcoma, high grade chondrosarcoma fibrosarcoma, angiosarcoma, leukemia and metastasis

Matrix Pattern

Osseous Matrix
- Bony trabeculae, radiodense struts (pathognomonic)
- Osteosarcoma, parosteal osteosarcoma, osteoblastoma, FD, fat necrosis

Cartilage Matrix
- Flecks, punctate, flocculated calcified foci.
- **Punctate**—When disruption is in zone of provisional calcification
- **Ring and arc**—Disrupted enchondral bone formation
- Enchondroma, osteochondroma

Periosteal Reaction

Continuous
- **Single lamella**
  - Healing fracture, Osteomyelitis
- **Solid periosteal**
  - Osteoid osteoma (smooth)
  Undulating
  - OM
  - Pulmonary osteoarthropathy

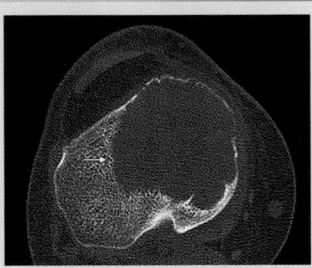

GCT [no marginal sclerosis]

> **important**
> NCCT—most valuable modality in detection of subtle matrix calcifications

> **important**
> (**-FD-shows thick sclerotic rim—Rind of orange)

> **important**
> **Benign tumor**—sharp inner and outer margin
> **Benign inflammatory condition**—sharp inner but fuzzy outer margin

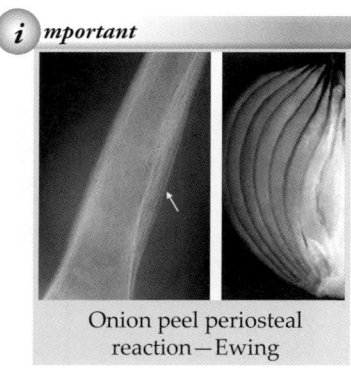

Onion peel periosteal reaction—Ewing

- **Multilamellated/onion peel** (Waxing waning course) (Figure)
    - OM
    - ABC
    - **Ewing's**
    - Osteosarcoma
- **Spiculated**
    - **Parallel spiculation**—hair on end
        - **Thalassemia**
        - Metastasis
        - Ewing's
        - Osteosarcoma
    - **Divergent/Sunburst** spicules
        - **Osteosarcoma**
        - Hemangioma
        - Osteoblastic metastasis
    - Various directions
        - Ewing's sarcoma

Interrupted/discontinuous (Aggressive)

- **Codman's Angle/Triangle**
    - Due to tumor, blood, edema, pus
    - Both malignant and benign
- **Buttress**
    - Slow growing tumor
- **Truncated lamella**
    - Neoplasm, virulent infection

Causes of Expansile Rib Lesions

Non-neoplastic

- FD
- Paget's
- Brown tumor
- OM
- Gaucher
- Thalassemia

Benign

- **FD (most common)**
- Exostosis, Enchondroma
- LCH
- GCT, ABC

- Neurofibroma
- Osteoblastoma
- Chondroblasto

Neoplastic

- Metastases (bronchus, kidney, prostate, breast)
- Lymphoma
- **Ewing's (most common malignant tumor of ribs)**
- **Neuroblastoma**
- Osteosarcoma MM/Plasmacytoma
- **Chondrosarcoma (calcified matrix) (most common)**
- PNET

Metastasis

- IOC for bone metastasis is bone scintigraphy (Tc-MDP is used) except in spine, where MRI is preferred. MRI is also IOC for extent of primary bony tumor
    - Most common-pattern-**hot lesions** scattered diffusely
- **Causes of False-negative** bone scintigraphy in a patient of bone metastasis
    - Avascular lesions
    - Rapidly growing pure osteoclastic lesions with no osteoblastic activity
    - Lesions with low bone turnover (MM and thyroid cancer)
- Causes of false positive results
    - Increase blood flow in osteoarthritis, trauma and inflammation

Findings on Bone Scan

- **Stress Fractures** → (Shows uptake also on blood phases with delayed phases)
- **Fatigue** → Repeated stress (normal bones)-**Fusiform increased radiotracer uptake**
- Insufficiency—Normal stress on abnormal bone
- **Sacral stress** fracture → **Honda sign-/'H' sign**
- **Shin splints** → Exercise induced pain/tenderness in posteromedial aspect of tibia → Linear **uptake on delayed phases-Oriented** longitudinally ((n) blood pool and blood flow unlike stress fractures)

> *important*
> MC-malignant bone tumor-Skeletal metastasis

> *important*
> Soft tissue lesion—Hyperintense-both on T1W & T2W images **Lipoma**

> *important*
> Osteomyelitis—shows increased activity on all three phases of bone scan

> *important*
> IOC for stress fracture of tibia → MRI
> IOC for B/C stress fracture → Bone scan

> *important*
> FDG-PETCT is IOC-for Assessing Treatment Response for Metastasis
> - Decrease in standard uptake value (SUV) suggests response to treatment

> **important**
> Bone scan remains positive for months even after treatment of acute osteomyelitis—cannot differentiate between healing from chronic active disease.

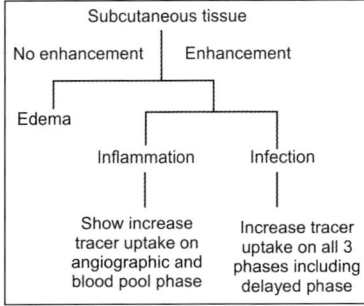

> **important**
> **Benign lesions showing uptake on SPECT**
> - Osteoid osteoma
> - Eosinophilic granuloma
> - ABC
> - Chondroblastoma
> - Enchondroma

> **important**
> KeiL – (Keinbock-lunate)
> KoNa – (Kohler-navicular)

> **important**
> Bone scan may be (normal) in 85% of cases in first 48 hours but then reduced activity (cold) for a variable period.

Paget's Disease
- 'V' shape advanced edge
- Clover, heart and micky mouse signs of uptake in vertebral bodies

Hyperparathyroidism
- **Super scan (most common)**
- Pseudofracture → focal

Renal Osteodystrophy
- Superscan with absent UB activity (due to renal failure)

AVN
- MRI-IOC
  - Bisphosphonate Therapy—Jaw
  - Keinbock's—lunate
  - Kohler's—Navicular

But bone scan (BS) detects AVN **earlier than MRI** (72 hours vs 6 days).

Reflex-Sympathetic Dystrophy
- Reduced blood flow and blood pool phase, **increased on delayed**.
- Periarticular uptake of radiotracer.

TUBERCULOSIS OF BONES

- **Sequestration and periostitis are not common and usually no sclerosis**
- Very small sequestrum
- Marginal erosions in weight bearing joints.
- Kissing sequestra
- **Rice bodies**
  - Synovial joints
  - Tendon sheaths
  - Bursae

Four Stages
- Inflammatory edema and exudates
- Necrosis and cavitation
- Destruction and deformation
- Healing and repair.

- **Hip tubercular arthritis** can arise in acetabulum, synovium, femoral epiphysis and metaphysis **(Babcock's triangle)**
  - Wandering acetabulum
  - Bird's beak appearance of femur
  - Mortar and pestle appearance (figure)
  - Breaking of Shenton's line
- **Knee TB**
  - **Triple deformity** in advanced cases, i.e. lateral, posterior and superior displacement of tibia on femur
  - Shoulder TB synovial lesions are rare in **shoulder** joint TB atrophic type without pus- **carries sica**
- **Frontal bone TB**
  - Button sequestrum
- **Pelvis TB**
  - **Weaver's bottom**
- **TB dactylitis**
  - Cystic expansion of short bones
  - **Spina ventosa** (spina-short, ventosa-expanded with air)
  - Plain radiography is the modality of choice for evaluation and follow-up
  - Differential diagnosis—**syphilitic dactylitis** →
    - Bilateral involvement
    - Symmetric involvement
    - **More periosteitis**   Seen in
    - Less soft tissue swelling   Syphilitic
    - Less sequestrations   dactylitis
- **TB of Tendon Sheath/Bursae**
  - Dumbbell-shaped swelling
  - Melon seed bodies
  - Rice bodies (serofibrinous stage)

> *important*
> Dense circumscribed blush in early arterial phase of angiography → **osteoid-osteoma**.

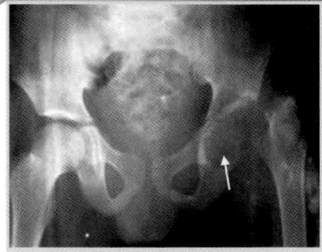

Wandering acetabulum—TB.

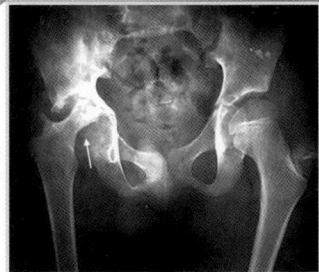

Tuberculosis of hip joint—mortar and pestle.

BONE AND JOINT INFECTION

Acute Osteomyelitis

- Osteomyelitis is most frequent at end plates d/t greater no. of arteries at this location.
- **Ist ordered investigation**—X-ray
  - Cortical irregularity
  - Periosteal reaction
  - Deep soft tissue swelling

> *important*
> Acute pyogenic arthritis is a complication of OM in infants (< 1 year) and in adults. In rest the physis block spread of infection to joint.

> **important**
> However in all cases of shoulder/hip joints due to periosteal spread into synovium due to metaphysical attachment of synovium or joint capsule.

> **important**
> Soft tissue swelling is the Ist radiographic sign of pyogenic arthritis/OM
> Earliest bone change 7-10 day after infection.

> **important**
> Cellulitis and OM show similar soft tissue changes, however in cellulitis, the bone is (n).

> **important**
> - Sickle cell disease:
>   - Prone to salmonella infection (cortical fissuring and tunneling).

> **important**
>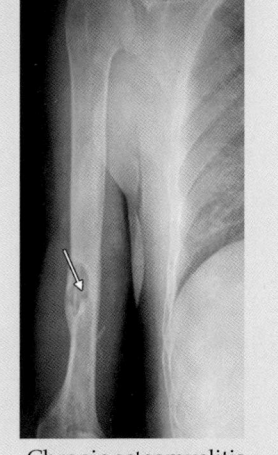
> Chronic osteomyelitis (dead dense bone)

- Demineralization
- X-ray-Earliest bone changes (7–10 days)
- USG
  - Deep soft tissue swelling is the earliest sign (2–3 days)
  - Periosteal elevation (hyperechoic line)
  - Subperiosteal fluid collection
  - Cortical breach.
- MRI
  - Investigation of choice for bone infection
  - Most sensitive investigation as it can pickup marrow edema within six hours
- Bone scintigraphy
  - Can be positive (1–3 day) earliest
  - Uptake on all three phases:
    - Blood flow (angiography),
    - Blood pool (capillary),
    - Delayed (2–4 hours) uptake in bone
- Gallium scan
  - 67Ga (gallium) bind to leukocyte and go to sites of inflammation
  - If gallium scan is congruent or hotter than Tc99 MDP, infection is implied.
  - If gallium scan is noncongruent or colder-no infection
  - Labeled leukocytes not useful for spinal infection as 50% or more of spinal osteomyelitis present as nonspecific areas of decreased or absent activity.

Chronic Osteomyelitis

- Cloacae
- Involucrum-3-week
- Sequestrum-4-week (dead dense bone) (Figure)
- Bony thickening and deformity
  No sclerosis however seen in skull OM.

Chronic OM of Garre

- Children (endosteal expansion of bone).

Brodie's Abscess—Lytic Bone Lesion with Sclerosed Margin

- Serpiginous tract/channel having sclerosed margin which marks the tract of infection

- Finger like extension in adjacent normal bone pathognomonic

Syphilis

Earliest change is in metaphysis with widening of zone of provisional calcification.
- Congenital Syphilis
  - Bilateral symmetrical destruction of medial end of proximal tibial metaphysis **(Wimberger's ring) Pathognomonic**
- Late Congenital Syphilis
  - Hutchinson teeth, mulberry molar
  - **Hot cross bun skull**
  - Thickening of upper half of tibia anteriorly → sabre tibia d/t **periosteitis (MC feature)**

Rubella OM

- **Celery stalk appearance**

Maduromycosis OM

- No pain
- No sequestrum
- No osteopenia
- Shaggy periostitis, reactive sclerosis/**melting snow appearance**
- **Dot and Dash appearance on MRI (Actinomycosis)**

Leprosy

- **Licked candy appearance**

TB SPINE (POTT'S SPINE)

- Begins in cancellous area
- **Paradiscal region**–MC site (less commonly in centrum or at anterior surface)
- Anterior wedging common in dorsal spine
- **Disc avascular**–hence involvement of disc is via direct spread from subchondral bone or beneath anterior or post longitudinal ligaments.
- Skip lesions

*Pyogenic infection on contrary causes more disk destruction.

> *important*
> **False Positive on Scintigraphy**
> - Degenerative disease
> - Healing fracture
> - Loose prosthesis
> But do not show uptake on early phases (I and IInd).

> *important*
> - Celery stalk appearance also seen in mucoid degeneration of anterior cruciate ligament on T2W/STIR images.

> *important*
> Wimberger's ring is seen in scurvy

> *important*
> Flowing wax appearance – melorrheostosis.

> *important*
> - Dot and Dash appearance also seen in cases of Multiple sclerosis on FLAIR images of MRI.

> **important**
> - **Spinal vertebral hydatid-** Usually unilocular with diverticulated cysts
> - Subarachnoid neurocysticerosis is MC type of spinal cysticerci.

MRI

- **IOC**—Better detection of skip lesions
- **Earliest detection** of Pott's spine is **on STIR/Post Contrast T_1W images**

FDG-PET

- Standard uptake values (SUV) > 2.5 for malignant but **up to '21' can be seen in tubercular infections**
- However uptake peaks at 60 minutes than decrease in infective/inflammatory lesions while does not decrease in malignant diseases.
- **FDG-PET + C-11 acetate** → latter accumulates only in malignant lesions.

CT

- Better to detect calcification
- **Epidural extent can be missed on plain CT due to beam hardening artifact**

> **important**
> On X-ray > 30–50% mineral must be lost before a radiolucent lesion becomes conspicuous.

Most Common Variety

- **Paradiscal/marginal/intervertebral/subarticular/metaphyseal lesions.**
- Disease process usually begins in anterior part of vertebral body.
- In dorsal spine the paraspinal abscess has fusiform appearance (**Bird's Nest appearance**).
- Abscess at the **dorsolumbar junction has an indistinct converging lower border (Petering abscess")**.
- Calcification: **Pathognomonic** of tubercular abscess (**tear drop shaped calcification**).
- Four Patterns of Destruction on CT
  - **Fragmentry (47%)-exploded vertebral bodies-MC**
  - Osteolytic (33%)
  - Subperiosteal (10%)
  - Well defined lytic with sclerotic margins (10%)
- Thick nodular rim of increased attenuation due to increase vascularity and hypercellular wall of the inflammatory cavity–**Rind sign**.
- Preserved disk space despite extensive bone destruction–**Floating disk sign**.

> **important**
> In posterior elements TB has predilection for → Pedicle and lamina
> Pyogenic disease-predilection for–facet joints.

> **important**
> Pyogenic spondylitis shows multiple small erosions like a 'Pepper Pot' with no calcification.

Healing TB

- Ivory vertebra
- Fusion of contiguous vertebrae considered surest sign of healing.

NONINFECTIVE INFLAMMATORY ARTHRITIS

RHEUMATOID ARTHRITIS

MC Inflammatory Arthritis

- Early changes → (Nonosseous) → USG and MRI
- Late changes → (osseous)
- Earliest
  - Joint space widening and soft tissue swelling (due to edema and swelling of synovium) and effusion
  - Best detected at 5th MCP joint
- Fusiform soft tissue swelling at-PIP and IInd to 5th MCP
- Swelling over ulnar styloid—due to involvement of extensor carpi ulnaris sheath
- Blurring and obliteration of pre-Achilles fat pad
- Blurring and thickening of the Achilles tendon.
- Osteopenia
  - Juxta articular—due to synovial inflammation
  - Generalized → Limitation of movement due pain.

Early X-Ray Change

- Juxta articular osteopenia
- Uniform narrowing of:
  - Distal radioulnar
  - Radiocarpal
  - Intercarpal joints
- Subluxations at Ist MCP and IP (**Hitchhiker's deformity**)
- Terminal phalangeal sclerosis
- **Lack of periosteal reaction—Hallmark of disease.**

Erosions

- **Most important diagnostic feature (indicates irreversible joint damage) which** contain inflamed synovium-enhance on postcontrast imaging

> *important*
> - T2W hyperintensity without T1W hypointensity in the cord → **cord edema**
> - with T1W hypointensity → **myelomalacia.**

> *important*
> **Gas within disk**
> - Brucellosis discitis (Hallmark)
> - Clostridial
> - Streptococcal
> Gas in degenerative disk vacuum phenomenon

> *important*
> MRI is IOC for early RA, as treatment is more effective, if administered early.

- Ball-catcher's view to see erosions
- USG more sensitive than radiographs for erosions
- Earliest sites
    - Bare areas between edge of articular cartilage and site of attachment of joint capsule.
    - Wrist, MCP and PIP MC at radialvolar aspect of head of 2nd and 3rd metacarpals are commonly involved.
    - **Fusion of carpal bones (latter)**
    - Posterosuperior aspect of calcaneum above the insertion of Achilles tendon.
    - Tarsal erosions less common in RA than seronegative spondyloarthropathies.
    - En face-Erosions appear cystic

> *important*
> DIP joints are spared in RA

> *important*
> No uniform joint space narrowing–Osteoarthritis.

> *important*
> Superior compartment involvement in c/o—OA

Hip

- Reduced medical joint space with medial migration of head of femur and **protrusion acetabuli**.

Late Changes of RA

- Subluxation with ulnar deviation at MCP joints
- **Boutonniere deformity** → flexion at PIP/extension at IP joints
- **Swan-Neck deformity** → extension at PIP/Flexion at DIP
- **Hitchhiker's thumb** → Flexion at MCP/extension at IP joint
- **Bayonet deformity** → Dislocation of the carpus
- **Hallux valgus** → Lateral deviation of toe
- Hallux sesamoids subluxation
- Flattening of transverse arch
- **Telescoping of bones/fingers**
- **Arthritis mutilans**
- **Bird's beak appearance**
    - Grass loss of bone at femoral head (also seen in TB hip).
- Resorption of distal clavicle
- Stress fracture
- Giant synovial cyst
- Ankylosis of carpal bones
- *Sec. O.A. in weight bearing* joints however with very less new bone formation.

Axial Skeleton

- Cervical spine—Most Commonly Involved
  - Osteoporosis/disc narrowing/end plate irregularity (More common in upper cervical vertebrae)
  - **Step ladder appearance due to facet joint erosions**
  - Atlanto-axial subluxation (> 2.5 mm adult; > 4 mm-child)
  - **Erosion of odontoid peg.**

Best Imaging for **RA** → **MRI** → Gold std for synovial imaging

- Increase of enhancement correlates with degree of inflammation
- Fibrotic pannus and pannus with hemosiderin deposit→low signal
- **Rice bodies**

> *important*
> **Arthritis mutilans**
> RA
> Erosive OA
> Multicentric reticulo-histiocytosis
> Psoriatic arthritis

JRA

- Fused cervical vertebrae
- Fusion of carpi (squashed carpi)
- Ballooned epiphysis (widened)
- Decrease soft tissue bulk.

> *important*
> Lung changes
> - **Effusion (MC)**
> - Pulmonary nodules
> - **ILD lower lobes**

ANKYLOSING SPONDYLITIS

Synovitis with predisposition to develop ankylosis via cartilage metaplasia, enchondral ossification, fibrosis/woven bone formation.

- Bilateral symmetrical sacroiliitis
  - (Earliest change-Loss or blurring of subchondral cortex)
- Rat bite erosions (iliac aspect)
- Spine
  - Romanus lesions (Erosions at corners-at attachment site of outer fibers of annulus fibrosis) (MRI)
  - **Shiny corner sign (On X-ray)**
  - Erosive spondylitis
  - Squaring of vertebrae (due to ALL/PLL thickening)
  - **Barrel-shaped vertebrae** (convex anterior border due to exuberant new bone formation)

- **Syndesmophytes** (Marginal/Symmetrical/fine/delicate)
- Bamboo spine
- **Calcification of i/v discs**
- **Dagger sign** (ossification of interspinous ligament)
- **Tram track sign** (ossification of facet joints)
- Enthesitis
- Spinal fractures (just beneath the end plates)
    - Traumatic (after spinal fusion) (unstable) (all three columns)
    - Stress (Cervico-thoracic/thoracolumbar junction) Sclerotic pseudoarthrosis with destruction of disk and vertebral end plates (**Andersson lesions**) (**Resemble infective discitis**)
- **Large posterior dural diverticulae-meningoceles**
- Arachnoiditis
- Atlantoaxial subluxation

- **Hip**
    - Concentric joint space reduction
    - Axial migration
    - Cuff like osteophytes
    - **Protrusio acetabuli**
    - Shaggy periostitis
- **Shoulder**
    - **Hatchet deformity** on humeral head d/t enthesitis of rotator cuff tendon.
    - Enthesitis → Ischial tuberosity (**Ischial whiskering**)

> *important*
> Rice bodies
> - RA
> - TB

> *important*
> Protrusio Acetabuli
> - RA
> - AS
> - Osteomalacia

Psoriatic Arthropathy (PA)

- Mono/oligoarticular with enteritis
- Peripheral/polyarticular like RA
- Axial like AS

Imaging Fracture

- Bone proliferation-**Bone density preserved**
- Fusiform soft tissue swelling (sausage digit)
- Marginal erosions which proceed toward joint along articular surface (**Surface erosion**)
- Proceed along the capsule away from joint along the metaphysis (**enthesitis erosion**)
- Proceed along the articular surface (surface erosion)

> *important*
> DIP joint are involved in psoriatic arthritis

- Pencil in cup deformity
- Mouse-ears sign (d/t bone proliferation)
- Resorption of terminal tufts
- Arthritis mutilans
- Opera glass hand
- Nonmarginal syndesmophytes
- B/L asymmetric sacroiliitis
- Paravertebral ossifications.

REITER'S SYNDROME

- U/L Asymmetric sacroiliitis
- Asymmetric syndesmophytes
- Calcaneal spurs (d/t lamellar or fluffy periostitis)

> **important**
> PA have asymmetric sacroiliitis with nonmarginal syndesmophytes unlike AS.

CRYSTAL DEPOSITION ARTHROPATHY

Gout

- Monosodium Urate Crystals
- Strong **'negative' birefringence**
- Sharply marginated, round to oval erosions oriented along long axis of bone, **sclerotic rim, overhanging edges**
- Initially periarticular extend to joint
- Tophi
    - Lumpy-Bumpy Soft Tissue
    - Saucerise Underlying Bone
- Chondrocalcinosis

CPPD Deposition

- In hyaline and fibrocartilage
- Weakly birefringent
- **Pseudogout** (intermittent acute attacks)
- Chondrocalcinosis
    - Triangular cartilage
    - Lunotriquetral ligament
    - Symphysis pubis
    - Rotator cuff

> **important**
> Chondrocalcinosis
> - Gout
> - CPPD
> - Chronic renal disease (hyperparathyroidism Primary)

Neuropathic Joint 5-Ds

- Disorganization, increased density, debris, destruction and deformity.

> **Important**
> **Triad of pseudogout**
> - Pain
> - Cartilage calcification
> - Joint destruction

DEGENERATIVE

- Cryomicrotomy/discography for radial tears.
- Vacuum phenomenon → air in degenerated disk
- Facetal arthropathy
  - More linked with pain than disk and
  - **CT better than MRI for early detection of facetal arthropathy**
- Air within vertebral body—**avascular necrosis of spine**
- Osteoporosis and osteoarthritis are inversely proportional.

Osteoarthritis (OA)

- **False profile view** for hip joint cartilage space.
- Subchondral cysts in acetabulum **(Egger's cysts)**
  - **Sunrise view and merchant view**→ femoropatellar joint
  - **Tooth Sign**→ hyperostotic changes at anterosuperior aspect of patella.
- Palpable Osteophytes
  - Bony nodules at PIP—**Bouchard's**
  - Bony nodule at DIP—**Heberden's nodes**
  - Wavey contours of base of distal phalanx—**Sea gull sign/gull wing sign**
  - OA of 1st metatarsophalangeal joint—**Hallux rigidus**
  - **Patella MC bone to be affected in OA**

METABOLIC DISEASE

1. Defects of osteoid formation—scurvy
2. Defects of mineralization—Rickets/osteomalacia
3. Altered bone resorption—Hyperparathyroidism
4. Decreased bone mass with no defect in mineralization/osteoid-osteoporosis

1. Defects of Osteoid Formation—Scurvy

- Osteoporosis
- White line of frankel (metaphyseal)
- Trummerfeld zone or scorbutic zone
- Wimberger's ring—small sharply defined epiphysis
- Pelkan's spur
- Subperiosteal hemorrhage

> **Important**
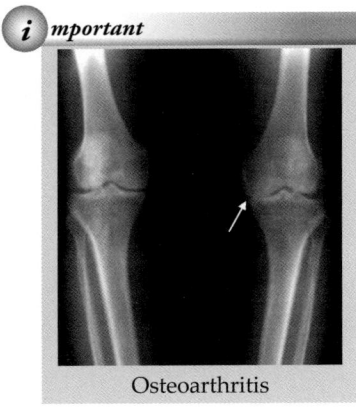
Osteoarthritis

2. Defect in Mineralization of Osteoid

- Rickets (child)/Osteomalacia (Adults)
- Incomplete mineralization of normal osteoid tissue
- Soft tissue swelling around growth plates due to hypertrophied cartilage.
- Disorganized zone of provisional calcification.

Rickets

- Increased non-calcified osteoid—Increased radiolucency
- **Osteopenia (MC X-ray finding although non-specific)**
- Changes earlier at distal radius & Ulna (Ulna > radius)
- Growth Activity
  - Costochondral junction > distal femur > proximal humerus > both ends of tibia > distal ulna > distal radius
- Widening, fraying and cupping—classical findings (Figure)
- Widening of growth plates (d/t bulky cartilaginous cells) (Earliest specific radiologic change)
- Irregular metaphyseal margins (paint brush metaphysis) d/t fraying & disorganization of the spongy bone.
- Widening and cupping of metaphysis (d/t **protrusion of bulky cartilaginous cells into poorly mineralized metaphysis**)
- **Osteopenic epiphysis** → irregular, indistinct borders and delayed appearance of ossification center.
- Rarefaction of shafts with coarse texture of cortex.
- Skeletal Deformities
  - **Skull** → posterior flattening, craniotabes (squaring of skull)
  - **Long bones** → bowing
  - **Ribs** → Rachitic rosary—d/t bulbous enlargement (indent the pleural surface/thymus)
  - **Spine** → scoliosis
  - **Pelvis** → Triradiate configuration—d/t protrusion of hip and spine
  - Fractures

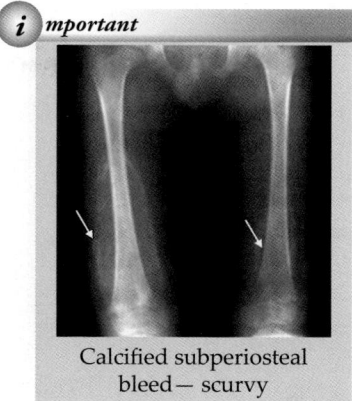

important

Calcified subperiosteal bleed— scurvy

important

Normal cupping in infants distal Ulna, both ends of fibula and distal tibia
Normal cupping never seen in bones of elbow

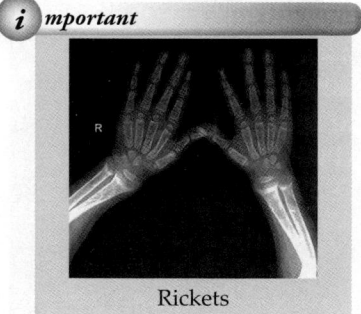

important

Rickets

> *important*

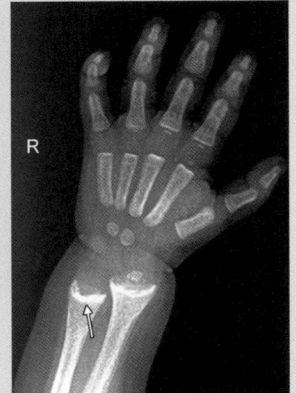

Healing rickets—dense zone of provisional calcification

> *important*
> Renal osteodystrophy- Rugger jersey spine/striped jersey-otosclerosis stage

> *important*

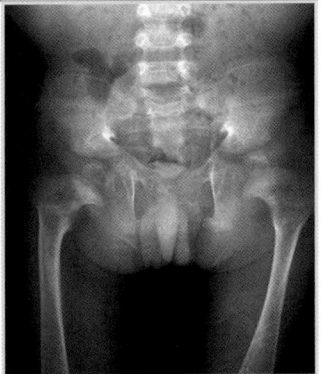

Triradiate pelvis—osteomalacia

> *important*
> - Trabeculae are coarse and indistinct osteomalacia
> - Trabeculae are thin & sharp osteoporosis
> - Uniform spinal deformity osteomalacia
> - Nonuniform spinal deformity osteoporosis

Signs of Healing Rickets

- Reappearance of dense zone of provisional calcification.
- Increase in cupping of healing metaphysis
- Recalcification of the subperiosteal osteoid
- Epiphyseal center becomes sharply defined.

Osteomalacia

- Defective mineralization of cortical & spongy bone.
- **Osteopenia (MC radiological sign)**
- Coarse indistinct trabecular pattern
- Thin cortices
- **Pseudofracture/looser's zone**/Milkman's fracture/ increment fractures/Umbauzonen **(at right angle to cortex)** (Mild sclerosis with absence of callus)
  - Axillary margins of scapula
  - Superior and inferior Pubic rami
  - Inner margins of the prox. femur
  - Posterior margins of the prox. ulna and fibula
  - Ribs
- Bone Scintigraphy for osteomalacia
  - Widening of mandible
  - Rachitic rosary sing
  - Tie sign of sternum
  - Pseudofracture sign
  - Prominent epiphysis of knee
- Bony Deformities
  - **Protrusio acetabuli**
  - Triradiate pelvis
  - Biconcave shape vertebral bodies (Cod fish vertebra)
  - Basilar invagination

3. Altered Bone Resorption

Hyperparathyroidism (HPT)

Primary HPT	Secondary HPT
• Consist of skeletal features of HPT only	• Skeletal features of HPT with features of renal osteodystrophy (Rickets/osteosclerosis)

Contd...

Contd...

Primary HPT	Secondary HPT
• Skeletal changes less florid	• More florid
• Sclerosis rarely seen	• Commonly seen sclerosis
• Brown tumors	• Less common
• Chondrocalcinosis	• Less common
• Soft tissue and vascular calcification are less common	• More common

- Bone resorption and substitutive fibrosis hallmark of disease
  - Subperiosteal
  - Intracortical (increased cortical **striations-Tunneling**) blurring of trabecular bone.
  - Endosteal
  - Subchondral
  - Trabecular surfaces
  - **Subperiosteal Resorption**
    - Earliest and best along radial aspect of middle phalanges of middle and index finger.
  - Trabecular bone resorption
    - Salt and pepper skull
  - Brown tumors/osteitis fibrosa cystica/von Recklinghausen disease
  - Condrocalcinosis
    - **Pri:** HPT
    - CPPD disease
    - Chronic renal disease
- **Renal osteodystrophy (Sec-HPT)**-In children metaphyseal changes with cortical erosions-rotting fence postappearance
- *The radiopharmaceutical of choice—99mTc sestamibi for parathyroid*

Hypoparathyroidism

- **Bony sclerosis (MC) finding**
- Calvarial thickening
- Band like areas of increased radiodensity in metaphysis
- **DISH-Diffuse idiopathic skeletal hyperostosis**
- Subcutaneous calcification
- **Basal ganglia calcification**

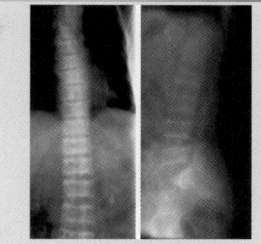

Renal osteodystrophy—rugger jersey spine, diffuse sclerosis

important
Secondary HPT
- **Sk**eletal changes
- **Sc**lerosis
- **So**ft tissue calcification

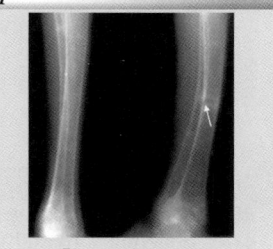

Looser's zone

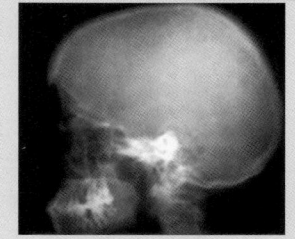

Salt and pepper skull

important
Other causes of basal ganglia calcification
- Fahr's (ferrocalcinosis)
- CO poisoning
- Toxoplasma
- CMV
- Radiation
- Pseudohypoparathyroidism

> **important**

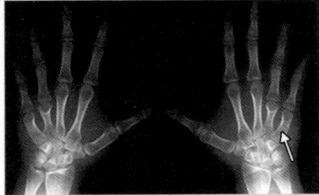

Short 4th and 5th metacarpals-pseudohypoparathyroidism

> **important**
> **Positive metacarpal sign**
> – Basal cell nevus syndrome
> – Multiple epiphyseal dysplasia
> – Beckwith-Wiedemann syndrome
> – Juvenile chronic arthritis
> – Sickle cell anemia
> – Turner's syndrome

> **important**
> **Bullet shaped vertebrae**
> – Congenital hypothyroidism
> – Achondroplasia
> – Metachromatic leukodystrophy

Pseudohypoparathyroidism

- **Shortening of 4th metacarpal (Metacarpal sign + if tangential line from heads of 4th & 5th MT intersect IIIrd**
- Exostosis (at 90 degrees to bones rather than away from joint)

Hypercortisolism

- Osteoporosis
- Accentuation of pri. trabeculae
- Increased density of superior and inferior endplates of collapsed vertebra d/t exuberant callus known as—**Marginal condensation**
- Osteonecrosis

Congenital Hypothyroidism

- Deformed and irregular epiphysis (epiphyseal dysgenesis)
- Wormian bones in skull
- Bullet shaped vertebrae
- Slipped capital femoral epiphysis

Thyroid Acropachy

After treatment by antithyroid drugs dense, solid, periosteal new bone with feathery margins along radial margins of metacarpals and phalanges in the diaphyseal region.

Turner's Syndrome

- Depression or slanting of medial tibial plateau with overgrowth of medial femoral condyle.
- Short 4th and 5th metacarpals.

Acromegaly

- Heel pad thickening
- Enlarged sella
- Hyperpneumatized maxillary sinuses
- Widening of mandibular angle
- Prominent joint space in hands
- **Arrow head appearance of distal phalanx**
- Large sesamoid index > 40
- Increased interstyloid distance
- Increased height of intervertebral discs

- Widened and elongated vertebral bodies
- Beaking of symphysis pubis

Fluorosis
- Osteosclerosis
- Thickening of the cortex
- Rose thorn appearance irregularity/fringed inferior margin of ribs
- Ligamentous calcification and ossification
- Ossification of interosseous membrane (Figure)
- Osteophytosis
- Paraspinal/intraspinal ligament ossification.

4. Decreased Bone Mass with no Defect in Mineralization/Osteoid-Osteoporosis

- Z score → age and gender matched
- T score → compared with standard young population

WHO define BMD on the basis of 'T' scores
- Normal-T ≥ – 1 SD of normal
- Osteopenia – 2.5 < T < – 1.0 T between – 1 to – 2.5 SD
- Osteoporosis T ≤ – 2.5 SD
- Severe osteoporosis T ≤ –2.5 SD with fragility fractures

Vanishing Bone Disease
- Gorham's disease
- Angiomatosis of bone
- Thick coarse trabeculae with lytic areas in between

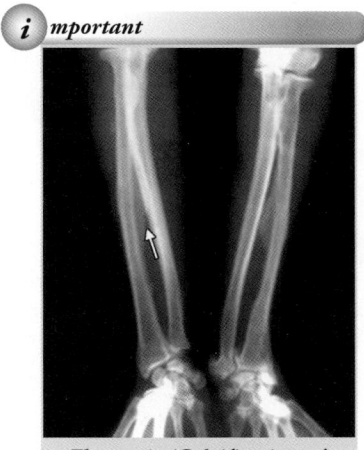

Fluorosis (Calcification of interosseous membrane)

BONE TUMORS

Enostosis/Bony Islands
- Dense intramedullary lamellar bone
- **Aligned along long axis of trabeculae**

Osteoid Osteoma
- Nidus <1 cm–cortical (MC)
- Medullary and subperiosteal (less sclerotic bone)
- IOC: CT > MRI
- Equilibrium phases of bone scintigraphy → double density sign.

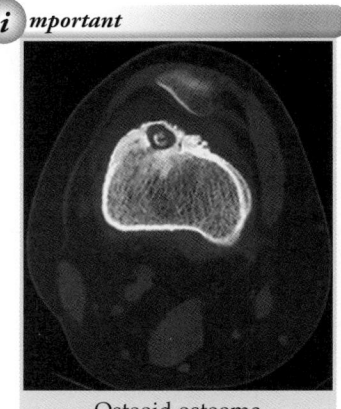

Osteoid osteoma

> **important**
> MRI → IOC for all bone tumors except osteoid osteoma where CT is better than MRI

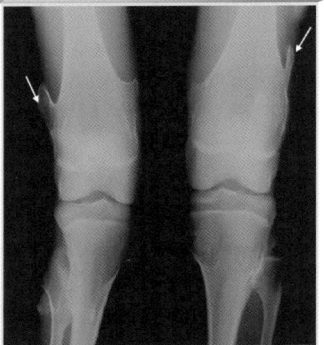

Osteochondroma diaphyseal aclasis.

> **important**
> Joint extension of tumor if hyaline cartilage is penetrated or tumor extends through capsule.

Osteoblastoma
- Nidus > 2 cm
- Less surrounding sclerotic halo

FCD
- Fibrous cortical defect-blister like expansion of cortex with thin shell

Osteochondroma
- Malignant
  - If grows after epiphyseal closure
  - Cartilage cap > 2.0 cm
- Diaphyseal aclasis (Figure)

Enchondroma
- **Ollier's disease** → multiple enchondromas
- Enchondromatosis with multiple hemangioma Maffucci's syndrome
- 'O'/ring sign → popcorn or annular calcification.

Fibrous Dysplasia
- + Precocious puberty-McCune-Albright syndrome
- Shepherd's Crook deformity of femur
- Leonine facies
- Expansion of medullary cavity with sclerotic **margin**
- Ground glass opacity on X-ray
- Increased uptake on radionuclide studies

Calvarial Hemangioma
- Sunburst appearance

Vertebral Hemangioma
- Corduroy on X-ray
- Polka dot on CT
- Hyperintense on both T1W and T2W-MRI.

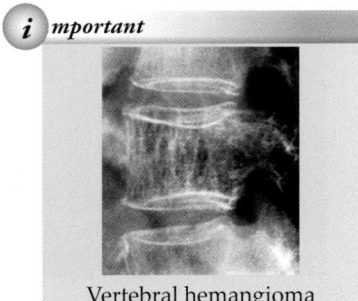

Vertebral hemangioma

Giant Cell Tumor (Osteoclastoma)
- Soap bubble appearance
- **Eccentric lytic without sclerotic rim after closure of epiphysis.**

Simple Bone Cyst (Unicameral Bone Cyst)

Majority (Prox. humerus)
- Fallen fragment sign (d/t cystic/fluid nature)
- Trap door sign (Figure)
- Rising bubble sign

Aneurysmal Bone Cyst

- Multiloculated expansile
- Cystic/ballooned out
- **Blood fluid level**

Eosinophilic Granuloma

- Punched out lytic lesion with bevelled margin (d/t unequal involvement of inner and outer table)
- Sclerotic focus (button sequestrum)
- Floating teeth sign in mandible
- Solitary collapsed vertebra in children

Osteosarcoma

- Commonest primary malignant bone tumor in the young
- Sunburst/Sunray pattern/spiculated periosteal reaction (Figure)
- Onion skin periosteal reaction
- Cumulus cloud appearance (d/t osteoid mineralization)
- **MRI-IOC**
- **Intracortical osteosarcomas are rarest**
  - Small lytic lesion surrounded by thickened cortex
  - D/d-Osteoid osteoma and osteoblastoma
- **Pneumothorax**
  - Metastasis of osteosarcoma in lung causes Pneumothorax
- **Juxtacortical/parosteal osteosarcoma**
  - Attached to the surface of the affected bone and has a tendency to encircle it
  - **MC site** → lower end of post. aspect of femur,
  - X-Ray: A well defined radiolucent line separates the tumor from the normal cortex

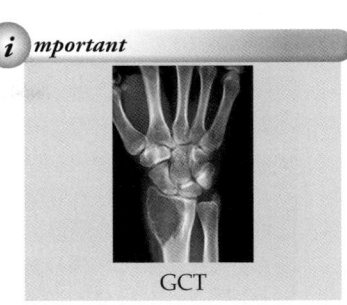

GCT

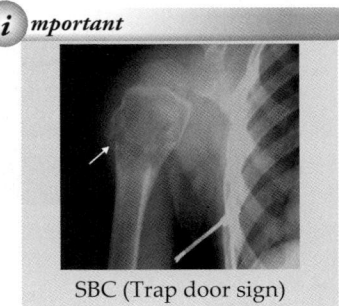

SBC (Trap door sign)

important
Blood fluid level can also be seen in
- Osteosarcoma (telangiectatic)
- GCT
- Osteoblastoma
- Chondroblastoma

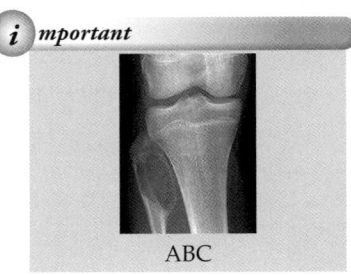

ABC

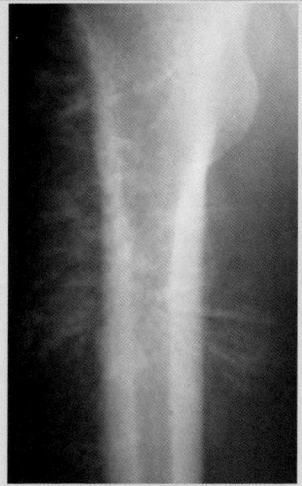

Osteosarcoma—sunray periosteal reaction

> **important**
> **Metastasis going beyond elbow and knee joints—BBC**
> - Bronchus
> - Bladder (urinary)
> - Colon

> **important**
> - Post-radiation sarcoma
>   - MC in pelvic/shoulder girdle
>   - MC → osteosarcoma
>   - IInd MC → malignant fibrous histiocytoma

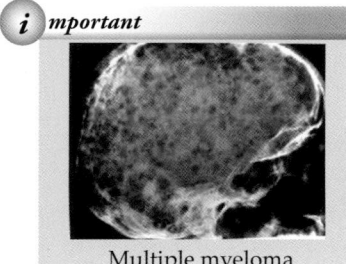

Multiple myeloma

- D/d- myositis ossificans (peripheral calcification)
- Parosteal o.sarcoma (central calcification)

Secondary Osteosarcoma (Mnemonic-FOPP)
- Fibrous dysplasia
- Ollier's disease
- Paget's disease
- Post-radiation osteosarcoma

Ewing's Sarcoma
- Central diaphyseal permeative lesion with wide zone of transition
- Saucerization
- Multilaminar (onion peel) periosteal result however incomplete laminar periosteal reaction is more common with marginal codman's triangle.
- Hair on end periosteal reaction can also be seen.
- MC pri. malignant tumor to metastasize to bone.

Chordoma
- Lytic destruction with calcification → Sacrum/basiocciput.

Multiple Myeloma
- MC primary malignant neoplasm of bone.
- Normal ALP and Phosphate
- Increased ALP, if healing
- Punched out lytic lesions (Rain drop lesion) (Figure)
- D/d—metastasis

Plasmacytoma
- **Medulla of bone**
- Geographic, radiolucent bone which is expansile with apparent trabeculation
- Differential Diagnosis
  - Metastasis
  - Chordoma
  - Brown tumor
  - Hemophilic pseudotumor
  - Hydatid cyst
  - FD
  - GCT

Multiple Myeloma	Metastasis
• Less common	• Post. elements more common
• I/V disc may involve	• Less likely
• Soft tissue mass associated with bony lesion	• Soft tissue ext. less common
• Mandible common site	• Rarely
• False 'negative' on radionuclide studies	• Radionuclide studies very sensitive
• ALP may be (n)	• ALP always raised
• Punched out	• Irregular lytic lesions

POEMS Syndrome

- Polyneuropathy
- Organomegaly (hepatosplenomegaly)
- Endocrinopathy (DM)
- M-proteins (plasma cell dyscrasia)
- Skin changes (hirsutism, pigmentation)

Metastasis

Predominantly Osteoblastic Metastasis

- Prostate (Figure)
- Carcinoid
- Stomach

Mixed Osteolytic and Osteoblastic

- Breast
- Lung

Osteolytic

- Hypernephroma (RCR) (Blow out metastasis)
- Thyroid

IOC for-metastatic workup is bony scintigraphy except in spine where MRI is preferred

Super scan

- Generalized increased bone activity with absent or reduced renal activity, e.g. diffuse osteoblastic metastatic disease

TRAUMA

Plain Radiography-Ist investigation
IOC → NCCT

> **important**
> Soap bubble app.
> – GCT
> – Angiosarcoma
> – Fibrosarcoma

> **important**
> Skeletal survey is better than bone scan as MM lesions are osteolytic with no-bone reaction

> **important**
> Metastasis can give:
> – Sunburst appearance
> – Simulating osteosarcoma

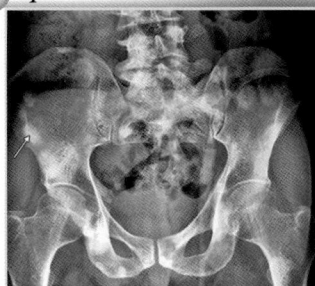

Predominantly osteoblastic metastasis from carcinoma prostate

> **important**
> ***FDG PET more sensitive and specific for bone metastasis than bone scintigraphy. ***NaF (Sodium fluoride) PET more sensitive to detect both osteolytic & osteoblastic metastasis.

> **important**
> CNS tumors and BCC of skin. Does not metastasize to bone- rest all tumors can metastasize to bone.

- Green Stick (Hickory Stick Fracture) d/t angulative force break on convex cortex with intact concave side
- Torus (Buckling)
  - Longitudinal **compressive** forces
  - Cortex bulges out

Fractures of Growth Plate/physis-salter-Harris Classification X-ray

- Type I: Through growth plate-**X-ray (n)**
  - II: Fracture through displaced growth plate along with metaphysis-**(MC)Thurston Holland-sign**
  - III: Through growth plate and epiphysis→**Intra-articular (need open reduction)**
  - IV: Though G.P., Meta and epiphysis
  - V: Crush/compressive fracture

Features of Nonunion

- Rounding of fracture edges
- Smoothening of margins with sclerosis
- Gap b/w two fragments
- Demonstration of mobility (on serial stress radiograph/fluoroscopy)
- **Lack of callus formation**
- Pseudoarthrosis

Upper Limb

- Anterior dislocation of shoulder
  - **Hill-Sach's defect** (Impaction of humeral head)
  - **Bankart's lesion** (avulsion of inferior glenoid labrum)
- Post. Dislocation
  - Light bulb sign on AP-X-ray
  - Tennis Racquet sign
- Inf. dislocation
  - Luxatio erecta — arm held in abduction

Fractures with Acronyms

- Fracture of Prox. ulnar shaft with dislocation of the radial head
  - Monteggia's Fracture Dislocation (MUS)

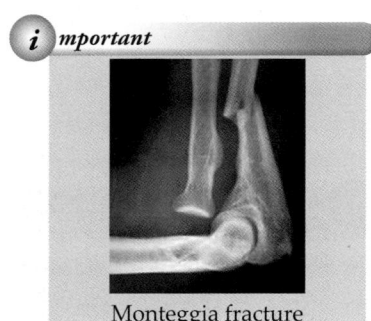

Monteggia fracture

- Isolated # of distal ulnar shaft → **Nightstick/Parry**
- Fracture of distal shaft of radius at junction of middle & distal third with dislocation of distal radioulnar joint
  - Galeazzi or Reversed Monteggia#
- Fracture of distal end of radius with post. angulation of distal fragment → **Colle's #**
  - Dinner Fork Deformity on Lateral View
- Fracture of distal radius with anterior angulation
  - Smith's fracture/Reversed Coll's fracture
- # Post. rim of distal radius→**Barton's #**
- # Anterior rim of distal radius→**Reverse Barton's**
- Radial styoid-**Chauffeur's fracture**
- #Scaphoid→AVN-X-ray view of choice → oblique view
- Avulsion fracture of triquetrum at attachment site of radiocarpal ligament → **Fischer's fractures**
- Scapholunate Dislocation
  - Terry Thomas sign
  - Signet ring sign (Small and circular scaphoid)
- Oblique intraarticular # of base of 1st metacarpal with dorsal and radial displacement of shaft → **Bennett's fracture**
- Comminuted Bennett's fracture→is **Ronaldo's #**
- Transvers # of neck of 5th MC with volar angulation- **Boxer's #**
- Avulsion chip # At insertion of extensor tendon- **Mallet finger**

Lower Limb

- # of lateral tibial plateau at attachment of iliotibial tract→Segond's #
- Undisplaced spiral # of shaft (<2 yrs) of tibia→ Toddler's #
- #Calcaneum→less/decreased Bohler's angle (N)-28-40 degrees)
- Lisfranc's dislocation at tarsometatarsal joints
- Chopart's dislocation-medial dislocation of talonavicular and calcaneo- cuboid joints of the foot.
- Fracture of the base of 5th metatarsal—John's fracture

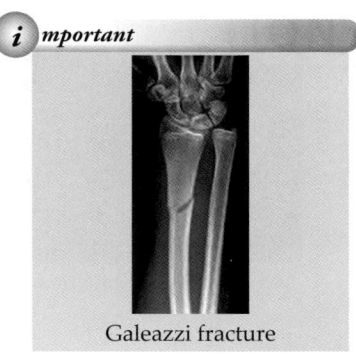
Galeazzi fracture

important
AVN-common sites are:
- Femoral head
- Scaphoid
- Humeral head
- Talus

important
–MRI is IOC for joints and soft tissue lesions

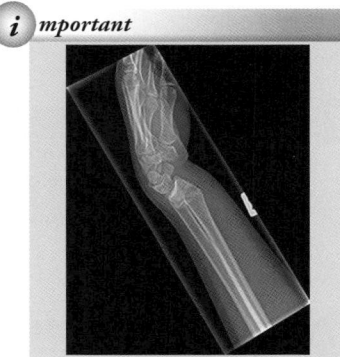
Colle's fracture

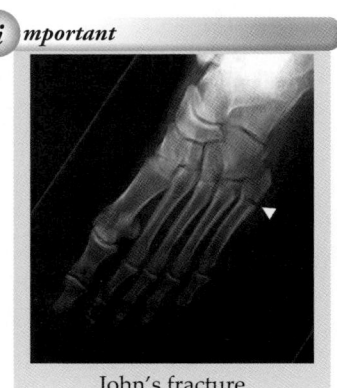
John's fracture

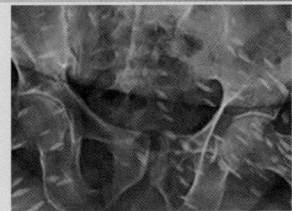
Cysticercosis of muscles

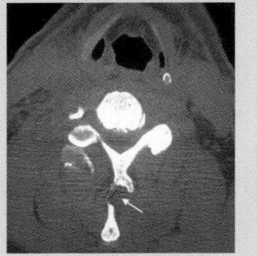
Clay shoveler's fracture

> **Important**
> - Fracture of C₇ spinous process–Clay Shoveler's fracture

> **Important**
> **AVN**
> - Prox. femoral epiphysis → Perthe's
> - Distal epiphysis of IInd MT → Freiberg's
> - Navicular → Kohler's
> - Lunate → Kienbock's

Soft Tissue

- Decrease radiodensity of soft tissue **(Fat and air)**
- Calcified cyst, oval, elongated along the long axis of muscle fiber–cysticercosis (Figure)
- Pipe stem calcification→phlebolith/vascular calcification
- Repeated trauma leads to bone formation at tendon/lig. Insertion sites
  - Adductor longus muscle → Rider's bone
  - Pellegrini-Stieda lesion → adductor tubercle of distal femur
  - Fencer's bone → brachialis muscle
  - Dancer's bone → soleus muscle
- Bursitis superficial to patella-**house maid's knee**
- Bursae superficial to olecranon-**Student's elbow**.

Spondylolisthesis

- Inverted Napoleon hat sign (on AP view)
- Beheaded Scottish terrier sign on oblique view spondylolysis-Scotty dog with collar

Tractional Injuries

Tibial tubercle	– Osgood Schlatter's
Distal pole of patella	– Sinding Larsen's
Os calcis	– Severs
Ring epiphysis of vertebra	– Scheuermann's
Capitulum	– Panner's
Scaphoid	– Preiser's

Injuries around Knee

Meniscal Injuries

- Radial/free edge tears
  - Cleft sign
  - Marching cleft sign
  - Ghost sign (absent meniscus)
  - Truncated triangle sign.
- Longitudinal Tears
  - Bucket handle tear (Double PCL sign)
  - Absent bow-tie on 2-successive sagittal images on MRI (Absent bow-tie sign).

ACL Tear
- Empty notch sign (MRI)
- Lax PCL (Question mark configuration)

Segond Fracture
- Anterolateral corner fracture of tibial plateau

O' Donoghue Triad
- ACL tear
- MCL disruption
- Medial meniscus tear

Pellegrini-Stieda Disease
- Calcification around the medial femoral condyle chronic partial/complete tears of MCL

Baker's Cyst
- b/w semimembranous and medial head of gastrocnemius.

Shoulder Labral Injury
- Perthes → Labrum injury + intact periosteum
- GLAD → Labrum + cartilage (Glenolabral articular disruption)
- ALPSA → Labrum + periosteal (stripping) (Antero-labroligamentous periosteal sleeve avulsion)
- **Bankart-periosteal rupture + labrum injury**
- HAGL-capsule and IGHC detached from humerus (Humeral avulsion of GHL)
- **Thick MGHL with absent anterosuperior → Buford complex** labrum

Avascular Necrosis of HIP
- MC MRI Appearance
  - Geographic/serpiginous circumscribed subchondral lesion
  - Double line sign on T2W images
  - Bright Band sign
  - Crescent sign (subchondral collapse)
- Mitchell's Classification
  - Class A: Adipose – Fat
  - B: Blood – Blood
  - C: sea – Water
  - D: Dense – Fibrosed

> **important**
> Elastographic techniques
> ARFI → acoustic radiation force impulse
> TE → Transient elastography

> **important**
> (N) oblique view Scottish dog appearance

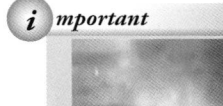

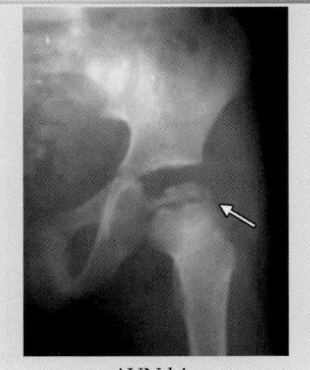

AVN hip

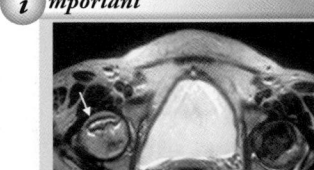

Double line sign—AVN hip

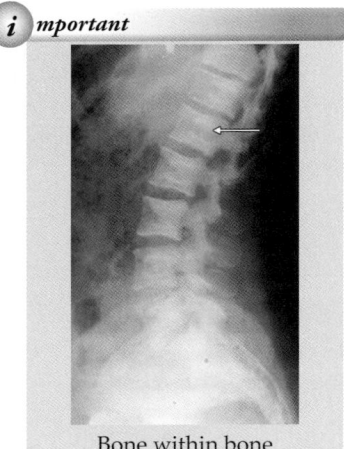

Bone within bone osteopetrosis

H shaped vertebrae
- Sickel cell disease
- Thanatophoric dwarfism

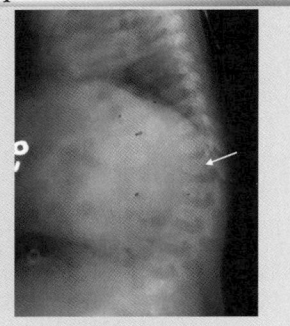

Bullet shape vertebrae

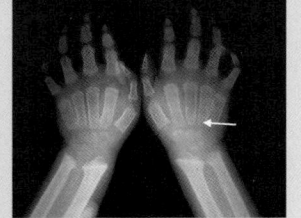

Proximal tapering of metacarpels- Mucopolysaccharidosis

- Radionuclide Study by 99Tc MDP Later
  - Photopenic zone
  - Doughnut sign—Due to reactive hyperemia/reparative response

Femoroacetabular Impingement

- **Cam impingement** → pistol grip deformity
- **Pincer impingement** → crossover sign

Erlenmeyer Flask Deformity

- Metaphyseal dysplasia
- Thalassemia
- Osteopetrosis
- Gaucher's disease

Paget's Disease

- Osteoporosis circumscripta
- Picture frame vertebra
- Cotton wool skull

Benign vertebral collapse	Malignant vertebral collapse
(n) signal intensity in nonfractured vertebrae	Ab (n) signal in other non-fractured vertebrae
Ab (n) signal parallels fracture	Ab (n) signal of entire fractured vertebra
Flat post. border of vertebra	Convex post: border of fractured vertebrae
No paravertebral mass	Occasional paravertebral mass
Ab (n) signal stabilizes with time	Progresses to destruction
Fluid sign present (also in osteoporotic collapse)	

ANEMIA

Thalassemia

- Diploic widening (occiput spared)
- **Hair on end**
- **Crew cut**
- **Hair brush**

Musculoskeletal Radiology

- Flask shaped femora
- Rodent facies
- Widened Intercondylar Notch-
  - Hemophilic arthropathy
  - JRA
  - TB

Ivory Vertebra

- Paget's
- Metastasis
- Lymphoma
- Infection

Vertebra Plana

- Eosinophilic granuloma (child)
- Metastasis/Melanoma
- Lymphoma
- TB/Trauma

Achondroplasia

- Champagne Glass pelvis (narrow Sacrosciatic notch)
- Trident hand
- Chevron sign-V shape notch in metaphysis
- Bullet shape vertebrae
- Post scalloping of vertebrae
- Tomb stone iliac blades

Mucopolysaccharidosis

- Oar shaped ribs
- Anterior beaking of vertebra central Morquios, anteroinferior Hurler's
- J Shaped sella
- Prox. tapering of metacarpals
- Simian pelvis

Pyknodysostosis

- Increase bone density
- Spool vertebra
- Obtuse angle of mandible
- Acroosteolysis
- Osteogenesis imperfecta
  - Diaphyseal fractures

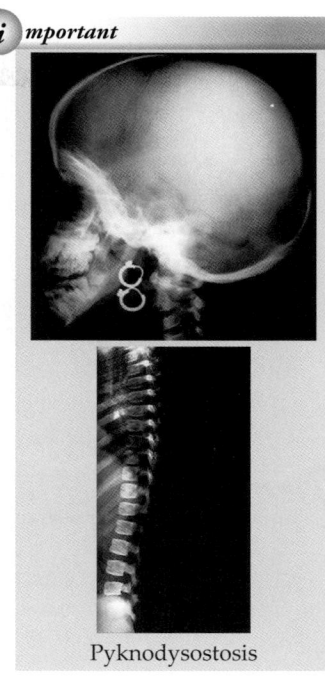

Pyknodysostosis

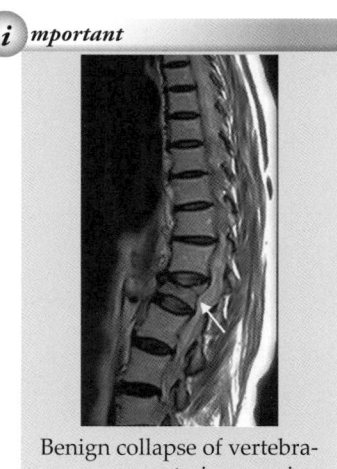

Benign collapse of vertebra-concave posterior margin

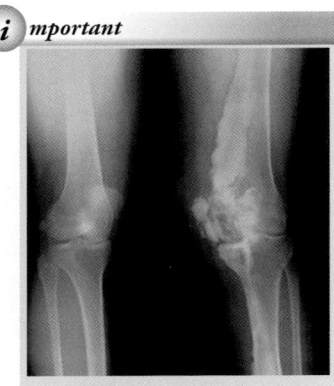

Melorheostosis → flowing wax

> *important*
> **Bone within bone appearance**
> – Sickle cell disease
> – Osteopetrosis

- Battered baby syndrome
  – Metaphyseal corner #
  – Post rib #
- **Melorheostosis**
  – Molten wax appearances/Candle dripping sign (Figure)
- Nail patella syndrome
  – Iliac horns.
- Thanatophoric dwarfism
  – H-shaped vertebra
  – **Telephone handle long bones**
  – Clover leaf skull

BREAST IMAGING

Screening Mammography

Mammogaraphy have 4 basic X-ray films two for each breasts which includes mediolateral oblique and craniocaudal views.

The standard mammogram (along with appropriate history-taking) makes up the entire screening mammogram. The indication for this examination is the search for

- **Occult carcinoma in an asymptomatic patient** (> 40 years)
- Breast lump in men
- Surveillance of breast following local excision.
- (Younger women have dense breast due to glandular tissue- low sensitivity for mammography)
- Mammography is the screening modality of choice for breast cancer as sometimes only microcalcification is the finding in DCIS.
- MRI is most sensitive to detect DCIS. (dynamic enhancement curves; Type-1 benign, type 2 is intermediate and type 3 curve signify malignancy)
- MRI is screening method of choice in patients with family history or BRACA/P53 mutations as need assessment at younger age where mammography is not sensitive
- Also MRI is preferred in patients with silicon implants.

Diagnostic Mammography

The diagnostic mammogram begins with the two-view standard mammogram.

Indications for diagnostic mammography are (1) a palpable mass or other symptom or sign (e.g. skin dimpling, nipple retraction, or nipple discharge that is clear or bloody) and (2) a radiographic abnormality on a screening mammogram. Additionally, patients with a personal history of breast cancer may be considered in the diagnostic category.

- Mammography is a part of triple assessment which includes—clinical assessment (history and examination), mammography or USG and histopathology which is used to confirm the diagnosis.

Features of breast lesion on mammography

Benign	Malignant
• Smooth marginated, low density, homogenous lesion	• Ill defined irregular margins with spiculations, high density, heterogenous lesion
• Macrocalcifications (> 0.5 mm) <5 in number (Lobular, rod like (duct ectasia), tram like (vascular) calcifications)	• **Microcalcifications (< 0.5 mm) >10 in number**
• Calcification with level in milk of calcium cyst	• Granular
• Egg shell curvilinear calcification in fat necrosis	• Casting calcification within ducts
• **Popcorn calcification in involuting fibroadenoma**	• **Pleomorphic**
• Punctuate (very small sharply defined, pin point like)	• **Fine heterogenous-rounded very thin but irregular shaped**
	• **Fine branching**

BIRADS: breast imaging reporting and data system— used to grade the breast lesion on mammography

Grade	Interpretation	Management
0	Incomplete evaluation	Complete it
1	Normal	Routine mammography
2	Benign	Routine mammography
3	Probably benign (<2% chances of malignancy)	Short follow up (6 months)

Contd...

Contd...

Grade	Interpretation	Management
4	Suspicious/intermediate (>2-90% chances of malignancy)	Biopsy
5	Highly suspicious (> 95% chances of malignancy)	Biopsy
6	Biopsy proven	Definitive treatment

Breast Ultrasonography

The indications for ultrasonography are:
- Mammographically detected mass, the nature of which is indeterminate
- A palpable mass that is not seen on mammography
- A palpable mass in a patient below the age recommended for routine mammography
- Guidance for intervention
- The augmented breast
- Breast inflammation
- Breast lump in male
- **Breast lump developing during pregnancy or lactation**

Ultrasonography is a highly reliable technique for differentiating cystic from solid masses. If criteria for a simple cyst are met, the diagnosis is more than 99% accurate.

A limitation of ultrasonography is that it is very operator dependent.

Features on USG

The benign lesions are usually well defined, smooth marginated, broader than taller, homogenous hypoechoic masses.

Malignant masses are heteroechoic masses, taller than broader, irregular, spiculated, infiltrating margins with necrosis and internal vascularity.

USG Elastography

It is a recent advancement of USG used to detect stiffness of tissue. Malignant masses have more stiffness than benign.

QUESTIONS

1. Molten-wax appearance is seen in:
   a. Osteoporosis
   b. Osteopoikilosis
   c. Melorheostosis
   d. Osteogenesis imperfecta
2. A person has an injury in the forefinger with glass and it is suspected that he has a retained piece of glass in his finger. What is the first investigation you will do?
   a. MRI
   b. CT scan
   c. Plain radiograph
   d. Ultrasonography
3. A 76-year-old man presents with lytic lesion in the vertebrae. X-ray skull showed multiple punched out lesions The diagnosis is:
   a. Metastasis
   b. Multiple myeloma
   c. Osteomalacia
   d. Hyperparathyroidism
4. Champagne glass pelvis is seen in:
   a. CDH
   b. Down's syndrome
   c. Cretinism
   d. Achondroplasia
5. Multiple punched-out lesions on skull X-ray is found in:
   a. Down's syndrome
   b. Hyperparathyroidism
   c. Multiple myeloma
   d. All of the above
6. In scurvy all the following radiological signs are seen except:
   a. Pelican spur
   b. Soap bubble appearance
   c. Zone of demarcation near epiphysis
   d. Frenkel's line
7. Pelkan spur is seen in:
   a. Rickets
   b. Scurvy
   c. Hemophilia
   d. All of the above
8. Wind swept deformity is seen in:
   a. Ankylosing spondylitis
   b. Scurvy
   c. Rheumatoid arthritis
   d. Rickets
9. Which of the following features on mammogram would suggest malignancy?
   a. Well defined lesion
   b. A mass of decreased density
   c. Areas of speculated microcalcifications
   d. Smooth borders
10. Investigation to diagnose stage-I carcinoma breast:
    a. B/L mammogram
    b. X-ray chest
    c. Bone scan
    d. Liver scan
11. The sensitivity of Mammography is low in young females because:
    a. Less glandular tissue and more fat
    b. Young females are less cooperative
    c. Young breasts have dense tissue
    d. Because of less fat content
12. Which of the following is the least useful for diagnosis of spondylolisthesis?
    a. CT
    b. MR
    c. X-ray lumbar spine-AP view
    d. X-ray lumbar spine-Lateral view
13. Beheaded scottish terrier sign is:
    a. Spondylosis
    b. Spondylolisthesis

c. Lumbar canal stenosis
d. Slipped disc

14. In spondylolisthesis following radiological features is seen:
    a. Scotty dog
    b. Scotty dog wearing a collar
    c. Beheaded scotty dog terrier sign
    d. Napoleon sign

15. Calcification around the joint is seen in:
    a. Pseudogout
    b. Hyperparathyroidism
    c. Rh. arthritis gout

16. Looser's zone is seen in:
    a. Osteogenesis imperfecta
    b. Osteopetrosis
    c. Osteomalacia
    d. Hypoparathyroidism

17. Bamboo spine is seen in:
    a. Ankylosing spondylitis
    b. RA
    c. Paget's disease
    d. All of the above

18. X-ray finding of osteomyelitis within 5 day is:
    a. Cystic swelling
    b. Soft tissue swelling
    c. New bone formation
    d. Sequestrum formation

19. Wormian bones are seen in all except:
    a. Hypothyroidism
    b. Down syndrome
    c. Turner syndrome
    d. Osteogenesis imperfecta

20. Bare orbit is/are seen in:
    a. NF-1
    b. Osteomyelitis
    c. VHL
    d. Tuberous sclerosis

21. Best radiographic view for fracture of C1, C2 vertebrae is:
    a. AP view
    b. Odontoid view
    c. Lateral view
    d. Oblique view

22. Which of the following is not true regarding ossified posterior longitudinal ligament (OPLL)?
    a. Most commonly involves 'thoracic spine
    b. Gradient echo MR sequence may overestimate the canal stenosis
    c. MRI is best for diagnosis
    d. Low signal intensity on all MR sequences

23. Multiple lytic lesions of skull with beveled edges are seen in:
    a. Eosinophilic granuloma
    b. Metastases
    c. Multiple myeloma
    d. Neuroblastoma

24. Sonographic finding of spina bifida:
    a. Ventriculomegaly
    b. Obliteration of cisterna magna
    c. Small BPD
    d. Abnormal curvature of cerebellum

25. Hair on end" appearance is seen in:
    a. Thalassemia
    b. Sickle cell anemia
    c. Hemochromatosis
    d. Megaloblastic anemia

26. Radiological findings of scurvy are A/E:
    a. Epiphyseal widening
    b. Metaphyseal porosis
    c. Metapyseal infarction
    d. Pelkan spur

27. Radiological feature of osteosarcoma is:
    a. New bone formation
    b. Sunray appearance
    c. Cotton wool appearance
    d. Osteoid formation

28. Radiographic appearance of Pindborg's tumor is:
    a. Onion-peel appearance
    b. Sunburst appearance
    c. Cherry-blossom appearance
    d. Driven-snow appearance

29. Expansile lytic lesion with fluid-fluid levels within the metaphysis of fibula seen on CT ailed MRI in an early adolescent female is typical of:
    a. Giant cell tumor
    b. Aneurysmal bone cyst
    c. Hemangioma
    d. Fibrous dysplasia

30. Not a radiological feature of rickets:
    a. Splaying of metaphysis
    b. Cupping of metaphysis
    c. Rachitic rosary
    d. Pelkan's spur

31. Which endocrine disorder is associated with epiphyseal dysgenesis?
    a. Hypothyroidism
    b. Cupping of metaphysis
    c. Addison's disease
    d. Hypoparathyroidism

32. A classical expansive lytic lesion in the transverse process of a vertebra is seen in:
    a. Osteosarcoma
    b. Aneurysmal bone cyst
    c. Osteoblastoma
    d. Metastasis

33. Best investigation for bone metastasis is:
    a. MRI
    b. CT
    c. Bone scan
    d. X-ray

34. An eight-year-old boy presents with back pain and mild fever. His plain X-ray of the dorsolumbar spine reveals a solitary collapsed dorsal vertebra with preserved disk spaces. There was no associated soft tissue shadow. The most likely diagnosis is:
    a. Ewing's sarcoma
    b. Tuberculosis
    c. Histiocytosis
    d. Metastasis

35. Chondrocalcinosis is seen with:
    a. Gout
    b. Osteoarthritis
    c. Pseudogout
    d. Septic arthritis

36. Investigation of choice for a lesion of temporal bone:
    a. CT
    b. MRI
    c. USG
    d. Plain X-ray

37. Codman's triangle is a feature of:
    a. Osteosarcoma
    b. Osteochondroma
    c. Osteoid osteoma
    d. Chondrosarcoma

38. Radiological mass shows sunray appearance is:
    a. Osteosarcoma
    b. GCT
    c. Osteomyelitis
    d. Ewing's sarcoma

39. A 40-year-old male patient on long-term steroid therapy presents with recent onset of severe pain in the right hip. Imaging modality of choice for this problem is:
    a. CT scan
    b. Bone scan
    c. MRI
    d. Plain X-ray

40. Which one of following is the earliest radiographic manifestation of childhood leukemia?
    a. Radiolucent transverse metaphyseal band
    b. Diffuse demineralization of bones
    c. Osteoblastic lesions in skull
    d. Parenchymal pulmonary lesions on chest films

41. Calcification of intervertebral disc is seen in:
    a. T.B. spine
    b. Prolapse of intervertebral disk (PID)
    c. Non-rheumatic ankylosis
    d. Rheumatic ankylosis

42. Postirradiation thyroid tumor is:
    a. Follicular Ca
    b. Papillary Ca
    c. Lymphoma
    d. Hurthle cell tumor

43. Calcification of meniscal cartilage is feature of:
    a. Achondroplasia
    b. Hyperparathyroidism
    c. Gaucher's disease
    d. Pseudogout

44. Which one of the following is a recognized X-ray feature of rheumatoid arthritis?
    a. Juxta-articular osteosclerosis
    b. Sacroiliitis
    c. Bone erosions
    d. Periarticular calcification

45. Bone density is best studied by
    a. CT scan
    b. DEXA scan
    c. MRI scan
    d. Bone scan

46. Earliest evidence of healing in rickets is provided by:
    a. S. Ca^{++}
    b. S. PO$_4^{3-}$
    c. Radiological examination of growing bone ends
    d. S. Alkaline Phosphate level

47. Splaying and cupping of the metaphysis is seen in:
    a. Rickets
    b. Scurvy
    c. Paget's disease
    d. Lead poisoning

48. Flaring of anterior ends of the ribs is characteristically seen in:
    a. Neurofibromatosis
    b. Scurvy
    c. Rickets
    d. Hypothyroidism

49. Best investigation for traumatic paraplegia:
    a. CT scan
    b. MRI
    c. X-ray spine
    d. Myelography

50. A small simple lytic lesion in X-ray of upper end of humerus. The diagnosis is ?
    a. Osteosarcoma
    b. Osteochondroma
    c. Unicameral bone cyst
    d. Osteoclastoma

51. Radiological features of scleroderma are A/E:
    a. Diffuse periosteal reaction
    b. Esophageal dysmotility
    c. Erosion of tip of phalanx
    d. Lung nodules

52. Fraying and cupping of metaphyses of long bones in a child does not occur in:
    a. Rickets
    b. Lead poisoning
    c. Metaphyseal dysplasia
    d. Hypophosphatasia

53. X-ray of which bone (s) would be diagnostic in hyperparathyroidism?
    a. Skull
    b. Phalanges
    c. Long bones
    d. Scapula
    e. Spine

54. Pathognomonic feature of hyperparathyroidism:
    a. Osteopenia
    b. Loss of Lamina dura
    c. Brown's tumor
    d. Subperiosteal resorption of phalanges

55. The gold standard for the diagnosis of osteoporosis is:
    a. Dual energy X-ray absorptiometry
    b. Single energy X-ray absorptiometry
    c. Ultrasound
    d. Quantitative computed tomography
56. Which of the following is not a cause of generalized increase in bone density in adults?
    a. Myelosclerosis
    b. Renal osteodystrophy
    c. Fluorosis
    d. Caffey's disease
57. Expansion of the contrast filled space in myelography is seen in:
    a. Intramedullary tumor
    b. Intradural extramedullary tumor
    c. Spinal dysraphism
    d. Extradural tumor
58. Heberden's nodes are found in:
    a. PIP joints in osteoarthritis
    b. DIP joints in osteoarthritis
    c. PIP joints in rheumatoid arthritis
    d. DIP joints in rheumatoid arthritis
59. Tufting of distal phalanx is characteristically seen in:
    a. Gout
    b. Psoriatic arthropathy
    c. Hypoparathyroidism
    d. Hyperparathyroidism
60. Increased bone density is seen in all except:
    a. Primary hyperparathyroidism
    b. Osteopetrosis
    c. Fluorosis
    d. Hypoparathyroidism
61. "Flowing wax" appearance on anterior and posterior borders of vertebrae with normal intervertebral disc space occurring due to ligament calcification is seen in:
    a. Ankylosing spondylitis
    b. Diffuse idiopathic skeletal hypertrophy
    c. Psoriatic spondyloarthropathy
    d. RA
62. X-ray shows soap bubble appearance at lower end of radius treatment of choice is:
    a. Local excision
    b. Excision & Bone grafting
    c. Amputation
    d. RT
63. Lytic lesion in skull are seen in following except:
    a. Multiple myeloma
    b. Metastasis bronchus
    c. Thalassemia
    d. Ca prostate
    e. Eosinophilic granuloma
64. Osteolytic metastasis is seen with:
    a. Lung   b. Kidney
    c. Thyroid   d. All of the above
65. A 70 years old female is on treatment with Alendronate for 7 years for osteoporosis. Now she complains of pain in right thigh. What is the next investigation to be performed?
    a. DEXA scan   b. X-ray
    c. Serum vitamin D levels
    d. Serum alkaline phosphate levels
66. Wimberger's sign is seen in?
    a. Scurvy   b. Rickets
    c. Congenital syphilis
    d. Osteomalacia
67. CT scan finding in carotid cavernous sinus fistula is:
    a. Enlarged superior ophthalmic vein
    b. Enlarged inferior ophthalmic vein
    c. Enlarged superior ophthalmic artery
    d. Enlarged inferior ophthalmic artery
68. Mammographic abnormality seen in CA breast is:
    a. Change in density
    b. Clusters of microcalcification

c. Change in architecture
d. All of the above

69. **Hallmark of breast malignancy on mammography:**
    a. Low-density lesion
    b. Smooth margin
    c. Clusters of microcalcification
    d. Popcorn calcification

70. **Which of the following features on mammogram would suggest malignancy?**
    a. Well defined lesion
    b. A mass of decreased density
    c. Areas of spiculated microcalcifications
    d. Smooth borders

71. **The sensitivity of mammography is low in young females because of:**
    a. Less glandular tissue and more fat
    b. Young females are less cooperative
    c. Young breast have dense tissue
    d. Because of less fat content

72. **On mammography following are the features of a malignant tumor except:**
    a. Spiculation
    b. Microcalcification
    c. Macrocalcification
    d. Irregular mass

73. **Which of the following does not contain fat on mammography?**
    a. Post-traumatic cyst
    b. Hamartoma
    c. Seborrheic keratosis
    d. Galactocele

74. **Investigation to diagnose stage-I carcinoma breast:**
    a. Bilateral mammogram
    b. X-ray chest
    c. Bone scan
    d. CT scan

75. **The most sensitive investigation for DCIS (ductal carcinoma in situ) of breast?**
    a. Mammography
    b. Ultrasound
    c. MRI
    d. PET scan

76. **Triple assessment for carcinoma breast includes:**
    a. History, clinical examination, biopsy/cytology
    b. Clinical examination, mammography, biopsy/cytology
    c. History, clinical examination, ultrasonography
    d. Observation, ultrasonography, biopsy/cytology

77. **Mammograph can be used in:**
    a. Early breast carcinoma
    b. Mastitis
    c. Fibroadenoma
    d. Phyllodes tumor

78. **Soft tissue mass in chest with rib erosion in X-ray is seen in all except:**
    a. Leukemia
    b. Ewing's sarcoma
    c. Multiple myeloma
    d. Osteosarcoma

79. **What is true regarding NIPT?**
    a. DNA is extracted from fetal cells circulating in maternal circulation.
    b. It is done on amniotic fluid
    c. It is done before 7 weeks
    d. It is done on fetal serum

80. **Fallen fragment sign is characteristic of**
    a. Aneurysmal bone cyst
    b. Simple bone cyst
    c. Giant cell tumor
    d. Osteosarcoma

Multiple Correct Answers

81. **A 2-year-old boy suffering from leukemia, following are the X-ray finding:**
    a. Osteolytic lesion in flat bones
    b. Metaphyseal osteoporosis
    c. Periosteal new bone formation
    d. Osteosclerosis of long bones
    e. Transverse line of dark band below the growth plate

82. **All are radiological features of sickle cell anemia except:**
    a. Vertebra plana
    b. Floating teeth
    c. Bone infarct
    d. Marrow hyperplasia
    e. Secondary osteomyelitis

83. **Radiological features of rickets include:**
    a. Narrowing of epiphysis
    b. Cupping of metaphysis
    c. Ricketic rosary
    d. Pelikan's spur

84. **Radio iodine is used in treatment of:**
    a. Papillary Ca thyroid
    b. Medullary Ca thyroid
    c. Follicular Ca thyroid
    d. Anaplastic Ca thyroid

85. **Fallen fragment sign is characteristic of:**
    a. Aneurysmal bone cyst
    b. Simple bone cyst
    c. Giant cell tumor
    d. Osteosarcoma

ANSWERS

1. Ans. c. Melorheostosis
2. Ans. c. Plain radiograph
3. Ans. b. Multiple myeloma
4. Ans. d. Achondroplasia
5. Ans. c. Multiple myeloma
6. Ans. b. Soap bubble appearance
7. Ans. b. Scurvy
8. Ans. d. Rickets > c. Rheumatoid arthritis
9. Ans. c. Areas of speculated microcalcifications
10. Ans. a. B/L mammogram
11. Ans. c. Young breasts have dense tissue
12. Ans. c. X-ray lumbar spine-AP view
13. Ans. b. Spondylolisthesis
14. Ans. c. Beheaded scotty dog terrier sign
15. Ans. a. Pseudogout
16. Ans. c. Osteomalacia
17. Ans. a. Ankylosing spondylitis
18. Ans. b. Soft tissue swelling
19. Ans. c. Turner syndrome
20. Ans. a. NF-1
21. Ans. b. Odontoid view
22. Ans. a. Most commonly involves 'thoracic spine
23. Ans. a. Eosinophilic granuloma
24. Ans. d. Abnormal curvature of cerebellum
25. Ans. a. Thalassemia
26. Ans. a. Epiphyseal widening
27. Ans. b. Sunray appearance
28. Ans. d. Driven-snow appearance
29. Ans. b. Aneurysmal bone cyst
30. Ans. d. Pelkan's spur.
31. Ans. a. Hypothyroidism
32. Ans. b. Aneurysmal bone cyst
33. Ans. c. Bone scan
34. Ans. c. Histiocytosis
35. Ans. c. Pseudogout
36. Ans. a. CT
37. Ans. a. Osteosarcoma
38. Ans. a. Osteosarcoma
39. Ans. c. MRI
40. Ans. a. Radiolucent transverse metaphyseal band
41. Ans. c. Non-rheumatic ankylosis
42. Ans. b. Papillary Ca
43. Ans. d. Pseudogout
44. Ans. c. Bone erosions
45. Ans. b. DEXA scan
46. Ans. c. Radiological examination of growing bone ends
47. Ans. a. Rickets
48. Ans. c. Rickets
49. Ans. b. MRI
50. Ans. c. Unicameral bone cyst
51. Ans. d. Lung nodules
52. Ans. b. Lead poisoning
53. Ans. b. Phalanges
54. Ans. d. Subperiosteal resorption of phalanges
55. Ans. a. Dual energy X-ray absorptiometry
56. Ans. d. Caffey's disease
57. Ans. b. Intradural extramedullary tumor
58. Ans. b. DIP joints in osteoarthritis
59. Ans. b. Psoriatic arthropathy
60. Ans. a. Primary hyperparathyroidism
61. Ans. b. Diffuse idiopathic skeletal hypertrophy
62. Ans. b. Excision & Bone grafting

63. **Ans. c.** Thalassemia **d.** Ca prostate
64. **Ans. d.** All of the above
65. **Ans. b.** X-ray
66. **Ans. c.** Congenital syphilis
67. **Ans. a.** Enlarged superior ophthalmic vein
68. **Ans. d.** All of the above
69. **Ans. c.** Clusters of microcalcification
70. **Ans. c.** Areas of speculated microcalcifications
71. **Ans. c.** Young breasts have dense tissue
72. **Ans. c.** Macrocalcification
73. **Ans. c.** Seborrheic keratosis
74. **Ans. a.** Bilateral mammogram
75. **Ans. c.** MRI
76. **Ans. b.** Clinical examination, mammography, biopsy/cytology
77. **Ans. a.** Early breast carcinoma
78. **Ans. a.** Leukemia
79. **Ans. a.** DNA is extracted from fetal cells circulating in maternal circulation.
80. **Ans. b.** Simple bone cyst

Multiple Correct Answers

81. **Ans. a.** Osteolytic lesion in flat bones **c.** Periosteal new bone formation **d.** Osteosclerosis of long bones **e.** Transverse line of dark band below the growth plate
82. **Ans. b.** Floating teeth
83. **Ans. b.** Cupping of metaphysis and **c.** Ricketic rosary
84. **Ans. a.** Papillary Ca thyroid **c.** Follicular Ca thyroid
85. **Ans. b.** Simple bone cyst

SECTION C

RADIOTHERAPY AND NUCLEAR SCANS

- Radiotherapy and Chemotherapy
- Nuclear Scans

CHAPTER 6

Radiotherapy and Chemotherapy

INTERACTION OF RADIATION WITH MATTER

- **Photoelectric Effect:** At low energies (30 to 100 keV), as in diagnostic radiology, the Photoelectric effect is important. In this process, the incident photon interacts with an electron in one of the outer shells of an atom (typically K, L, or M). If the energy of the photon is greater than the binding energy of the electron, then the electron is expelled from the orbit with a kinetic energy that is equal to the energy of the incident photon minus the binding energy of the electron.

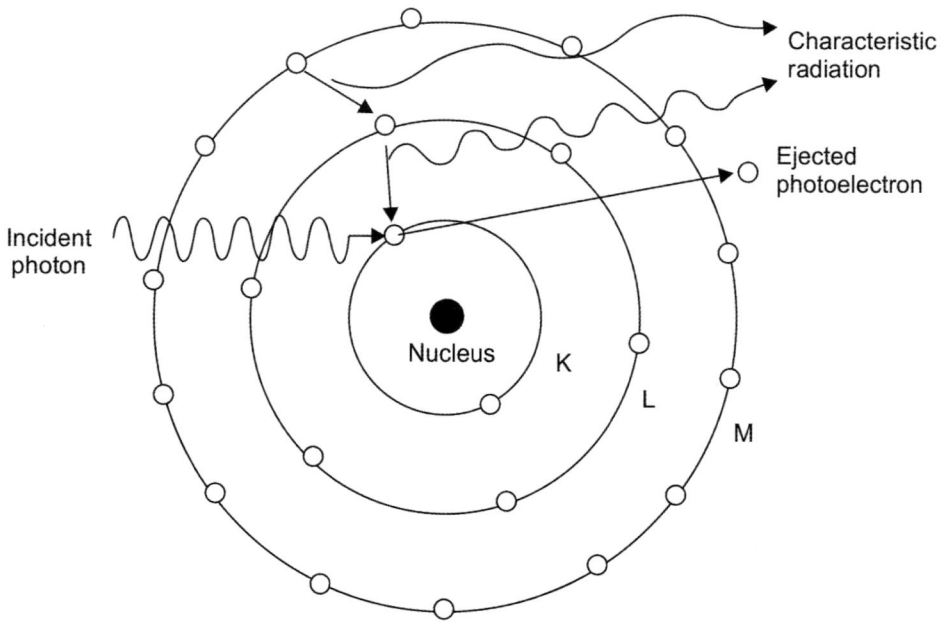

Features of Photoelectric Effect	
Most likely to occur	a. With inner-shell electrons b. With tightly bound electrons c. When X-ray energy is just higher than electron-binding energy
As X-ray energy increases	a. Increased penetration through tissue without interaction b. Less photoelectric effect relative to Compton effect c. Reduced absolute photoelectric effect
As atomic number of absorber increases	Increases proportionately with the cube of the atomic number Z^3
As mass density of absorber increases	Proportional increase in photoelectric absorption

- **Compton Effect:** At higher energies, as used in therapeutic radiology, the **Compton effect** dominates. In this process, the incident photon interacts with an electron in an orbital shell. Part of the incident photon energy appears as kinetic energy of electrons and the residual energy continues as a less energetic deflected photon.

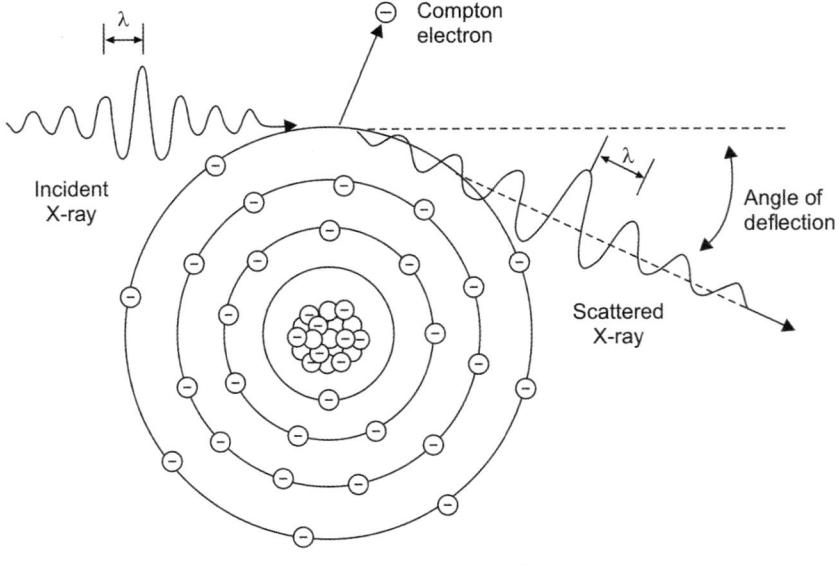

$\lambda < \lambda'$

Comptom effects reduces the contrast in an X-ray image

Features of Compton Scattering	
Most likely to occur	a. With outer-shell electrons b. With loosely bound electrons
As X-ray energy increases	a. Increased penetration through tissue without interaction b. Increased Compton Scattering relative to Photoelectric effect
As atomic number of absorber increases	No effect on Compton scattering
As mass density of absorber increases	Proportional increase in Compton scattering

1. The X-rays may be absorbed or scattered by the atomic electrons. In the absorption process (photoelectric absorption), the X-ray is completely absorbed, giving all of its energy to an inner shell atomic electron, which is then ejected from the atom and goes on to ionize other atoms in the immediate vicinity of the initial interaction.
2. In the scattering process (Compton scattering), the X-ray ricochets off an atomic electron, losing some of its energy and changing its direction. The recoiling electron also goes on to ionize hundreds of atoms in the vicinity. **Electrons from both processes go on to ionize many other atoms, and are responsible for the biological Damage produced by X-rays.**

Photoelectric effect	Compton effect
• Inner shell e⁻	• Outer shell e⁻
• Incident energy is completely absorbed	• Incident energy is partially absorbed
• X-ray energy: 70 kVp	• X-ray energy: 140 kVp
• Incidence increases with increase in atomic no	• No effect
• Radiography	• CT scan

- **Pair Production:** At energy levels above 1.02 MeV, the photons may be absorbed through **Pair production**. In this process, both a positron and an electron are produced in the absorbing material. A positron has the same mass as an electron but has a positive instead of a negative charge. The positron travels a very short distance in the absorbing medium before it interacts with another electron. When that happens, the to energy, with the emission of two photons in exactly opposite directions.

RADIOTHERAPY

It is the treatment of various body ailments using radioactive sources. It is based on the interaction of ionizing particles with tissues at the molecular level.

Mechanism of Action

- Ionization of molecules by breaking the chemical bonds
- Direct DNA damage

Properties of Commonly Used Isotopes

Isotope	Half-life	Use
Tc99m	6 hours	Radionuclide scan
Ra-226	1622 years	For brachytherapy but not used nowadays
Co-60	5.26 years	Teletherapy & brachytherapy
Cs-137	30 years	Teletherapy & brachytherapy
Ir-192	74.2 days	Brachytherapy
I-125	60.2 days	Brachytherapy
I-123	13.2 hours	For thyroid scan (not available in India)
I-131	8 days	Systemic therapy for well differentiated thyroid cancer
P-32	14 days	Brachytherapy
Au-198	2.7 days	Brachytherapy
18FDG	110 Minutes	PET SCAN

Modes of Radiotherapy

- Teletherapy **(External beam radiation therapy)—most commonly used therapy**
- Brachytherapy
    - Interstitial
    - Intracavitary
    - Mold
- Systemic radiotherapy

Teletherapy

Generation of energy particles at some distance from the patient.

- Commonly used source for Teletherapy are **Cobalt – 60** and CS-137
- **Linear accelerators (currently best source for teletherapy)**
    - Capable of generating X-rays along with electrons.
    - Most patients are treated with megavoltage X-rays or gamma rays (photons), which are penetrating whereas electron beam is usually used for superficial tumors.
- Neutrons and proton

Inverse Square Law

The intensity of radiation from any source decreases by the square of the distance from the source.

Thus, if the radiation source is 10 cm above the skin surface and the tumor is 10 cm below the skin surface, the intensity of radiation in the tumor will be 25% of the intensity at the skin.

Types of External Beam Therapy

- Orthovoltage or deep X-ray therapy (200–400 kV)
- Megavoltage therapy (2 to 8 million volts)
- Supervoltage therapy

Megavoltage therapy is preferred over orthovoltage therapy because of following advantages:

- **Skin sparing effects:** with orthovoltage X-rays, maximum dose is received by skin surface, whereas with high voltages, maximum dose is at some distance beneath skin; the skin is thus spared from high dose
- Greater penetration of beam
- Differential absorption in tissues; Greater penetration of energy in target volume
- Improved collimation; Very low scatter

Uses of X-ray Beam

- 4- to 6-MeV X-rays or cobalt 60 gamma for tumors of head and neck, usually located at a depth of 7–8 cm.
- 15- to 25-MeV X-rays for cancers 12 to 15 cm deep, such as cancer of the prostate or uterine cervix.

Uses of Electron Beam

Poorer skin-sparing properties than photon beams
- 6-MeV electrons are commonly used for cancers of the skin or lip
- 6- to 9-MeV electrons for cervical lymph nodes over the spinal cord
- 9- to 12-MeV electrons for cancers of the buccal mucosa
- 15- to 18-MeV electrons for cancers of the tonsillar area or parotid gland.

Brachytherapy

Radioactive sources are placed within or close to the target volume.
- **Interstitial Brachytherapy**: These sources can be placed directly into the tumor and surrounding tissues, e.g. prostate cancer
- **Intracavitary Brachytherapy:** within body cavities, e.g. gynecological malignacies
- **Mold Brachytherapy:** onto epithelial surfaces, ocular malignancy.

Brachytherapy Implants are of Two Types

Temporary implants (long-lived isotopes)	Permanent implants (short-lived isotopes)
Radium 226	Cesium 133
Cesium 137	Gold 198
Iridium 192	Iodine 125
	Palladium 103 yttrium

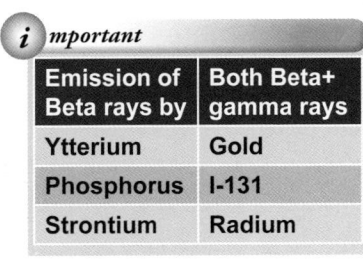

important

Emission of Beta rays by	Both Beta+ gamma rays
Ytterium	Gold
Phosphorus	I-131
Strontium	Radium

Systemic Radiotherapy

- I-131 for well differentiated thyroid cancer
- P-32 for Polycythemia Rubra vera

Dosing Pattern

- Conventional fractionation (usually 5 days a week (Monday to Friday)

- Hyperfractionation RT: multiple doses of radiation (b.i.d. or t.i.d.) can be given to exploit the radiobiological advantages. Used in head and neck cancers and carcinoma of lung.
- Accelerated RT: over a shorter period of time; head and Neck cancer
- **CHART** regimen: **Continuous hyperfractionated accelerated radiotherapy; used in** non-small cell lung cancer
- Hypofractionation RT; palliation of advanced cancers; painful bone metastasis.

Types of Radiotherapy Treatment
Radical radiotherapy:
- Early stages of cancers at an aim to cure.
- The common tumors treated are:
  - Vocal cord cancer of larynx
  - Nasopharynx
  - Cancer of uterine cervix
  - Skin cancers
  - Bladder cancers
  - Breast cancers
  - Prostate cancers

Radical radiotherapy should be considered in patients with localized lung cancer if surgery is contraindicated or refused. It is suitable for less than 5% of patients. Criteria for eligibility are as follows:
- Tumors 5 cm or less in maximum dimension
- Age less than 70 years
- Good general medical condition
- Adequate pulmonary function
- Non-small cell histology

Adjuvant radiotherapy:
- To improve the results of other treatment usually surgery and ultimately survival
  - Before surgery (preoperative radiotherapy),
  - After surgery (postoperative radiotherapy),
  - During surgery (intraoperative radiotherapy
  - Combination of preoperative and postoperative radiotherapy (sandwich radiotherapy)
- Commonly used in
  - Rectal cancers

- Head and neck cancers
- Breast cancers
- Brain tumors
- Most frequently used in postoperative set up.

Intraoperative radiotherapy (IORT):
- Very simple technique where radiation are delivered to the tumor bed after the removal of the tumor.
- Electrons are most commonly used for intraoperative radiotherapy.
- IORT seem to improve local control figures in retroperitonel soft-tissue sarcomas, pancreatic cancers, and other abdominopelvic tumors where external radiation is not feasible in view of higher normal tissue complications. It is also used in Breast cancer.

Preoperative radiotherapy:
- Carcinoma cervix
- Rectal cancer
- Inoperable non-small cell lung Ca

Postoperative radiotherapy:
- Poorly differentiated tumors
- Positive tumor margins
- More depth of infilteration
- Positive nodes
- Multifocal tumors

Concurrent chemoradiotherapy:
- Anti-neoplastic drugs like cisplatinum, 5FU and hydroxyurea when given in conjunction with radiotherapy, enhance the efficacy of radiation.
- When radiation given concurrently with chemotherapy the cancer cell kill increases twofold.

Commonly used in organ preservation techniques in
- Anal canal cancer, bladder cancer, esophageal cancer, nasopharyngeal cancer and cervical cancers

Radiosensitizers	Radioprotectors
Metronidazole, misonidazole	Amifostine
Hyperbaric oxygen	Pentoxyphyline
Cisplatin	Il-1
5 FU	GM-CSF
Gemcitabine	
hydroxyurea	
CYCLOPHOSPHAMIDE IS NOT	

Chemosensitivity of Tumors

Highly Chemosensitive

- Teratoma testis
- Hodgkin's disease
- Non-Hodgkin's disease (high grade)
- Wilm's tumors
- Choriocarcinoma
- Acute lymphoblastic leukemia (ALL)

Relatively Insensitive

- Gastric carcinoma
- Bladder carcinoma
- Squamous cell carcinoma (head, neck)
- Soft tissue sarcoma
- Cervical carcinoma

Moderately Chemosensitive

- Ovarian cancer
- Small cell carcinoma lungs
- Non-Hodgkin's disease (low grade)
- Breast carcinoma
- Myeloma
- Acute myeloid leukemia (AML)

Extremely Resistant

- Melanoma
- Squamous cell carcinoma lungs
- Large bowel carcinoma

Multi-modal (Holistic) Approach

- Many anticancer treatments are joined together to attack cancer cell in many ways called *multi-modal (holistic) approach* in cancer treatment.
- *Radiotherapy and surgery interval is kept between 4 to 6 weeks except for Wilms' tumor where radiotherapy should be started on 10th day.*
- *In Wilms'* tumor initially nephrectomy is done then local radiotherapy on the 10th day and subsequently chemotherapy (VAC) for 12–24 months.
- The other tumors treated by combined approach includes:
  - locally advanced breast cancer
  - cancer endometrium
  - soft tissue sarcoma.

Palliative Radiotherapy

- Cure is not possible

Used for:
- Painful bony metastasis (8 gy in single dose is preferred)
- Multiple brain metastasis
- SVC obstruction

Curative therapy	Palliative therapy	Preventive therapy
• Hodgkin's disease • Head and neck cancer (larynx, oral cavity, pharynx) prostate cancer • Gynecologic cancers (vagina, cervix) • Esophagus • Skin	• Relief of bone pain from metastatic disease • Control of brain metastases • Reversal of spinal cord compression superior vena caval obstruction shrinkage of painful masses • Opening of threatened airways	Development of leptomeningeal disease and brain metastases in acute leukemia and lung cancer

Modification/Advances in Radiotherapy

3D CRT (Conformal RT)
- To reduce radiation dose to the normal healthy tissue
- A CT scan is done first
- Planning of the field to be irradiated is done
- Skin marking is done for ensuring the same area is irradiated every time
- Used for tumors closed to important radiosensitive organ and structure of the body
    - Prostate cancer
    - Esophageal cancer
    - Lung cancer
    - Bladder cancer
    - Pancreatic cancer

INTENSITY-MODULATED RADIOTHERAPY (IMRT)

- Uses a multi-leaf collimator to shape the treatment area precisely to fit to the tumor shape.
- Microscopic cancer cells just outside the treatment area may not be destroyed.
- IMRT found useful in the treatment of small brain tumors, and head and neck cancers. It is best suitable for carcinoma of prostate.

STEREOTACTIC RADIOSURGERY

- High precision, stereotactically guided delivery of large dose of radiation in a single fraction
- Gamma knife' consisting of multiple cobalt-60 radioactive sources or X-rays from **linear accelerator.**

It is used for treating following lesions:
- Solitary cerebral metastasis
- Arteriovenous malformation
- Small meningiomas
- Schwannomas
- Pituitary adenomas

PROTON BEAM

- Proton beam therapy exploits subatomic particles with mass rather than X-rays to deliver radiation dose. It has gained increasing interest primarily due to its advantageous physical property. When passing through tissue, a proton deposits increasing dose slowly until reaching a sharp increase (Bragg peak) at its maximum depth of penetration, eliminating the exit dose seen with photons. Proton beam therapy seems to be promising, as it allows high dosages of radiation delivery to region near critical structures, but it has limited availability and its costs are high. It is not available in India. The Bragg peak is a pronounced peak on the Bragg curve which plots the energy loss of ionizing radiation during its travel through matter. For protons, α-rays, and other ion rays, the peak occurs immediately before the particles come to rest. This is called Bragg peak. When a fast charged particle moves through matter, it ionizes atoms of the material and deposits a dose along its path. A peak occurs because the interaction cross section increases as the charged particle's energy decreases. Energy lost by charged particles is inversely proportional to the square of their velocity, which explains the peak occurring just before the particle comes to a complete stop. The phenomenon is exploited in particle therapy of cancer, to concentrate the effect of light ion beams on the tumor being treated while minimizing the effect on the surrounding healthy tissue.

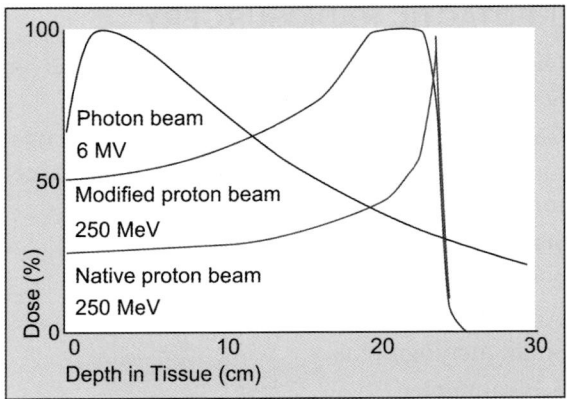

Proton therapy is being used to treat tumors in these areas of the bodies with good results
1. Lung
2. Prostate
3. Brain
4. Liver
5. Breast
6. Esophagus
7. Rectum
8. Skull base sarcomas
9. Pediatric brain tumors
10. Head and neck
11. Eye melanomas

SIDE EFFECTS OF RADIOTHERAPY FATIGUE

- Most common radiation side effect is dermatitis
- Depends upon the field size, fraction size and the total dose of radiation.

Early reacting tissues	Late reacting tissues
• Rapidly dividing cells	• Slowly dividing cells
• Mucosa and hematopoietic cells	• Stable cells like kidney, and brain
• Greater potentiality to regenerate	• Cannot regenerate
• Sub-lethal radiation damage	• Effects of radiation damage are permanent
• Immediately after radiotherapy	• 6 Months to years following radiotherapy

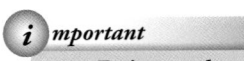

important

Fatigue > dermatitis

Contd...

Contd...

Early reacting tissues	Late reacting tissues
• e.g. Radiation sickness • Mucositis and sore throat • Diarrhea • Cystitis • Vomiting • Fall in blood counts	• Rectal bleeding • Hematuria • Osteoradionecrosis • Radiation nephritis

Acute Effect of Total Body Radiation

System affected	Dose	Time of death post exposure
Hematopoietic syndrome	2–8 gray	Weeks
Gastrointestinal syndrome	5–12 gray	Days
Cerebrovascular syndrome	20–100 gray	24–48 hours

GUIDE TO THE RELATIVE RADIOSENSITIVITY OF TISSUE

	Most	Least
Stage of cell cycle	G2M > M	S
Organ	Ovary, testis	Vagina>bone>cns
Tissue	Gonads, bone marrow	Nervous tissue
Cell type (Law of Bergonie and Tribondeau)	Undifferentiated, well nourished highly metabolically active	Quiescent
Blood cell	Lymphocyte	Platelet
Retinal layer	Retinal vessel endothelium	Retinal pigmented epithelium > ganglion cell layer

GUIDE TO THE RELATIVE RADIOSENSITIVITY OF TUMORS

Highly radiosensitive (WELMS)	Highly resistant (HOMP)
Wilms' tumor	Hepatoma
Ewing's sarcoma	Osteosarcoma

Contd...

Contd...

Highly radiosensitive (WELMS)	Highly resistant (HOMP)
Lymphoma	Melanoma
Myeloma	Pancreatic Ca
Seminoma/dysgerminoma	

FOLLOW-UP OF CANCER PATIENT RECEIVING RADIOTHERAPY

- Reappearances of the disease within 6 months are called residual disease
- Reappearances of the disease after 6 months are called recurrent disease
- Follow-up is usually done
  - Every 2 months × 2 years
  - Every 3 months × 3 years
  - Every 6 months × 5 years
  - Every year × 10 years

TREATMENT OF VARIOUS MALIGNANCIES

Surgery alone—treatment of choice:

- Lower esophagus, stomach, colon
- Pancreas
- Kidney
- Thyroid
- Melanoma
- Hcc
- Keratoacanthoma

Radiotherapy – the treatment of choice:

- Oral cavity, lip, tongue, cheek
- Nasopharynx, oropharynx and hypopharynx
- Nasal cavity
- Larynx
- Skin cancers (except melanoma)
- Cervix
- Bladder (except t1)
- Testis – seminoma
- Hodgkin's disease – early disease
- Nhl – early disease
- Medulloblastoma (following surgical resection)
- Astrocytomas (grades 3 and 4)

- Retinoblastoma

Chemotherapy – the treatment of choice:

- Acute and chronic leukemias
- HD (advanced)
- NHL (advanced)
- Testicular teratoma
- Choriocarcinoma
- Small cell lung cancer
- Rhabdomyosarcoma
- Neuroblastoma

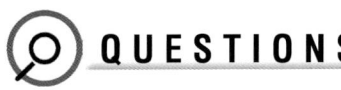

QUESTIONS

1. All of the following are pure beta emitters except:
   a. Yttrium-90
   b. Phosphorus-32
   c. Strontium-90
   d. Samarium-153
2. Amifostine is a:
   a. Radiosensitizer
   b. Radioprotector
   c. Radiomodifier
   d. Radio modulator
3. Stereotactic radiotherapy is used in:
   a. Miliary tuberculosis
   b. Stage I lung carcinoma
   c. Lymphangitis carcinomatosa
   d. Carcinoma base of tongue with positive lymph nodes
4. For radiotherapy an isotope is placed in or around cancer site. It is called as:
   a. Brachytherapy
   b. Teletherapy
   c. External beam therapy
   d. Intensity-modulated radiotherapy
5. That is atomic number:
   a. Proton
   b. Electrons + protons
   c. Proteins + neutrons
   d. Protons + protons
6. Substance with same atomic number but different mass number:
   a. Isotope
   b. Isobar
   c. Atom
   d. Mineral
7. Principle used in radiotherapy is:
   a. Cytoplasmic coagulation
   b. Ionization of molecules
   c. DNA damage
   d. Necrosis of tissue
8. Ionization radiation acts on tissue leading to:
   a. Linear acceleration injury
   b. Excitation of electron from orbit
   c. Formation of pyramidine dimer
   d. Thermal injury
9. Functional basics of ionizing radiation depends on:
   a. Pyramidine base pairing
   b. Removal of orbital electron
   c. Linear energy transfer
   d. Adding orbital electron
10. Most sensitive structure in cell for radiotherapy is:
    a. Cell membrane
    b. Mitochondrial membrane
    c. DNA
    d. Enzymes
11. Which of the following statements best describes 'Background Radiation'?
    a. Radiation in the background of nuclear reactors
    b. Radiation in the background during radiological investigations
    c. Radiation present constantly from natural sources
    d. Radiation from nuclear fallout
12. Principles of linear accelerators are used in:
    a. X-rays
    b. Gamma rays
    c. Alpha rays
    d. Infrared rays
13. Brachytherapy is:
    a. Radiotherapy with the source of radiation outside the body well at a distance
    b. External beam radiation therapy

c. Radiation source used in body cavities or implated directly into the tissues
d. Per oral radiation therapy

14. Most commonly used rays for radiotherapy:
    a. X-rays
    b. γ-rays
    c. α-rays
    d. β-rays

15. The major difference between X-rays and light is:
    a. Energy
    b. Mass
    c. Speed
    d. Type of wave

16. Which one of the following has the maximum ionization potential?
    a. Electron
    b. Proton
    c. Helium ion
    d. Gamma Photon

17. Which of the following is the most penetrating beam?
    a. Electron beam
    b. 6 MV photons
    c. 18 MV photons
    d. Proton beam

18. Most harmful to individual cell:
    a. X-rays
    b. α-particles
    c. p-particles
    d. Gamma rays

19. For the treatment of deep seated tumors, the following rays are used:
    a. X-rays and Gamma-rays
    b. Alpha rays and Beta-rays
    c. Electrons and positrons
    d. High-power laser beams

20. Which of the following is used for permanent interstitial implant brachytherapy?
    a. Boron
    b. Cesium-131
    c. Phosphorus
    d. Iridium

21. Most common skin manifestation seen after 2 days of radiation therapy is:
    a. Erythema
    b. Atopy
    c. Hyperpigmentation
    d. Dermatitis

22. For teletherapy setup, all are used except:
    a. Iridium 127
    b. Cobalt 60
    c. Simulator
    d. Computer

23. Which is used in teletherapy and brachytherapy both:
    a. Iridium 127
    b. Cobalt 60
    c. Palladium
    d. Iodine 131

24. Radioactive phosphorus is used in the treatment of:
    a. Polycythemia vera
    b. Thyroid metastasis
    c. Multiple myeloma
    d. Embryonal cell carcinoma

25. Which of the following elements is obsolete in radiotherapy?
    a. Radium 226
    b. Cobalt 60
    c. Iridium 192
    d. Cesium 137

26. MC cancer due to radiation:
    a. Leukemia
    b. Bronchogenic Ca
    c. Thyroid Ca
    d. Breast cancer

27. Stereotactic radiosurgery uses all except:
    a. Proton
    b. Electron
    c. Linear accelerator
    d. Gamma knife

28. Isotopes used in relief of metastatic bone pain includes:
    a. Strontium 89
    b. I-131
    c. Gold-198
    d. P-32
    e. Rhenium-186

29. The technique employed in radiotherapy to counteract the effect of tumor motion due to breathing is known as:
    a. Arc technique
    b. Modulation
    c. Gating
    d. Shunting

30. Hyperfractionation radiotherapy is used in the management of:
    a. Lung cancer
    b. Breast cancer
    c. Seminoma
    d. Ovarian cancer

31. Most radiosensitive tissue of body among the following is:
    a. Bone marrow
    b. Spleen
    c. Kidney
    d. Brain

32. Low-dose radiation causes:
    a. Lung cancer
    b. AML
    c. Cervical cancer
    d. Glioma
    e. Meningioma

33. Postradiation transverse myelitis usually presents at white urine after radiation therapy:
    a. 1–2 weeks   b. 1–2 months
    c. 4–6 months   d. 1 year

34. The maximum permissible radiation exposure per year recommended by NCRP for radiation worker is:
    a. 3 rad   b. 8 rad
    c. 10 rad   d. 50 mSv

35. Point A and point B Manchester location are important for treatment of which cancer:
    a. Cervix   b. Vagina
    c. Ovary   d. Uterus

36. Maximum recommended external beam radiation therapy dose for a case of carcinoma cervix is:
    a. 80 Gy   b. 70 Gy
    c. 50 Gy   d. 35 Gy

37. Photodynamic therapy with lematoporphyrins and light is increasingly used in treatment of:
    a. Ovary Ca   b. Skin Ca
    c. Colon Ca   d. All of the above

38. The ideal timing of radiotherapy for Wilms' tumor after surgery is:
    a. Within 10 days
    b. Within 2 weeks
    c. Within 3 weeks
    d. Any time after surgery

39. At t = 0. there are 6×10^{23} radioactive atoms of a substance, which decay with a disintegration constant equal to 0.01/sec. What would be the initial decay rate?
    a. 6×10^{23} b. 6×10^{22}
    c. 6×10^{21} d. 6×10^{20}

40. All are features of radiation except:
    a. Biological
    b. Photographic
    c. Fluorescent
    d. Nonpenetrating

41. Most stable radio-isotope among the following:
    a. 0-18   b. C-I4
    c. P-32   d. I-125

42. Which is not a deep heat therapy?
    a. Short wave diathermy
    b. Infrared
    c. USG
    d. Microwave

43. Radiation produces its effect on tissue by:
    a. Coagulation of cytoplasm
    b. Increasing the temperature
    c. Charring of nucleoprotein
    d. Hydrolysis

44. Gray equals:
    a. 100 rad
    b. 1000 rad
    c. 10000 rad
    d. 10 rad

45. Curie is unit of:
    a. Radiation exposure
    b. Radiation absorption
    c. Radioactivity
    d. All of the above

46. Which of the following radioactive isotopes is not used for brachytherapy?
    a. Iodine-125
    b. Iodine-131
    c. Cobalt-60
    d. Iridium-192
47. Isotope used in radioactive iodine uptake is:
    a. I131
    b. I123
    c. I125
    d. I127
48. All of the following radioisotopes are used as systemic radionucleides except:
    a. Phosphorus-32
    b. Strontium-89
    c. Iridium-192
    d. Samarium-153
49. Which one of the following radio-isotopes is not used as permanent implant?
    a. Iodine-125
    b. Palladium-103
    c. Gold-198
    d. Cesium-137
50. Radioisotopes are used in the following techniques except:
    a. Mass spectroscopy
    b. RIA
    c. ELISA
    d. Sequencing of nucleic acid
51. Which of the following radioisotopes is commonly used as a source for external beam radiotherapy in the treatment of cancer patients?
    a. Strontium-89
    b. Radium-226
    c. Cobalt-59
    d. Cobalt-60
52. Longest half life is seen in:
    a. Radon
    b. Radium
    c. Uranium
    d. Cobalt
53. The half life of Cobalt-60 is:
    a. 3.4 years
    b. 5.2 years
    c. 1.2 years
    d. 2.3 years
54. Half life of I131 is:
    a. 4 hours
    b. 8 days
    c. 4 days
    d. 10 days
55. The half life of Technetium is:
    a. 6 hours
    b. 12 hours
    c. 24 hours
    d. 26 hours
56. Radiation emits by Ir-192:
    a. 0.5 Mev
    b. 0.6 Mev
    c. 0.66 Mev
    d. 0.666 Mev
    e. 0.47 Mev
57. Phosphorus-32 emits:
    a. Beta particles
    b. Alfa particles
    c. Neutrons
    d. X-rays
58. Most suitable radioisotope of Iodine for treating hyperthyroidism is:
    a. I123
    b. I125
    c. I131
    d. I132
59. Maximum dose of radiation per year in a human which is safe is:
    a. 1 rads
    b. 5 rads
    c. 10 rads
    d. 20 rads
60. Maximum permissible radiation dose in pregnancy is:
    a. 0.5 rad
    b. 1.0 rad
    c. 1.5 rad
    d. 5 rad
61. Most sensitive tissue to radiaton is:
    a. Liver
    b. Gonads
    c. Spleen
    d. Skin
62. The cell most sensitive to RT:
    a. Neutrophil
    b. Lymphocyte
    c. Basophil
    d. Platelet
63. The radiation tolerance of whole liver is:
    a. 15 Gy
    b. 30 Gy
    c. 40 Gy
    d. 45 Gy

64. Most radiosensitive stage:
    a. S phase   b. G1 phase
    c. G2 phase   d. G2M phase
65. Photon transferring some of its energy to electron is:
    a. Photoelectric effect
    b. Bremsstrahlung effect
    c. Compton effect
    d. Ionization
66. Photoelectric effect is:
    a. Interaction between high energy incident photon and the inner shell electron
    b. Interaction between the low energy incident photon and the inner shell electron
    c. Interaction of the incident photon with the nucleus
    d. Interaction between a photon and electric current
67. Ionising radiation is most sensitive in:
    a. Hypoxia
    b. S phase
    c. G2M phase
    d. Activating cell
68. Most radiosensitive stage of cell cycle:
    a. G1 phase
    b. G2M interphase
    c. Early S phase
    d. Late S phase
    e. M phase
69. What is radioresistant?
    a. Cartilage
    b. Seminoma
    c. Ewing's sarcoma
    d. GI epithelium
70. Which of the following is the most radiosensitive tumor?
    a. Ewing's tumor
    b. Hodgkin's disease
    c. Carcinoma cervix
    d. Malignant fibrous histiocytoma

71. Most radiosensititive ovarian tumor is:
    a. Serus cystadenoma
    b. Dysgerminoma
    c. Dermoid cyst
    d. Teratoma
72. Most radiosensitive brain tumor is:
    a. Astrocytoma
    b. Ependymoma
    c. Medulloblastoma
    d. Craniopharyngioma
73. Most radiosensitive tumor is:
    a. Brenner's tumor
    b. Dysgerminoma
    c. Mucinous cystadenoma
    d. Teratoma
74. All are highly radiosensitive except:
    a. Osteogenic sarcoma
    b. Lymphoma
    c. Ewing's sarcoma
    d. Seminoma
75. Most radiosensitive testicular tumor is:
    a. Yolk sack tumor
    b. Embryonal cell tumor
    c. Teratoma
    d. Seminoma
76. Most radiosensitive lung CA is:
    a. Sqamous cell
    b. Small cell
    c. Adeno cell
    d. Large cell
77. The most radiosensitive tumor among the following is:
    a. Bronchogenic carcinoma
    b. Carcinoma parotid
    c. Dysgerminoma
    d. Osteogenic sarcoma
78. Which of the following malignant tumors is radioresistant?
    a. Ewing's sarcoma
    b. Retinoblastoma
    c. Osteosarcoma
    d. Neuroblastoma

79. Most radiosensitive tumor of the following is:
    a. Ca Kidney
    b. Ca Colon
    c. Ca Pancreas
    d. Ca Cervix
80. Tumor responding best to radiation includes the following:
    a. Melanoma
    b. Dysgerminoma
    c. Teratoma
    d. Choriocarcinoma
81. All are chemosensitive except:
    a. Small Cell CA
    b. Ca Cervix
    c. Ewing's tumor
    d. Malignant melanoma
82. Radiation exposure during infancy has been linked to which of the following carcinomas:
    a. Breast   b. Melanoma
    c. Thyroid   d. Lung
83. Least amenable to screening is:
    a. Breast CA
    b. Cervix CA
    c. Lung CA
    d. Oral cavity CA
84. Craniospinal irradiation is used in the treatment of:
    a. Oligodendroglioma
    b. Pilocytic astrocytoma
    c. Mixed oligoastrocytoma
    d. Medulloblastoma
85. Prophylactic cranial irradiation is not indicated in treatment of:
    a. Small cell Ca of lung
    b. ALL
    c. Hodgkin's lymphoma
    d. NHL
86. Prophylactic intracranial irradiations are given in:
    a. Small cell Ca of lung
    b. Testicular Ca
    c. Ca breast
    d. Ca stomach
87. Stereotactic radiosurgery is a form of:
    a. Radiotherapy
    b. Radioiodine therapy
    c. Robotic surgery
    d. Cryosurgery
88. Gamma knife:
    a. Steel knife
    b. Used for cutting tumors in difficult location
    c. Cobalt is used
    d. Recovery delayed
89. Radiation therapy to hypoxic tissues may be potentiated by the treatment with:
    a. Mycostatin
    b. Metronidazole
    c. Methotrexate
    d. Melphalan
90. For which malignancy is Intensity Modulated Radiotherapy (IMRT) the most suitable?
    a. Lung   b. Prostate
    c. Leukemias   d. Stomach
91. All are radiosensitizers except:
    a. 5-Fu
    b. BUDR
    c. Cyclophosphamide
    d. Hydroxyurea
92. Which of the following is not an indication of RT in pleomorphic adenoma of parotid?
    a. Involvement of deep lobe
    b. Second histologically benign recurrence
    c. Microscopically positive margins
    d. Malignant transformation
93. For mobile tumor of vocal cord treatment of choice is:
    a. Surgery
    b. Chemotherapy

c. Radiotherapy
d. None

94. What dose of radiation therapy is recommended for pain relief in bone metastases?
   a. 8 Gy in one fraction
   b. 20 Gy in 5 fractions
   c. 30 Gy in 10 fractions
   d. Above 70 Gy

95. In which malignancy is postoperative radiotherapy minimally used?
   a. Head and neck
   b. Stomach
   c. Colon
   d. Soft tissue sarcomas

96. Radioprotective drug is:
   a. Paclitaxem   b. Vincristine
   c. Amifostine   d. Etoposide

97. Intercavitatory radiotherapy is treatment modality for:
   a. Ca Cervix   b. Ca esophagus
   c. Ca Stomach d. Renal cell Ca

98. Point B in treatment of Ca cervix corresponds to:
   a. Mackenrodt's ligament
   b. Obturator lymph node
   c. Ischial tuberosity
   d. Round ligament

99. A patient with cancer received extreme degree of radiation toxicity. Further history revealed that the dose adjustment of a particular drug was missed during the course of radiotherapy. Which of the following drugs required a dose adjustment in that patient during radiotherapy in order to prevent radiation toxicity?
   a. Vincristine
   b. Dactinomycin
   c. Cyclophosphamide
   d. 6-Mercaptopurine

100. Amifostine protects all of the following except:
   a. CNS
   b. Salivary glands
   c. Kidneys
   d. GIT

101. Which of the following is used in the treatment of differentiated thyroid cancer?
   a. I-131   b. Tc-99
   c. P_{32} d. MIBG

102. Most common presentation of radiation carditis is:
   a. Pyogenic Pericarditis
   b. Pericardial Effusion
   c. Myocardial Fibrosis
   d. Atheromatous Plaque

103. Most common hormone deficiency seen after intracranial radiation therapy:
   a. Prolactin
   b. Gonadotropins
   c. ACTH
   d. Growth hormone

104. Photoelectric effect can be best described as an:
   a. Interaction between high energy incident photon in the outer shell electron
   b. Interaction between low energy incident photon and the outer shell electron
   c. Interaction of the high energy incident photon and the outer shell electron
   d. Interaction between a low energy incident photon and the inner shell electron

105. Phase of the cell cycle which is most sensitive to radiation:
   a. S   b. G1
   c. G2M   d. G0

106. Which of the following statements is true:
   a. γ-rays are produced from linear accelerator

b. γ-rays are produced by orbital electrons
c. X-rays are produced from Co-6O
d. X-rays and γ-rays have similar

107. Photon transferring some of its energy to electron is:
a. Photoelectric effect
b. Bremsstrahlung effect
c. Compton effect
d. Ionization

108. Which is provided by linear accelerator
a. Electron
b. Neutron
c. Proton
d. Infrared rays

109. Phosphorous 32 emits:
a. Beta particle
b. Alpha particle
c. Neptron
d. X-rays

110. Radioresistant tumor is:
a. Ewing's sarcoma
b. Retinoblastoma
c. Osteosarcoma
d. Neuroblastoma

111. All of the following modalities can be used for in situ ablation of liver secondaries, except:
a. Ultrasonic waves
b. Cryotherapy
c. Alcohol
d. Radiofrequency

112. Most commonly used isotope for treatment of bone cancer:
a. Pb86   b. I-125
c. Cr-51   d. Sr-89

113. Radioactive substance emits the following except:
a. Gamma   b. Beta
c. Alpha   d. X-rays

114. For teletheraphy, isotopes commonly used are:
a. 1-123   b. Cs-137
c. CO-60   d. Tc-99
e. Ir-191

Multiple Correct Answers

115. Used in radiotherapy:
a. I-131   b. Co-60
c. Ir-192   d. I-125

116. Artificial radioisotopes:
a. Radium   b. Uranium
c. Plutonium   d. Iridium
e. Cobalt

117. Radioactive isotopes that are used in treatment of cancer are:
a. Cesium
b. Cobalt
c. Carbon
d. Technetium
e. Nitrogen

118. Isotopes used for radiotherapy:
a. Radon   b. Cobalt-60
c. Iridium d. Cesium

119. Organs sensitive to radiation are:
a. Gonad
b. Bone marrow
c. Liver
d. Fat
e. Nervous tissue

120. Radiosensitive tumors are:
a. Seminoma
b. Lymphoma
c. Sarcoma
d. Ewing's sarcoma
e. Leukemia

121. Advantage of brachytherapy:
a. Noninvasive
b. Less radiation hazard to normal tissue
c. Maximum radiation to diseased tissue
d. Can be given in all malignancies
e. Doesn't require trained personnel

122. Radiotherapy is used for which stage-I cancer?
    a. Colon
    b. Larynx
    c. Anterior 2/3 of tongue
    d. Lung
    e. Stomach

123. Intraoperative RT is given in:
    a. Ca Cervix
    b. Ca Breast
    c. Ca Pancreas
    d. Ca Thyroid

124. Emergency radiotherapy is given in:
    a. Superior vena cava syndrome
    b. Pericardial tamponade
    c. Increased ICP
    d. Spinal cord compression

125. Late effects of radiation therapy:
    a. Mucositis
    b. Enteritis
    c. Nausea and vomiting
    d. Pneumonia
    e. Somatic mutations

126. Radionucleotide(s) used in external beam therapy:
    a. Iodine-131   b. Co-60
    c. Cs137   d. Ra226
    e. lr192

127. Stereotactic surgery is used for treatment of:
    a. Brain tumor
    b. Lung carcinoma
    c. Cervix cancer
    d. Renal carcinoma

128. Features of interstitial radiotherapy are all except:
    a. Only used in head and neck
    b. Damage to normal tissue
    c. Temporary or permanent
    d. Only iridium used
    e. Used for easily accessible organ

129. Radiosensitizer drug(s) is/are:
    a. Misonidazole b. Actinomycin D
    c. Oxygen   d. Hyperthermia
    e. Amifostine

130. Radium emits which of the following radiations:
    a. Alpha rays   b. Beta rays
    c. Gamma rays   d. X-rays
    e. Neutrons

131. Tumor(s) most responding to radiotherapy:
    a. Sarcoma   b. Seminoma
    c. Lymphoma   d. Leukemia

132. High energy accelerator produces:
    a. X-ray   b. Electron
    c. Gamma rays   d. Neutron
    e. Proton

Recently Asked Question

133. Half life of Ir-192 is:
    a. 74 days   b. 60 days
    c. 60 hours   d. 74 hours

134. Linear accelerator is used to provide:
    a. Protons   b. Neutrons
    c. Electrons
    d. Electrons and X-rays

135. Bragg's peak effect is due to:
    a. Gamma Rays b. Proton
    c. Sound waves d. X-rays

136. Stereotactic radiotherapy is used for the treatment of:
    a. Stage 1 lung cancer single lesion
    b. Lymphangitis carcinomatosis
    c. CA base tongue with positive lymph nodes
    d. Miliary metastasis

137. After radical resection of chordoma, it should be best treated with which form of radiotherapy?
    a. Photons   b. Neutrons
    c. Protons   d. Electrons

ANSWERS

1. **Ans. d.** Samarium-153
2. **Ans. b.** Radioprotector
3. **Ans. b.** Stage I lung carcinoma
4. **Ans. a.** Brachytherapy
5. **Ans. a.** Proton
6. **Ans. a.** Isotope
7. **Ans. b.** Ionization of molecules (b > c)
8. **Ans. b.** Excitation of electron from orbit
9. **Ans. b.** Removal of orbital electron; **c.** Linear energy transfer (b > c)
10. **Ans. c.** DNA
11. **Ans. c.** Radiation present constantly from natural sources
12. **Ans. a.** X-rays
13. **Ans. c.** Radiation source used in body cavities or implated directly into the tissues
14. **Ans. a.** X-rays
15. **Ans. a.** Energy
16. **Ans. c.** Helium ion
17. **Ans. c.** 18 MV photons
18. **Ans. b.** α-particles
19. **Ans. a.** X-rays and Gamma-rays
20. **Ans. b.** Cesium-131
21. **Ans. a.** Erythema
22. **Ans. a.** Iridium 127
23. **Ans. b.** Cobalt 60
24. **Ans. a.** Polycythemia vera
25. **Ans. a.** Radium 226
26. **Ans. a.** Leukemia
27. **Ans. b.** Electron
28. **Ans. a.** Strontium 89
29. **Ans. c.** Gating
30. **Ans. a.** Lung cancer
31. **Ans. a.** Bone marrow
32. **Ans. b.** AML

For decades, researchers have been trying to quantify the risks of very low doses of ionizing radiation—the kind that might be received from a medical scan, or from living within a few tens of kilometres of the damaged Fukushima nuclear reactors in Japan. So small are the effects on health—if they exist at all—that they seem barely possible to detect. A landmark international study has now provided the strongest support yet for the idea that long-term exposure to low-dose radiation increases the risk of leukaemia, although the rise is only minuscule (K. Leuraud et al. Lancet Haematol. http://doi.org/5s4; 2015).

ICRP recommendations, which most national radiation-protection agencies follow, already call for monitoring of individuals whose annual exposure is likely to exceed 6 mSv. They restrict exposure to 20 mSv annually over 5 years, with a maximum of 50 mSv in any one year. Researchers found that 531 of the workers died from leukaemia during the average 27 years they spent in the industry; the data suggest that 30 of those deaths could be attributed to the radiation. Even in this large study, there was no direct evidence that workers who had accumulated extremely low doses of radiation (below a total of 50 mSv) had an increased risk of leukaemia, says Olsen. But a mathematical extrapolation of the data suggests that each accumulation of 10 mSv of exposure raised a worker's risk of leukaemia by around 3%, compared to the average risk of the group of workers in the study.

33. **Ans. d.** 1 year
34. **Ans. d.** 50 mSv
35. **Ans. a.** Cervix
36. **Ans. c.** 50 Gy

    The risk of major complications is increased when the dose of whole-pelvic radiation exceeds 40 Gy at 2 Gy per fraction or 45 Gy at 1.8 Gy per fraction. There is no clear evidence that fraction sizes of less than 2 Gy significantly decrease the rate of late complications, although daily fractions of 1.8 Gy may reduce the severity of acute radiation effects when large treatment fields or concurrent chemotherapy is used. Although 40–45 Gy is usually sufficient to control microscopic tumor in the pelvis, additional treatment must be given to control gross disease. ICRT is used to deliver a high dose to cancer in the cervix; enlarged pelvic nodes or lateral parametrial tumor may lie beyond the high-dose range of ICRT (intracavitary radiation therapy) but may be given additional treatment with small external-beam fields.

    Jhingran, A, Eifel, P, Glob. libr. women's med.,
    (ISSN: 1756-2228) 2008; DOI 10.3843/GLOWM.10234

37. **Ans. b.** Skin cancer

    Photodynamic therapy (PDT) is a treatment that involves the use of a light-sensitive medication and a light source to destroy abnormal cells.

    It can be used to treat some skin and eye conditions, as well as certain types of cancer.

    On their own, the medication and light source are harmless, but when the medication is exposed to the light, it activates and causes a reaction that damages nearby cells.

    This allows small abnormal areas of tissue to be treated without the need for surgery.

    PDT can be used to treat abnormalities in parts of the body a light source can most easily reach, such as the skin, eyes, mouth, oesophagus (light reaches by endoscope) and lungs.

38. **Ans. a.** Within 10 days
39. **Ans. c.** 6×10^{21}
40. **Ans. d.** Nonpenetrating
41. **Ans. a.** 0-18
42. **Ans. b.** Infrared
43. **Ans. c.** Charring of nucleoprotein
44. **Ans. a.** 100 rad
45. **Ans. c.** Radioactivity
46. **Ans. b.** Iodine-131
47. **Ans. b.** I123
48. **Ans. c.** Iridium-192
49. **Ans. d.** Cesium-137
50. **Ans. c.** ELISA
51. **Ans. d.** Cobalt-60
52. **Ans. c.** Uranium
53. **Ans. b.** 5.2 years
54. **Ans. b.** 8 days
55. **Ans. a.** 6 hours
56. **Ans. e.** 0.47 Mev
57. **Ans. a.** Beta particles
58. **Ans. c.** I131
59. **Ans. b.** 5 rads
60. **Ans. a.** 0.5 rad
61. **Ans. b.** Gonads
62. **Ans. b.** Lymphocyte
63. **Ans. c.** 40 Gy
64. **Ans. d.** G2M phase
65. **Ans. c.** Compton effect
66. **Ans. b.** Interaction between the low energy incident photon and the inner shell electron

67. **Ans. c.** G2M phase
68. **Ans. b.** G2M interphase
69. **Ans. a.** Cartilage
70. **Ans. a.** Ewing's tumor
71. **Ans. b.** Dysgerminoma
72. **Ans. c.** Medulloblastoma
73. **Ans. b.** Dysgerminoma
74. **Ans. a.** Osteogenic sarcoma
75. **Ans. d.** Seminoma
76. **Ans. b.** Small cell
77. **Ans. c.** Dysgerminoma
78. **Ans. c.** Osteosarcoma
79. **Ans. d.** Ca Cervix
80. **Ans. b.** Dysgerminoma
81. **Ans. d.** Malignant melanoma
82. **Ans. c.** Thyroid
83. **Ans. c.** Lung CA
84. **Ans. d.** Medulloblastoma
85. **Ans. c.** Hodgkin's lymphoma
86. **Ans. a.** Small cell Ca of lung
87. **Ans. a.** Radiotherapy
88. **Ans. c.** Cobalt is used
89. **Ans. b.** Metronidazole
90. **Ans. b.** Prostate
91. **Ans. c.** Cyclophosphamide
92. **Ans. d.** Malignant transformation
93. **Ans. c.** Radiotherapy
94. **Ans. a.** 8 Gy in one fraction
95. **Ans. b.** Stomach
96. **Ans. c.** Amifostine
97. **Ans. a.** Ca Cervix
98. **Ans. b.** Obturator lymph node
99. **Ans. b.** Dactinomycin
100. **Ans. a.** CNS
101. **Ans. a.** I-131
102. **Ans. b.** Pericardial Effusion
103. **Ans. d.** Growth hormone
104. **Ans. d.** Interaction between a low energy incident photon and the inner shell electron
105. **Ans. c.** G2M
106. **Ans. d.** X-rays and γ-rays have similar properties
107. **Ans. c.** Compton effect
108. **Ans. a.** Electron
109. **Ans. a.** Beta particle
110. **Ans. c.** Osteosarcoma
111. **Ans. a.** Ultrasonic waves
112. **Ans. d.** Sr-89
113. **Ans. d.** X-rays
114. **Ans. b.** Cs-137

Multiple Correct Answers

115. **Ans. a.** I-131, **b.** Co-60, **c.** Ir-192 **d.** I-125
116. **Ans. d.** Iridium, **e.** Cobalt
117. **Ans. a.** Cesium, **b.** Cobalt
118. **Ans. a.** Radon, **b.** Cobalt-60, **c.** Iridium, **d.** Cesium
119. **Ans. a.** Gonad, **b.** Bone marrow, **c.** Liver
120. **Ans. a.** Seminoma, **b.** Lymphoma, **d.** Ewing's sarcoma
121. **Ans. b.** Less radiation hazard to normal tissue, **c.** Maximum radiation to diseased tissue
122. **Ans. b.** Larynx, **c.** Anterior 2/3 of tongue, **d.** Lung
123. **Ans. b.** Ca Breast, **c.** Ca Pancreas
124. **Ans. a.** Superior vena cava syndrome, **b.** Pericardial tamponade, **c.** Increased ICP, **d.** Spinal cord compression
125. **Ans. b.** Enteritis, **d.** Pneumonia, **e.** Somatic mutations
126. **Ans. b.** Co-60, **c.** Cs137, **e.** Ir192
127. **Ans. b.** Lung carcinoma
128. **Ans. a.** Only used in head and neck, **b.** Damage to normal tissue, **d.** Only iridium used

129. **Ans. a.** Misonidazole, **b.** Actinomycin D, **c.** Oxygen
130. **Ans. a.** Alpha rays, **b.** Beta rays, **c.** Gamma rays
131. **Ans. b.** Seminoma, **c.** Lymphoma, **d.** Leukemia
132. **Ans. a.** X-ray, **b.** Electron and **e.** Proton

Answers of Recently Asked Questions

133. **Ans. a.** 74 days
134. **Ans. d.** Electrons and X-rays
135. **Ans. b.** Proton
136. **Ans. a.** Stage 1 lung cancer single lesion
137. **Ans. c.** Protons

CHAPTER 7

Nuclear Scans

Nuclear Medicine

Nuclear scans are different from radiological scans as in nuclear medicine studies, a radiopharmaceutical substance is administered, that is known to target a certain organ or organs. Its distribution is then examined to determine any pathologic condition in that particular organ.

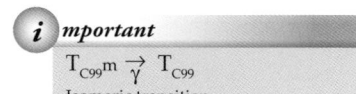

important

$T_{C99}m \xrightarrow{\gamma} T_{C99}$
Isomeric transition

Radiological studies	Nuclear scans
Predominantly uses X-rays	Gamma rays for imaging
Outside to inside	Inside to outside
Anatomical scans	Physiological/functional scans
E.g. CT scan	Bone scan

Most commonly used Radionuclide is Tc 99m

- Technetium-99m fulfills criteria of an ideal radio-nuclide.
- **Short half life of 6 hours**
- **Predominant emission of gamma rays of energy 140-keV**
- Tc-99m is obtained from the parent 99Mo (67-hour half-life)
- Taken up by salivary glands, choroid plexus, thyroid gland, gastric mucosa, and functioning breast tissue.
- Can cross placenta

Gamma camera, aka anger's camera is used to capture gamma photons generated by the radionuclide in the patient. It converts photons into a light pulse and subsequently into a voltage signal. This signal is used to form an image of the distribution of the radionuclide.

Radionuclide Scans

1. **Renal Scan**
   - **DTPA** (Diethylene triamine Penta acetic acid) is excreted through glomerular filtration and is the agent of choice for assessment of;
     - GFR
     - Vesicoureteral reflux
     - Perfusion
     - Obstructive uropathy
   - **Tc–99m Mercaptoacetyltriglycine** (MAG3) is a better agent for measurement of renal function as it has some tubular excretion as well but it is costly.
   - **Tc–99m DMSA** (dimercaptosuccinic acid) is suitable for imaging of; functioning cortical mass, pseudotumor versus the lesion. It is also the agent of choice for evaluation of scar in the kidney. It is also the agent of choice for differential renal function.
   - **I-131 OIH (Orthoiodohippurate)**-Largely replaced by Tc –99m MAG3 used for evaluation of Renal tubular function/effective renal plasma flow.

important
Metastasis from renal cell cancer doesn't show activity on bone scan as they are purely lytic.

2. **MDP Bone scan**
   - Used to evaluate cancer spread to osseous sites.
   - Sensitive but relatively nonspecific
   - False positive in healing fractures, arthritis, Paget's disease.

   Three-phase bone scan (99mTc-MDP): Characteristic finding in osteomyelitis: increased uptake in all three phases of scan.
   - Highly sensitive in acute infection.

3. **Meckel's scan**
   Pertechnetate is taken up by the gastric mucosa and is the agent of choice for evaluation of ectopic gastric mucosa of Meckel's diverticulum.

4. **GI nuclear imaging:**
   - Tc 99m RBC scintigraphy localize bleeding sites in patients with brisk hemorrhage so can be used to pick up intermittent bleeding.
   - The sensitivity is more than catheter angiography with bleeding rate as low as 0.05 mL/min can be picked up.

5. **V-P (Ventilation-perfusion) scan**

   Radioisotope scan in the form of V-P (Ventilation-perfusion) scan is the 2nd line **investigation** for the diagnosis of pulmonary thromboembolism. CT angiography is the investigation of choice for diagnosis of pulmonary embolism.

6. **Heart imaging**

   Multiple-gated blood pool imaging (MUGA), also known as, Equilibrium radionuclide angiography,
   - Provides an accurate, reproducible method for assessment of LV function.
   - Most commonly used when echocardiography is technically difficult or when poor LV function requires accurate quantitation.
   - **Involves the imaging of 99mTc-labeled** albumin or red cells that are uniformly distributed throughout the blood volume.

   Requires that the heart rate be reasonably constant.

   a. **Advantages of MUGA scan are:**
      - Higher information density than 1st pass method
      - Assessment of pharmacological effect possible
      - "Bad beat" rejection possible
   b. **Disadvantages of MUGA scan are:**
      - Significant background activity
      - Inability to monitor individual chambers
      - Plane of AV valve difficult to identify

7. **Biliary Scintigraphic Scan**

   Hepatic Iminodiacetic acid scan **(HIDA Scan)** is a biliary scintigraphic scan. Tc-99m acetanilide iminodiacetic acid analogs are HIDA agents and depending on their lipophilicity, there is a trade-off between renal excretion & hepatic uptake (HIDA is least lipophilic).

8. **Thyroid Scan**

   I^{123} is a preferred agent due to short half life and only gamma emission. In India, Tc 99m is used due to nonavailability of I^{123}.
   - Hot nodule → Adenoma and thyroid carcinoma (extremely rare)
   - Cold thyroid nodule → Inflammatory mass, Benign tumor and Malignant tumor

---

important
MRI is the most accurate investigation to assess ventricular function

important
a. **Myocardial Ischemia & viability can be studied:**
   i. **Directly** with myocardial perfusion imaging by
      - Thallium–201 chloride SPECT imaging
      - Tc-99m sestamibi/tetrofosmin SPECT imaging
      - PET
   ii. **Indirectly** with ventricular function imaging by
      - Multigated acquisition scan **(MUGA)**
      - First pass radionuclide coronary Angiography
   iii. **Simultaneous** assessment of myocardial perfusion + ventricular function by
      - First pass radionuclide angiography + gated **SPECT** perfusion imaging

important
FDG PET is considered to be the best noninvasive technique to assess cardiac viability.

important
Applications and indications of HIDA scan includes:[Q]
- Acute cholecystitis (**Gold standard**) USG is preferred nowadays for diagnosis because of the ease of performance
- Congenital biliary atresia (Excretion of the dye) in the duodenum rules out biliary atresia; May be false positive in severe neonatal hepatitis.
- Biliary leak evaluation
- Biliary-enteric fistula
- Chronic GB dysfunction

9. **Brain scan**
   - **Brain Tumors**
     - Localized defect on SPECT imaging in Both primary and metastatic brain lesions
     - **In the differentiation** of recurrent malignant glioma from radiation necrosis
   - **Epilepsy**
     - For evaluation of focus of intractable epilepsy like mesial temporal sclerosis which is the most common pathology
     - **PET imaging using** FDG is the method of choice for evaluating metabolism, whereas SPECT imaging with 99mTc perfusion agents, such as HMPAO or ECD, appears to be the method of choice for evaluation of perfusion status.

10. **Positron Emission Tomography (PET)/18-F DG PET SCAN**
    - Positron is a positively charged electron. No Tc is used in the PET scan.
    - Fluorine-18 (F-18) is most commonly preferred. To make the agent to go specifically to the site of interest, F-18 is coupled with deoxyglucose which gets more concentrated in malignant cells as they have much more metabolic demand compared to normal cells.
    - 18 F is a Positron emitter which interacts with an electron and cause the release of gamma-radiation (photons) upon collision with tissue. It is this gamma emission that is detected in the PET scanner.
    - **Basic principle:** Coincidence detection of paired high energy (511KeV) annihilation gamma photons from **positron emitting radionuclides** like carbon-11, nitrogen-13, oxygen-15 and fluorine-18.^{Q}
    - **PET camera:** Routine gamma camera is not used for PET imaging. PET detectors are made up of special material, called **BGO (Bismuth germinate) crystals**, which sensitively and specifically detects the high energy (511 kev) gamma photons produced after electron and emitted positron combine with each other.

important
$t_{1/2}$ of FDG is 110 minutes

important
Tumor cell proliferate GLUT-3 receptor on their cell surface which has high affinity for Glucose

a. **Advantages of PET:**
   - It is a 'unique tool' to study and quantify physiological and pathological function of human tissues and organs.
   - Imaging modality that permits noninvasive in vivo examination of metabolism (biochemical imaging), blood flow, electrical activity and neurochemistry:
   - Most accurate noninvasive method of detecting and evaluating most cancers.

b. **Clinical Applications of PET:**
   1. Oncology;   2. Neurology;   3. Cardiology
1. Oncologic (Glucose and oxygen utilization of tumors measured)
   - Lung cancer and pancreatic cancer
   - Differentiation of incidentalomas from metastasis in adrenals
   - Breast cancer
   - Colon cancer recurrence
   - LN metastasis from head and neck cancer Residual/recurrent tumor versus neurosis
   - Response to chemoradiation
   - Lymphoma staging
2. Neurology
   - Quantification of cerebral blood flow
   - Functional imaging of brain.
3. Cardiology
   - Myocardial Perfusion of the heart using Rubidium-82 tracer
   - Myocardial Perfusion of the heart using Ammonia N-13 tracer
   - Myocardial Viability using FDG: Hibernating myocardium uses glucose for metabolism

PET tracer (molecule)	Molecular mechanism of tumor uptake	Preliminary clinical data on future applications in oncology
[18F] fluoroethyl-l-tyrosine (FET)	Amino acid transport system	Clinical management of cerebral gliomas
11C-methionine (MET)	Amino acid transport system	Clinical management of cerebral gliomas

Contd...

Contd...

PET tracer (molecule)	Molecular mechanism of tumor uptake	Preliminary clinical data on future applications in oncology
C11-choline	Cell membrane synthesis targeting related to upregulation of choline kinase associated with cancer	Enhanced sensitivity and accuracy for the preoperative staging of prostate cancer in pelvic lymph nodes in prostate cancer
18F-FMISO (nitroimidazoles)	Nitroimidazoles are reduced to RNO2 radicals. bind covalently to intracellular macromolecules and remain within hypoxic cells	GBM, head and neck cancers. Hypoxia-specific treatment in patients with head and neck cancer
Ga-68-DOTATATE and others	SSTR uptake	Neuroendocrine tumor imaging and targeted therapy
18F-FES	Hormone receptor A binding through protein bound to albumin or SSBP (also known as sex hormone-binding globulin) to ER	ER imaging in breast cancer for prognosis, and prediction of response to hormone therapy
C-11 acetate	Uptake dependant on FAS expression in tumors	Prostate cancer for detection of recurrence
68Ga PSMA	Binding to PSMA	Androgen independence, metastasis in prostate cancers
18F-galacto-RGD and 18FAH111	Target the integrin molecule $\alpha v \beta 3$	Assessment of angiogenesis-inhibiting drugs

(FAS: Fatty acid synthase, ER: Estrogen receptor, PSMA: Prostate-specific membrane antigen, SSBP: Sex steroid-binding protein, SSTR: Somatostatin receptor, PET: Positron emission tomography).

Radioisotope (radiopharmaceutical)	Half-life	Imaging type
Indium-111 (In-111 pentetreotide), (In-111 DTPAOC), (In-111-DOTA-lanreotide), (In-111-DOTA-NOC-ATE), (In-111-DOTA-BOC-ATE)	2.8 days	SPECT
Technetium 99 m Tc-labeled hydrazinonicotinyl-Tyr3-octreotide (HYNIC-TOC)	6h	SPECT
Iodine-123 (I-123-Octreotide)	13 h	SPECT

Contd...

Contd...

Gallium-68 (Ga-68-DOTATATE) (Ga-68-DOTATOC) (Ga-68-DOTANOC)	68.3 min	PET
Copper-64 (Cu-64-DOTATATE)	12.7 h	PET
Fluorine-18 (F-18 FP-gluc-TOCA)	109.8 min	PET

(PET: Positron emission tomography, SPECT: Single-photon emission computerized tomography).

 important

The major application of ^{18}F-DOPA PET is in oncology, for the evaluation of neuroendocrine tumors. Neuroendocrine tumors have an increased L-DOPA decarboxylase activity and therefore show marked ^{18}F-DOPA uptake on PET examinations.

Clinical problem	Imaging technique	Radiopharmaceutical	Biological behavior
1. Head			
Epilepsy (presurgical localization)	Ictal SPECT	^{99m}Tc HMPAO	Uptake proportional to blood flow
	Cerebral metabolism PET	^{18}F fluorodeoxyglucose	Marker of glucose metabolism
	Interictal PET	^{18}F fluorodeoxyglucose	Marker of glucose metabolism
Dementia	Cerebral perfusion SPECT	^{99m}Tc HMPAO	Uptake proportional to blood flow
Cerebrovascular accident	Cerebral perfusion SPECT	^{99m}Tc HMPAO	Uptake proportional to blood flow
Hydrocephalus, CSF rhinorrhea, Encephalitis	Cerebrospinal fluid (CSF) study	^{111}In DTPA (intrathecal)	Marker of CSF flow.
	Blood–brain barrier (BBB) study	^{99m}Tc HMPAO	Passage across disrupted BBB
2. Neck			
Hyperparathyroidism (presurgical localization)	Parathyroid scintigraphy	^{99m}Tc MIBI	Differential expression of p-glycoprotein between parathyroid adenoma and thyroid
Thyrotoxicosis		^{123}I sodium iodide	Active uptake (^{123}I and ^{99m}Tc) followed by organification (^{123}I)
Thyroid nodule, Ectopic thyroid	Thyroid scintigraphy	^{99m}Tc pertechnetate	
Dry mouth (connective tissue disease)	Salivary gland study	^{99m}Tc pertechnetate	Secretion in saliva

Contd...

Contd...

Clinical problem	Imaging technique	Radiopharmaceutical	Biological behavior
3. Musculoskeletal system			
Tumor / Fracture / Avascular necrosis	Bone scintigraphy	^{99m}Tc polyphosphate compounds	Osteoblastic response (+ vascularity on early phases)
Arthropathy			
Lymphedema	Lymphoscintigraphy	^{99m}Tc nanocolloid	Lymphatic uptake and trapping
Metabolic bone disease			
Painful prosthesis / Osteomyelitis	Bone scintigraphy + white cell or gallium scintigraphy	^{99m}Tc polyphosphate	Osteoblastic activity
		^{99m}Tc- or ^{111}In-leucocytes	Leucocyte migration
		^{67}Ga gallium citrate	Binds to transferrin and leaks into extravascular space
4. Cardiovascular system			
Pulmonary embolism	Ventilation/perfusion (V/Q) scan	^{123}I fatty acids	
		Perfusion: ^{99m}Tc albumin	Pulmonary arteriole blockade
		Macroaggregates	
		Ventilation: ^{99m}Tc aerosols	Distributes in lungs in proportion to gas regional ventilation
		^{133}Xe gas, ^{81m}Kr gas	
Chest pain	Myocardial perfusion scan	^{201}Tl (thallous chloride)	K+ analogue indicating perfusion (ischemic heart disease) (delayed uptake reflects viability)
		^{99m}Tc isonitriles	Cationic complexes taken up by myocytes in proportion to blood flow
		^{99m}Tc teboroxime	Lipophilic compound which accumulates by diffusion
		^{99m}Tc phosphines	Uptake proportional to blood flow

Contd...

Contd...

Clinical problem	Imaging technique	Radiopharmaceutical	Biological behavior
Cardiac failure	Cardiac ventriculography (gated study)	^{99m}Tc red blood cells	Blood pool label
	Myocardial viability study	^{18}F fluorodeoxyglucose	Demonstrates shift from metabolism of fatty acids to glucose
Congenital heart disease	Quantitative shunt study	^{99m}Tc red blood cells	Blood pool label
5. Pulmonary system			
Solitary pulmonary nodule	Tumor imaging	^{18}F fluorodeoxyglucose	Marker of glucose metabolism
Occult lung disease (alveolitis)	Alveolar permeability study	^{99m}Tc DPTA aerosol	Passage across alveolar membrane into blood
6. Gastrointestinal system			
Ectopic gastric mucosa	Meckel's diverticulum scintigraphy	^{99m}Tc pertechnetate	Active uptake by ectopic gastric mucosa
Difficulty in swallowing	Esophageal transit and reflux	^{99m}Tc sulfur colloid	Transit of labeled material
Gastrointestinal hemorrhage	GI bleed study	^{99m}Tc sulfur colloid	Blood pool label extravasating into bowel
		^{99m}Tc labeled red cells	
Diarrhea (inflammatory bowel disease)	White cell scintigraphy	^{99m}Tc leucocytes	Leucocyte migration
Vomiting (gastroparesis)		^{99m}Tc sulphur colloid in egg (solid phase)	
	Gastric emptying study		Compartmental localization of labeled material
Dumping		^{111}In DTPA in orange juice (liquid phase)	
Ectopic splenic tissue	Splenic scintigraphy	Heat damaged ^{99m}Tc labeled red blood cells	Splenic trapping of damaged cells
Focal liver lesion (hemangioma)	Red blood cell study	^{99m}Tc labeled red blood cells	Red cell pooling

Contd...

Contd...

Clinical problem	Imaging technique	Radiopharmaceutical	Biological behavior
Cholecystitis Biliary dyskinesia			
	Hepatobiliary study	^{99m}Tc iminodiacetic acid derivatives	Uptake by hepatocytes and excretion into bile
Biliary atresia			
Bile leak (postoperative)			
Abdominal sepsis		^{99m}Tc	Leucocyte migration
	White cell or gallium scintigraphy		
Pyrexia of unknown origin		^{67}Ga gallium citrate	Binds to transferrin and leaks into extravascular space
7. Urological, adrenal and genitourinary systems			
Hypertension (renovascular disease)	Captopril renography	^{99m}Tc MAG3	Captopril-induced change in renal transit time and/or function
Renal tract obstruction	Diuresis renography	^{99m}Tc DTPA	Glomerular filtration
		^{99m}Tc MAG3	Proximal tubular secretion
Renal scarring	Static renal scintigraphy	^{99m}Tc DMSA	Glomerular filtration and proximal tubular uptake
Vesicoureteral reflux	Indirect micturating cystogram	^{99m}Tc MAG3	Compartmental localization
Adrenal medullary tumor	Adrenal study	^{123}I MIBG	Uptake by noradrenaline transporter
Adrenal cortical tumor	Adrenal study	^{123}I iodocholesterol	Incorporation into hormone metabolism
8. Cancer			
Skeletal metastases	Bone scintigraphy	^{99m}Tc polyphosphate	Osteoblastic response
Thyroid cancer	Whole body iodine scintigram	^{131}I sodium iodide	Uptake by Na/I transporter
Space occupying lesion in brain (SOL)	Tumor imaging	^{201}Tl (thallous chloride)	K+ analogue indicating perfusion

Contd...

Contd...

Clinical problem	Imaging technique	Radiopharmaceutical	Biological behavior
		^{18}F fluorodeoxyglucose	Marker of glucose metabolism
Soft tissue mass (sarcoma)	Tumor imaging	^{201}Tl (thallous chloride)	K+ analogue indicating perfusion
		^{18}F fluorodeoxyglucose	Marker of glucose metabolism
Tumor staging / Tumor recurrence / Tumor response assessment	Tumor imaging	^{18}F fluorodeoxyglucose	Tumor glucose metabolism
Neuroblastoma	MIBG scintigram	^{123}I MIBG	Uptake by noradrenaline transporter
Tumor hypoxia	Hypoxia imaging	^{18}F fluoromisonidazole	Trapped in hypoxic cells
Sentinel node detection	Lymphoscintigraphy	^{99m}Tc nanocolloid	Lymphatic uptake and trapping
Insulinoma			
Somatostatin receptor study / Carcinoid tumor		^{111}In pentetreotide (Octreotide®)	Binds to somatostatin receptors

QUESTIONS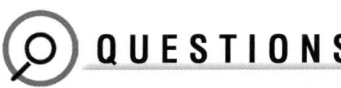

1. On 3 phase ^{99m}Tc- MDP bone scan, which of the following bone lesions will show least osteoblastic activity?
    a. Paget's disease
    b. Osteoid osteoma
    c. Fibrous dysplasia
    d. Fibrous cortical defect

2. Bone scan in multiple myeloma shows:
    a. Hot spot
    b. Cold spot
    c. Diffusely increased uptake
    d. Diffusely decreased uptake

3. Investigation of choice for locating parathyroid gland:
    a. Tc thallium substraction scan
    b. CAT scan
    c. USG
    d. Angiography

4. Gamma camera in nuclear medicine is used for:
    a. Organ imaging
    b. Measuring the radioactivity
    c. Monitoring the surface contamination
    d. RIA

5. Increased radioisotope uptake is seen in A/E:
    a. Primary bone tumor
    b. Osteomyelitis
    c. Paget's disease
    d. Pseudoarthrosis

6. Distribution of functional renal tissue is seen by:
    a. DMSA
    b. DTPA
    c. MAD3-Tc99
    d. I^{123} iodocholesterol

7. Vesicoureteric reflux is demonstrated by using:
    a. DMSA
    b. DTPA
    c. MAG3-Tc99
    d. I^{123} iodocholesterol

8. GFR is measured with which of the following?
    a. Iodohippurate b. ^{99m}Tc– DTPA
    c. ^{99m}Tc – MAG3 d. ^{99m}Tc-DMSA

9. Impaired renal function is assessed by:
    a. MAG3   b. Iodohippurate
    c. DMSA Scan   d. DTPA

10. Renal GFR is best measured by:
    a. ^{99m}Tc DMSA
    b. ^{99m}Tc pyrophosphate scan.
    c. ^{99m}Tc DTPA
    d. Creatinine clearance.
    e. ^{99m}Tc albumin scan.

11. Amount of I^{131} used for thyroid scan is?
    a. 5 Microcuries b. 50 Microcuries
    c. 50 Milicuries d. 500 Milicuries

12. In pancreatic scanning radioisotope used is:
    a. Cr51   b. Se75
    c. Tc99   d. I131

13. Which one of the following is the most preferred route to perform cerebral angiography?
    a. Transfemoral route
    b. Transaxillary route
    c. Direct carotid puncture
    d. Transbrachial route

14. Reversible ischemia of the heart is detected by:
    a. Angiography
    b. Thallium201-scan
    c. MUGA
    d. Resting echocardiography

15. ⁹⁹ᵐTc is derived from:
    a. Str-99   b. Mo-99
    c. Str-90   d. Mo-90
16. The half-life of ⁹⁹ᵐTc:
    a. 6 hours   b. 12 hours
    c. 24 hours   d. 48 hours
17. Dysprosium-16 is used for:
    a. Pituitary tumor ablation
    b. Resection of cerebral metastases
    c. Synovectomy in intractable arthritis
    d. Treatment of painful bone metastases
18. Multiple gated radionuclide cardiac MUGA scan is used for:
    a. Testing drug toxicity on myocardium
    b. Myocardial perfusion assessment
    c. Testing ventricular function
    d. Detecting myocardial aneurysm
19. Radioactive iodine used in radio-immunoassay:
    a. I-123   b. I-125
    c. I-131   d. I-133
20. Regarding cardiovascular imaging, false is:
    a. Perfusion agents: ⁹⁹ᵐTc-mibi, 201tl
    b. Viability agents : 18fdg, 201tl
    c. Multigated cardiac function muga: ⁹⁹ᵐTc-RBCS
    d. Infarct agents: ⁹⁹ᵐTc-pertectinate
    e. Angio-venography: ⁹⁹ᵐTc-RBCS
21. Commonly used agent for liver nuclear scan:
    a. ⁹⁹ᵐTc-sulfur colloid
    b. ⁹⁹ᵐTc-disida
    c. ⁹⁹ᵐTc-rbc   d. ⁹⁹ᵐTco4
22. In the nuclear bone scan all the following disorders will show up as 'hot spots' except:
    a. Metastasis to bone
    b. Multiple myeloma
    c. Osteomyelitis
    d. Hyperparathyroidism
23. Double density sign:
    a. Osteoclastoma b. Osteoma
    c. Osteosarcoma   d. Osteoid osteoma
24. Acute myocardial infarct scintigraphy is done with:
    a. Thallium   b. Gallium
    c. Neodymium
    d. Tc stannous pyrophosphate
25. Local pain can be treated with the following except:
    a. Portable MRI
    b. Diathermy
    c. Ultrasound therapy
    d. Transcutaneous electrical stimulation
26. Radionuclide scans are useful in following except:
    a. GI bleed   b. Cholecystitis
    c. Intrabdominal abscess
    d. Local staging of tumors
27. Radiation induced necrosis of brain—most sensitive:
    a. CT   b. MRI
    c. PET   d. Biopsy
28. Gastroparesis is most commonly diagnosed with:
    a. MRI abdomen
    b. Multidetector CT
    c. Scintigraphic scan
    d. High frequency ultrasound
29. Bilateral symmetric increased uptake on salivary gland scintigraphy is seen in:
    a. Sjogren's syndrome
    b. Pleomorphic adenoma
    c. Abscess   d. Calculi
30. Which of the following has the ability to identify ischemic or hibernating myocardium?
    a. ⁹⁹ᵐTc labeled compounds
    b. CT scan
    c. Gated single photon emission computed tomography
    d. Echocardiography

31. Contraindications to V/Q scanning include all the following except:
    a. Asthma
    b. Severe heart failure
    c. Right to left cardiac shunt
    d. Severe pulmonary hypertension

32. Best investigation to distinguish radiation necrosis from recurrence of a brain tumor:
    a. DWMRI with AOC mapping
    b. HMPAO SPECT
    c. MR spectroscopy
    d. PET scan

33. Positron emission tomographic (PET) scanning is useful in evaluation of the following except:
    a. Mycotic aortic aneurysm
    b. Solitary pulmonary nodules
    c. Staging lung cancer
    d. Lymph node involvement by malignancy

34. Brain SPECT utilizes:
    a. Radium   b. Technetium
    c. Plutonium   d. Barium

35. Most common radionuclide used for bone scan:
    a. I-123   b. Tc-99
    c. Cr-51   d. Sr-89

36. Investigation of choice in parathyroid pathology is:
    a. CT scan   b. Gallium scan
    c. Thallium scan
    d. Tc-thallium subtraction scan

37. Radionuclide scan done for parathyroid adenoma is:
    a. Sestamibi
    b. Iodine-123 scan
    c. 99m-Tc-sulphurcolloid
    d. Galliun scan

38. Investigation of choice in parathyroid pathology is:
    a. CT Scan
    b. Gallium Scan
    c. Thallium Scan
    d. Tc-Thallium substraction scan

39. The most accurate investigation for assessing ventricular function is:
    a. Multislice CT
    b. Echocardiography
    c. Nuclear scan
    d. MRI

40. Best Noninvasive test to assess cardiac viability is:
    a. Echo cardiography
    b. MRI
    c. Thallium scan
    d. FDG PET

41. Inherent soft tissue resolution is most poor with:
    a. CT   b. PET
    c. MRI   d. USG

42. Which tumor doesn't show activity on FDG PET?
    a. Typical Carcinoid
    b. Atypical carcinoid
    c. Large cell Neuroendocrine tumor
    d. Small cell cancer

43. Technetium-99m is most widely used and ideal isotope in diagnostic nuclear medicine because of all the following characteristics EXCEPT:
    a. Its half-life is six days
    b. It decays by a process by the virtue of which it emits gamma and low energy electrons, without high-energy beta emission.
    c. The low-energy gamma rays it emits easily escape the human body and are accurately detected by gamma camera.
    d. It can form traces by being incorporated into many biologically active substances so that it concentrates in the organs of interest.

ANSWERS

1. **Ans d.** Fibrous cortical defect
2. **Ans. d.** Diffusely decreased uptake
3. **Ans. a.** Tc thallium substraction scan
4. **Ans. a.** Organ imaging
5. **Ans. d.** Pseudoarthrosis
6. **Ans. a.** DMSA
7. **Ans. b.** DTPA
8. **Ans. b.** ^{99m}Tc-DTPA
9. **Ans. a.** MAG-3
10. **Ans. c.** ^{99m}Tc DTPA
11. **Ans. b.** 50 Microcuries
12. **Ans. b.** Se75
13. **Ans. a.** Transfemoral route
14. **Ans. b.** Thallium201-scan
15. **Ans. b.** Mo-99
16. **Ans. a.** 6 hours
17. **Ans. c.** Synovectomy in intractable arthritis
18. **Ans. a.** Testing drug toxicity on myocardium, **c.** Testing ventricular function
19. **Ans. a.** I-123
20. **Ans. d.** Infarct agents: ^{99m}Tc-pertectinate
21. **Ans. a.** ^{99m}Tc-sulfur colloid
22. **Ans. b.** Multiple myeloma
23. **Ans. d.** Osteoid osteoma
24. **Ans. d.** Tc stannous pyrophosphate
25. **Ans. a.** Portable MRI
26. **Ans. d.** Local staging of tumors
27. **Ans. c.** PET
28. **Ans. c.** Scintigraphic scan
29. **Ans. a.** Sjogren's syndrome
30. **Ans. a.** ^{99m}Tc labeled compounds
31. **Ans. a.** Asthma
32. **Ans. d.** PET scan
33. **Ans. a.** Mycotic aortic aneurysm
34. **Ans. b.** Technetium
35. **Ans. b.** Tc-99
36. **Ans. d.** Tc-thallium substraction scan
37. **Ans. a.** Sestamibi
38. **Ans. d.** Tc-thallium substraction scan
39. **Ans. d.** MRI
40. **Ans. d.** FDG PET
41. **Ans. b.** PET
42. **Ans. a.** Typical Carcinoid

    Neuroendocrine tumors of the lung arise from the Kulchitsky cells that are normally present in the bronchial mucosa and share the common neuroendocrine morphologic features including organoid nesting, palisading, rosettes, or a trabecular growth pattern. They can be classified clinically, radiologically, and pathologically into four subtypes: typical carcinoid, atypical carcinoid, LCNEC, and SCLC. Typical and atypical carcinoids represent low-grade and medium-grade malignancies, respectively, whereas large cell and small cell neuroendocrine carcinomas represent high-grade malignancies. Carcinoid tumors are isointense on T1-weighted MR images and hyperintense on T2-weighed images, with prominent enhancement. They have somatostatin receptors and can be identified on radiolabeled somatostatin analog indium 111 octreotide scans. Newer PET agents like Ga 68-DOTA TATE and other analogues have also improved the sensitivity of picking up these lesions. Carcinoid tumors with malignant potential show increased fluorodeoxyglucose (FDG) uptake at positron emission tomography (PET)/CT due to high metabolic activity. Thus, a patient with an established lung carcinoid can opt for conservative management if there is little or no FDG uptake at PET/CT.

43. **Ans. a.** Its half-life is six days

SECTION D

SPECIAL SECTION

- Few Thumb Rules in Radiology
- Image-Based Questions
- AIIMS New Pattern Questions with Answers

Few Thumb Rules in Radiology

- Bone fractures/congenital deformities—IOC-NCCT
- Osteomyelitis—MRI
- Bone tumors—MRI
- Bone metastasis—bone scan
- NCCT is IOC for bone fractures, stone (except gallstones – IOC is USG), air and acute cerebral bleed
- MRI is IOC for all skull and spine pathologies even the spinal bony metastasis.
- CT is IOC for most of the chest pathologies except pancoast tumor (MRI is IOC)
- CT is IOC for most mediastinal pathologies except posterior mediastinal pathologies like—Neuroenteric enteric cyst and neurogenic tumors (MRI is IOC)

INVESTIGATION OF CHOICE

- Multiple Bone Metastasis–Bone scan
- Spine Metastasis—MRI
- Avascular necrosis—MRI
- Bone Density/Osteoporosis-DEXA (Dual energy X-ray absorptiometry)
- Aneurysm/AV Fistula—Angiography
- Dissecting Aneurysm (Stable)-CTA (Unstable)—Transesophageal USG
- Pericardial Effusion-Echocardiography
- Loculated pericardial effusion—MRI > CT
- Minimum Pericardial Effusion—Echocardiography
- Ventricular Function—MRI
- Pulmonary Embolism—CT angiography (IOC) > Pulmonary Angiography (Gold standard) > V/Q Scan
- Interstitial lung disease (Sarcoidosis)—HRCT
- Bronchiectasis—HRCT scan
- Solitary Pulmonary Nodule—High resolution CT (HRCT)
- Posterior Mediastinal Tumor—MRI
- Pancoast Tumor (Superior Sulcus Tumor)–MRI
- Minimum Ascites/Pericardial effusion/Pleural effusion–USG
- Posterior Cranial Fossa–MRI
- Acute hemorrhage—NCCT
- Chronic hemorrhage—MRI
- Intracranial space occupying Lesion—MRI
- Primary brain tumour—contrast MRI (Gold standard however remains to be biopsy)

- Metastatic brain tumor—(Gadolinium) contrast enhanced MRI
- Temporal Bone—HRCT
- SAH Diagnosis—NCCT
- SAH etiology-4 vessel Angiography > CT Angiography (Gold standard is DSA)
- Nasopharyngeal angiofibroma—CECT scan. MRI for intraocular and intracranial extent
- Acoustic neuroma—Gadolinium enhanced MRI
- Obstetrics—USG
- Calcifications—NCCT
- Blunt abdominal Trauma—CECT Except unstable pt
- Acute necrotizing pancreatitis—CECT
- GERD-24 hour pH manometer > endoscopy
- Dysphagia-Endoscopy (1st investigation usually barium study)
- Congenital hypertrophic pyloric stenosis—USG
- Extrahepatic biliary atresia—perioperative cholangiogram. IOC–HIDA scan
- Obstructive Jaundice/GB Stones—USG
- Diverticulosis—barium enema
- Diverticulitis—CECT scan
- Renal TB (early)–IVP, (Late)—CECT
- Posterior urethral valve—MCU
- Ureteric stone—noncontrast CT
- Renal artery stenosis—Percutaneous angiography (Gold standard). (IOC–MR Angio)
- Discrete swelling (solitary nodule) of thyroid—FNAC

Radiological Appearance of Heart in Various Diseases
- Fallot's tetralogy: Boot shaped heart
- Tricuspid atresia: Box shaped heart
- TAPVC (total anomalus pulmonary venous connection): Snow man appearance, 8 shaped heart, cottage loaf appearance (Supracardiac)
- Constrictive pericarditis: Egg in cup
- Pericardial effusion: water bottle, pear shaped.
- Pulmonary hypertension: Jug handle
- Transposition of vessels: egg shell cracking/egg on side
- Hilar dance on fluoroscopy is seen in cases of ASD and Bronchiectasis
- Sitting duck sign is seen in—persistent truncus arteriosus

Emergency Radiotherapy is Given in—SANS
- S—Superior vena cava syndrome
- A—Acute epidural spinal cord compression
- N—Neoplastic cardiac tamponade
- S—Severe hypercalcemia

IMP Effective Doses (MSEV)

- **Chest (single PA film)**   **0.02**
- Skull   0.07
- Thoracic spine   0.7
- Lumbar spine   1.3
- Hip   0.3
- Pelvis   0.7
- Abdomen   1.0
- IVU   2.5
- Barium follow through   3
- Barium enema   7
- CT Head   2.3
- CT Chest   8
- CT abdomen or pelvis   10

IMP HU Values

Substance	HU value
Air	– 1000
Fat	– 50 to – 100
Water	0
Muscle	10-40
Blood	~60
Contrast	130
Bone	>400

IMP Half-Life

- *Isotope*   *Half life*
- Tc99   6 hours
- I123   13 hours
- I125   60 days
- I131   8 days
- I132   2.3 hours
- P32   14 days
- Co60   5.2 years
- Ra226   1622 years

- 18 FDG   110 minutes
- Ir192   74 days

Rigler's measurement and Eyeler's ratio are used to-differentiate LV enlargement from RV enlargement

Gold standard investigation for increased intracranial pressure—subarachnoid probe.

SIGNS OF SYSTEMIC RADIOLOGY

Neuroradiology

- Banana sign (antenatal US) — Refers to a banana-shaped configuration of the cerebellum. Associated with neural tube defects.
- Spalding sign — Overlapping cranial sutures. Sign of fatal demise on prenatal ultrasound.
- Tau sign (MRI) — Persistent trigeminal artery
- Bat wing appearance (MRI brain) — Appearance of 4th ventricle that may be seen with Joubert syndrome.
- Empty delta sign — Sign of intracranial dural sinus thrombosis on CECT
- Eye of the tiger sign — Low signal intensity circumscribing the globus pallidus in patients with Hallervorden-Spatz disease.
- Boxcar ventricles — Appearance of frontal horns that may be seen in Huntington's disease.
- Strawberry skull — Appearance of skull that may be seen on fetal US with trisomy 18
- Figure of eight (MRI brain) — Appearance of the brain in lissencephaly
- Mount Fuji sign (CT brain) — Tension pneumocephalus
- 'Salt and pepper' appearance on MRI — Paraganglioma
- Molar tooth sign (CT/MRI brain) — Joubert syndrome
- Salt and pepper skull — Hyperparathyroidism
- Starry sky sign CT — Appearance that may be seen with neurocysticercosis.
- Cloverleaf skull — Appearance of the skull that may be seen with thanatophoric dysplasia
- Tear drop sign (Orbits) — Blowout fracture
- Hot cross bun — Multisystem atrophy cerebellar type
- Humming bird sign — Progressive supra nuclear palsy

Cardiothoracic Radiology

- Figure 3 sign (CXR) — Appearance of the aorta that may be seen in patients with coarctation of the aorta.
- Comet tail sign — Produced by the distortion of vessels and bronchi that lead to an adjacent area of round atelectasis.
- Cob web appearance — False lumen in aortic dissection
- Bulging Fissure sign (CXR) — Klebsiella pneumonia.
- Egg on a string' heart — TGA

Few Thumb Rules in Radiology

- Crazy-Paving sign (HRTC lung) — Nonspecific appearance consisting of linear network or reticular pattern with areas of ground-glass opacification. Classically associated with pulmonary alveolar proteinosis.
- Epicardial fat pad sign — Sign of a pericardial effusion.
- Feeding vessel sign (CT chest) — Sign of pulmonary septic emboli. Can be seen with lung metastases. At times in wegener's granulomatosis.
- Sitting duck' heart — Persistent truncus arteriosus
- Bat wing appearance (chest) — Classic chest radiography finding for pulmonary edema.
- Finger in glove sign — Sign of mucous plugging seen with allergic bronchopulmonary aspergillosis.
- Golden 's' sign (CXR) — Right upper lobe atelectasis created by a central mass.
- Signet ring sign (chest CT) — Sign of bronchiectasis.
- Lambda sign (gallium-67 citrate scan) — Uptake in the hilar and paratracheal lymph nodes gives the appearance of a lambda. This is seen in sarcoidosis.
- Juxtaphrenic peak sign (CXR) — Tenting of the diaphragm that may be seen with right upper lobe atelectasis.
- Luftsichel sign (CXR) — "air cresent". Sign that may be seen with left upper lobe atelectasis.
- Naclerio's v sign (CXR) — V shaped lucency that may be seen over the left lower mediastinium in pneumomediastinum.
- Saber-Sheath trachea — Appearance of trachea that may be seen with COPD.
- Panda Sign — On a Gallium-67 citrate scan, uptake in the lacrimal and salivary glands gives the appearance of a panda. This is suggestive of sarcoidosis.
- Sandstorm appearance (CXR) — Pulmonary alveolar microlithiasis.
- Hampton's hump — Triangular opacity secondary to infarction in the periphery of the lung distal to a pulmonary embolism.
- Snowstorm pattern (CXR) — Silicosis
- Stripe sign — On a v/q scan, subpleural activity in a region of decreased pulmonary perfusion. Sign is used to rule out pulmonary embolism.
- Westermark's sign (CXR) — Regional pulmonary oligemia secondary to pulmonary embolism.
- Snowman's heart — Supracardiac total anomalous pulmonary venous connection.
(Figure of '8' or cottage loaf heart)

Gastrointestinal Radiology

- Ball-on-tee sign — Sign of papillary necrosis on IVU.
- Bowler's hat sign (ba enema) — Colonic polyp
- Carman's meniscus sign (ba meal) — Malignant gastric ulcer.
- Central dot sign (Doppler) — Sign of Caroli's disease.
- Champagne sign — Specific but not commonly seen ultrasound finding for emphysematous cholecystitis.
- Tip of the iceberg sign — Ultrasound sign that may be seen with mature cystic teratomas.
- Apple core lesion (ba enema) — Circumferential narrowing of the lumen secondary to colon cancer.
- Comet sign — Sign to differential a phlebolith from a ureteral stone. Calcified phlebolith represents the comet nucleus and the adjacent, tapering, noncalcified portion of the vein is the comet tail (also see soft-tissue rim sign).
- Medusa-lock sign — Round worm infestation
- Corkscrew esophagus — Diffuse esophageal spasm and presbyesophagus
- Lobster claw sign (IUV) — Sign of papillary necrosis.
- Paintbrush appearance — Linear striations of contrast material opacifying collecting tubules that may be seen with medullary sponge kidney.
- Double track sign — Appearance of hypertrophic pyloric stenosis that may be seen on upper GI series.
- Football sign (CXR) — Pneumoperitoneum (seen on supine radiographs).
- Frostburg's reverse '3' sign — Carcinoma head of pancreas (hypotonic duodenography)
- Lead pipe colon (ba enema) — Narrowing of colon with loss of haustra that may be seen in patients with ulcerative colitis.
- Picket fence — Appearance of bowel that may be seen on small bowel series with whipple disease or gastrointestinal amyloidosis.
- Coffee bean sign — Sigmoid Volvulus.
- Molar tooth sign (CT cystogram) — Perivesicular extravasation of contrast on CT cystogram in a patient with extraperitoneal bladder rupture.
- Corkscrew sign (upper GI series) — Midgut volvulus
- Moulage sign (enteroclysis) — Effaced loop of bowel that may be seen on a small bowel series in sprue.
- Nubbin sign — Reflux nephropathy involving the lower pole of a duplicated collecting system.
- Nutmeg liver — Pattern of liver enhancement seen with passive congestion.

- Keyhole sign (USG) — US appearance that may be seen with posterior urethral valves.
- Parallel track sign — Pattern of uptake that may be seen on bone scan in patients with hypertrophic osteoarthropathy.
- Starry sky sign — US appearance that may be seen with hepatitis.
- Shoulder sign (ba meal) — Appearance of hypertrophic pyloric stenosis that may be seen on upper GI series.
- Pearl necklace sign — MRI sign that may be seen with adenomyomatosis.
- Rosary sign — CT sign that may be seen with adenomyomatosis.
- Sandwich sign — Bulky lymphoma encasing mesenteric vessels.
- Target sign — CHPS.
  Intussuception.
  Hepatic candidiasis and liver metastases.
- Umbrella sign (on BMFT) — Sign of IC TB
- Soft-Tissue Rim Sign — Appearance of a ureteral edema surrounding a calculus. Helps differentiates a calculus from a phlebolith (also see comet sign).
- String of beads sign — Small bowel obstruction
- Whirlpool sign — US sign of midgut volvulus in a neonate.
- String sign — Ileocaecal TB, hypertrophic pyloric stenosis, Crohn's disease (seen on upper GI series).
- Tit sign — Appearance of hypertrophic pyloric stenosis that may be seen on upper GI series.
- Snowstorm pattern (ob/gyn) — US pattern for a molar pregnancy.
- Spider web — Appearance of collateral vessels that may be seen on hepatic venography in Budd-Chiari syndrome.

Musculoskeletal Radiology

- Sausage digit — Psoriasis
- Dagger sign — Ankylosing spondylitis
- Bamboo spine — Ankylosing spondylitis
- Blade of grass sign — Paget's disease (seen in leg bones)
- Linguine sign (MRI breast) — MRI sign that may be seen in patients with intracapsular breast implant rupture.
- Blood fluid levels (MRI) — Abc
- Sail sign — Elbow effusion
- Sandwich vertebra — Sclerotic end plates that may be seen with osteopetrosis.
- Bone bruise sign — Acl tear
- Hair on end skull — Hemolytic anemia/Thalassemia
- Bone in Bone'/Endobone sign — Osteopetrosis
- Crowded carpal sign — Volar perilunar dislocation

- Button Sequestrum — Eosinophilic granuloma
- Canoe paddle ribs — Appearance of ribs that may be seen with mucopolysaccharidoses.
- Saber shin — Appearance of tibia that may be seen with syphilis.
- Picture frame vertebral body — Paget disease.
- Celery stalking — Irregular appearance of metaphyses in patients with rubella. Also used to describe metaphyses in patients with osteopathia striata.
- Champagne-glass pelvis — Achondroplasia
- Scottie dog sign — On oblique radiographs, the posterior elements form the appearance of a scottie dog. Spondylolysis can have the appearance of a collar around the neck.
- Bullet carpal bones — Appearance of carpal bones that may be seen with mucopolysaccharidoses.
- Brim sign — Paget's disease
- Rugger Jersey Sign — Chronic renal failure
- C Sign — Subtalar coalition
- Deep lateral femoral notch sign — Acl tear
- Fallen fragment sign — Unicameral bone cyst
- FBI Sign — Lipohemarthrosis
- fish vertebra — Osteopenia
- Flaring of anterior ends of ribs — Rickets
- Fragment-In-Notch Sign — Bucket-handle tear of the menisci
- Groundglass appearance — Fibrous dysplasia of bone
- H-Shaped Vertebra — Sickle cell anemia
- Tumbling Bullet Sign — Post-traumatic bone cyst
- Trolley-Track Sign (X-ray) — Ankylosing spondylitis
- Lemon sign (antenatal US) — Refers to shape of calvarium associated with spina bifida.
- Half Moon Sign — Absent in posterior dislocation of the shoulder
- Lace like pattern (X-ray) — Pattern that may be seen with sarcoid arthropathy.
- Corduroy vertebral body — Appearance of thickening trabeculations seen in vertebral hemangiomas. (polka-dot sign on CT).
- Lacunar skull — Appearance of skull that may be seen in infants with Chiari ii malformation.
- Breast in a breast sign — Term used to describe fibroadenolipomas.
- Lateral capsular sign — Acl tear - segund fracture
- Metacarpal sign — Short 4th metacarpal
- Pedestal sign — Loosening prosthesis
- Bow Tie sign (MRI knee) — Discoid meniscus
- Crescent sign (X-ray) — Avascular necrosis

- Pencil in cup deformity — Erosion pattern of digits that may be seen in patients with psoriatic arthritis.
- Drooping shoulder sign — Inferior subluxation of the shoulder
- Cotton wool skull — Paget's disease
- Shepard's Crook Deformity — Appearance of proximal femur that may be seen with fibrous dyplasia.
- Snowstorm pattern (breast) — US pattern for breast implant rupture.
- Trough Line — In posterior shoulder dislocation, frontal radiographs reveal two nearly parallel lines in the superomedial aspect of the humeral head.
- Spade shaped tufts — Shape of tufts that may be seen with acromegaly.
- Vacuum Phenomenon (CT/MRI) — Degenerative disk disease
- Step-Off Vertebral Body Sign — Sickle cell, Gaucher's disease
-
- Trident hand — Appearance of hands that may be seen with achondroplasia.
- Wimberger's ring sign — A circular, opaque radiologic shadow surroundsing epiphyseal centers of ossification in patients with scurvy.
- Swan neck deformity — Rheumatoid arthritis
- Telephone receiver shaped femora — Appearance of femora that can be seen with thanatophoric dysplasia.

Few Important Discoveries in Radiology

- Antoine Henri Bacquerel — Radioactivity
- Charles Dotter — Image guided medical procedures; Father of Interventional Radiology
- David E. Kuhl — Positron Emission Tomography (PET)
- Ernest Rutherford — Alpha/beta particles, neutrons; Father of Nuclear Physics
- Godfrey Hounsfield — Computed Tomography (CT) scan
- Ian Donald — Ultrasonography (USG); Father of Obstetric Ultrasound
- John Caffey — Father of Pediatric Radiology
- Laterbeur and Mansfield — MRI (Nobel Prize in Medicine)
- Wilhelm Roentgen — X-rays (Nobel Prize in Physics); Father of Diagnostic Radiology
- Edward purcell — Discovery of Nuclear Magnetic Resonance

Image-Based Questions

1. Which of the following imaging has maximum radiation exposure?
   a.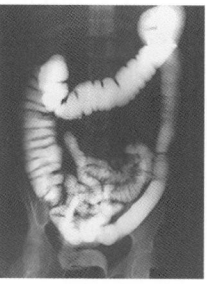
   b.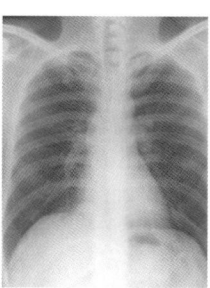
   c.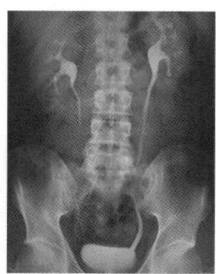
   d.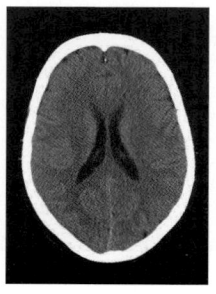

2. What investigation is being shown in the image below?

   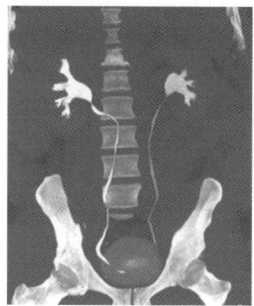

   a. IVP
   b. CT urography
   c. MR urography
   d. DTPA scan

3. Identify the marked structure in the following image?

   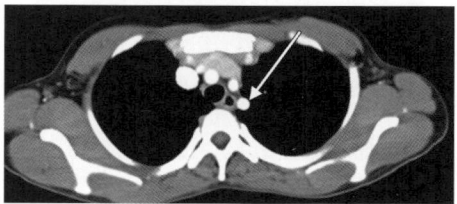

   a. Ascending aorta
   b. Descending aorta
   c. Left subclavian artery
   d. Superior vena cava

4. Identify the investigation.

   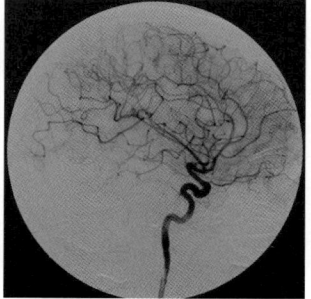

a. CT angiography
b. MR angiography
c. Catheter angiography
d. Doppler

5. Identify the investigation shown below.

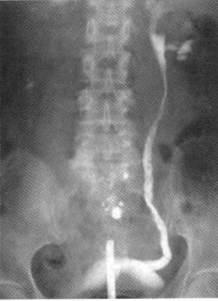

a. Renal angiogram
b. Antegrade pyelogram
c. Intravenous urogram
d. Retrograde ureterogram

6. Identify the investigation shown below?

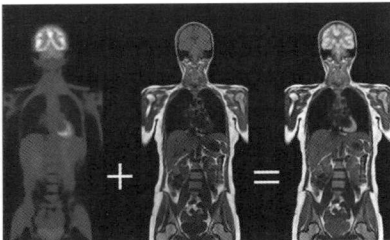

a. PET CT
b. PET MRI
c. SPECT
d. Functional MRI

7. What is the most probable diagnosis of the below given image is?

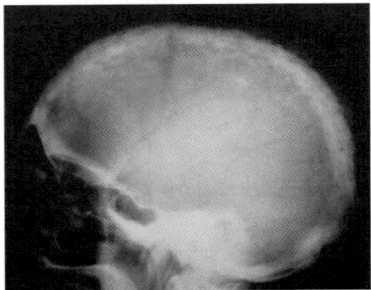

a. Multiple myeloma
b. Paget's disease
c. Hyperparathyroidism
d. Eosinophilic granuloma

8. A 45-year-old female presents with sudden severe onset of headache. There is evidence of neck rigidity but no fever. A CT was done and shown below. An angiography will most likely reveal the aneurysm from which vessel?

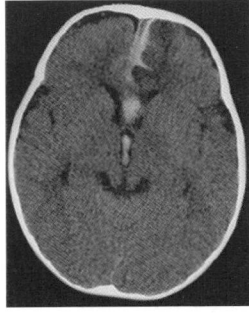

a. Right middle cerebral artery
b. Anterior communicating artery
c. Right anterior cerebral artery
d. Left anterior cerebral artery

9. A child had an episode of seizure and fell unconscious. The child was referred to a neurologist who prescribed for MRI head with spectroscopy as shown in the image below. What is the diagnosis?

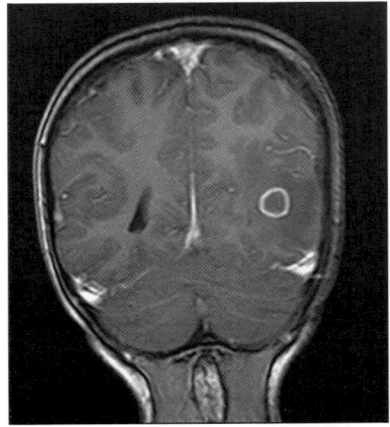

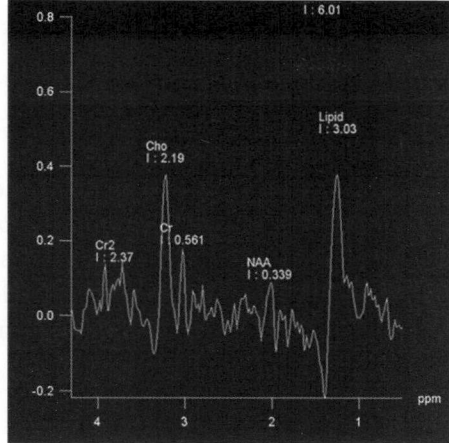

a. Tuberculoma
b. Metastasis
c. Abscess
d. Neurocysticercosis

10. A 42-year-old man presents to the doctor with c/o nervousness, sweating, tremulousness and weight loss. A thyroid scan is performed on the patient and image is shown below. The patient's findings are most consistent with which of the following disorders?

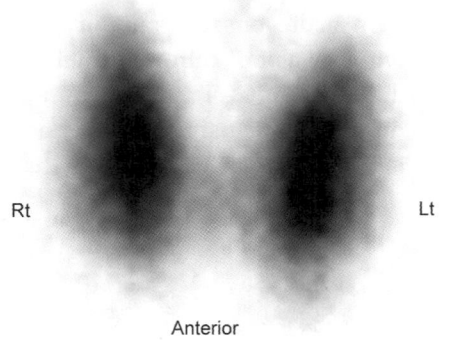

a. Hypersecreting adenoma
b. Grave's disease
c. Lateral aberrant thyroid
d. Papillary carcinoma thyroid

11. What is the most likely diagnosis of following image?

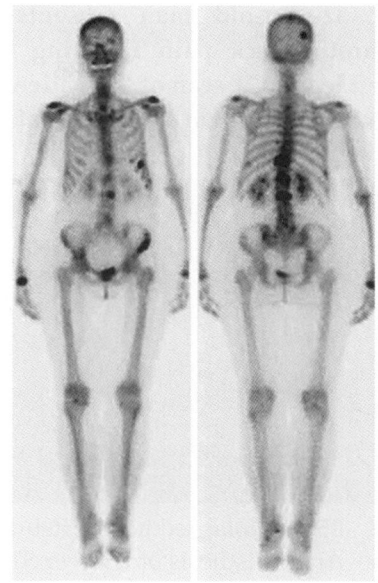

a. Hyperparathyroidism
b. Multiple myeloma
c. Skeletal metastasis
d. Stress fracture

12. A 27-year-old patient presented with back pain. On radiograph of the spine, this incidental finding is seen. Diagnosis?

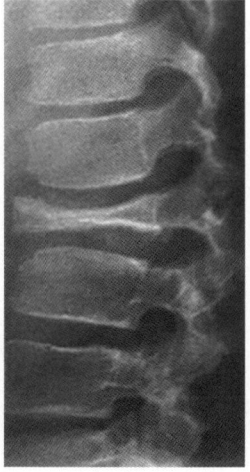

a. Hemangioma
b. Metastasis
c. Myeloma
d. Eosinophillic granuloma

13. A 32-year-old man presents with chronic back pain radiating to the left leg. A CT scan of the patients was done and shown below. What is the diagnosis?

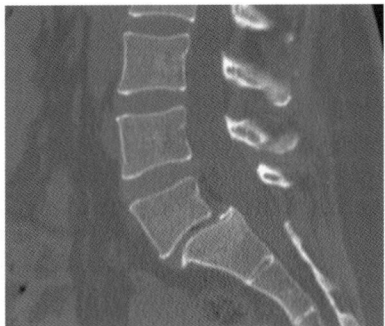

   a. L5-S1 prolapsed intervertebral disc
   b. Anterolisthesis of L5 over S1
   c. Retrolisthesis of S1 over L5
   d. Tethered cord

14. A patient of road traffic accident presented with fracture tibial condyles with knee joint swelling and effusion. NCCT of the patient reveals large joint effusion with fluid level with mean attenuation of contents in upper layer as '-95.5HU'. What is the slice orientation of CT scan image provided and diagnosis.

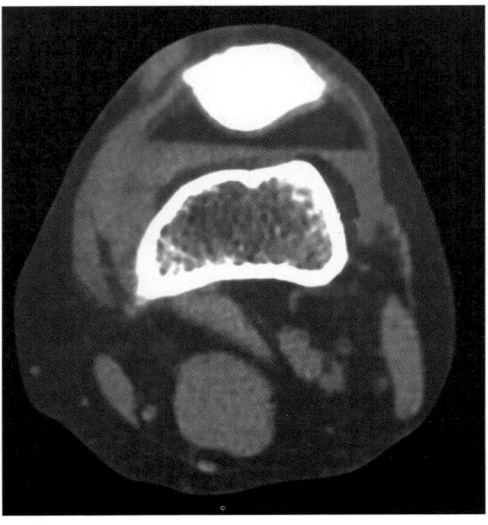

   a. Axial slice, pneumoarthrosis
   b. Axial slice, lipohemarthrosis
   c. Coronal slice, pneumoarthrosis
   d. Coronal slice, lipohemarthrosis

15. A child presented with features of acute onset intestinal obstruction with pain, vomiting and blood per rectum. Resident in the casualty advised ultrasound abdomen, which revealed following. What is the diagnosis and sign known as:

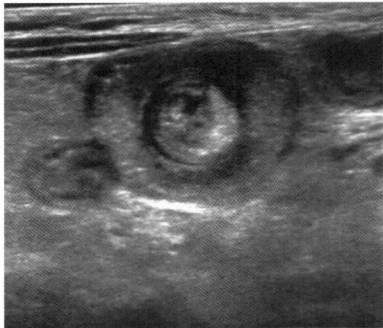

   a. IHPS, cervix sign
   b. Intussusception, dough nut sign
   c. Intussusception, target sign
   d. Worm infestation, hay fork sign

16. A patient presented in the emergency with acute onset respiratory distress, which was not relieving by bronchodialators. NCCT chest was advised due to inconclusive chest X-ray. What is the diagnosis?

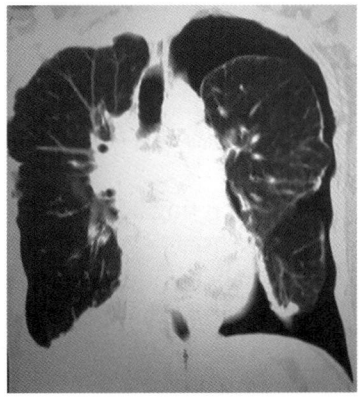

a. Pulmonary edema
b. Pleural effusion
c. Pneumothorax
d. Bronchiectasis

17. A patient presented with restricted movement of left shoulder after fall from a height. What is the diagnosis of the X-ray shoulder of the patient.

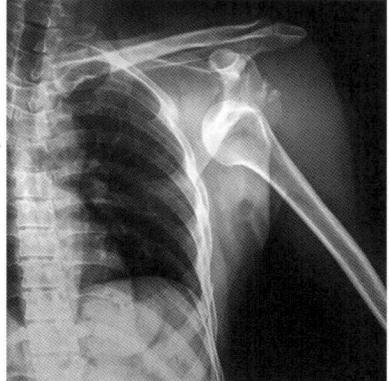

a. Posterior dislocation of shoulder
b. Luxatio erectia
c. Subcoracoid anterior shoulder dislocation
d. Simple bone cyst of head of humerus

18. A patient presented with vague abdominal pain in OPD. CECT abdomen was prescribed by the treating surgeon, which revealed an incidental focal hypodense lesion of '-50HU' mean attenuation in the right kidney. What syndrome the patient is most likely to be associated with:

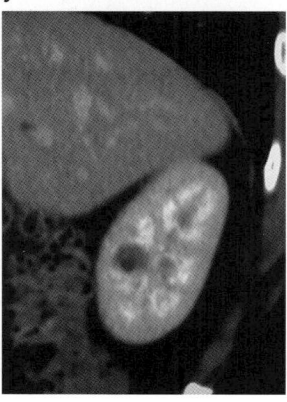

a. VHL
b. NF-1
c. Tuberous sclerosis
d. ADPCKD

19. An old patient presented with acute onset abdominal pain. Abdominal X-ray revealed gross pneumoperitoneum. All of the signs of pneumoperitoneum are seen in the X-ray provided except:

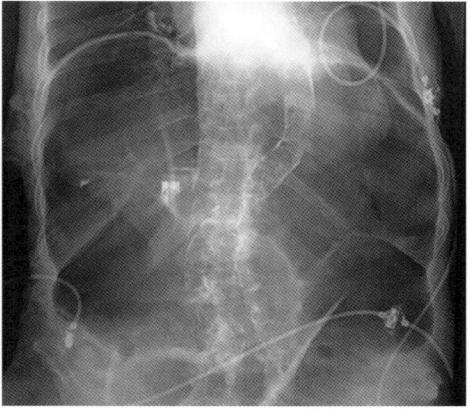

a. Gas under diaphragm
b. Falciform ligament sign
c. Cupola sign
d. Football sign

20. A young female with silicon implants in the breast presented after fall from height with vague pain in the breast. What is the study shown and what is the diagnosis?

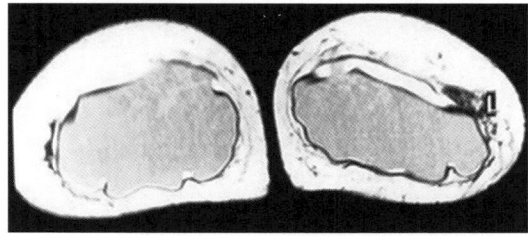

a. MRI, ruptured left silicon implant
b. MRI, ruptured right silicon implant
c. Mammography, ruptured right silicon implant
d. Mammography, ruptured left silicon implant

21. A child of rickets on treatment presented for follow-up visits to the pediatrician. What the X-ray reveals:

    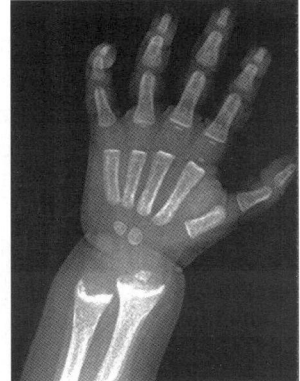

    a. Widening of growth plate
    b. Fraying
    c. Ring epiphysis
    d. Dense metaphysial line of healing rickets

22. Chest X-ray of an adult male presented with respiratory distress. What is the diagnosis?

    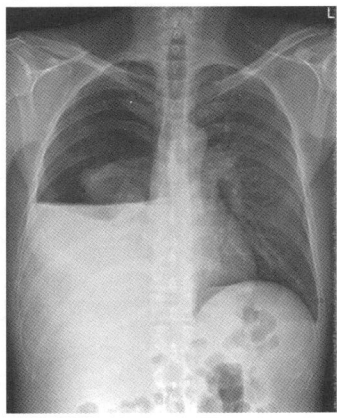

    a. Hydropneumothorax
    b. Pleural effusion
    c. Pneumothorax
    d. Consolidation of right lower lobe

23. A 28 years old female presented with knee pain in the orthopedics OPD. She did not have fever or constitutional symptoms. X-ray knee was advised. What is the diagnosis?

    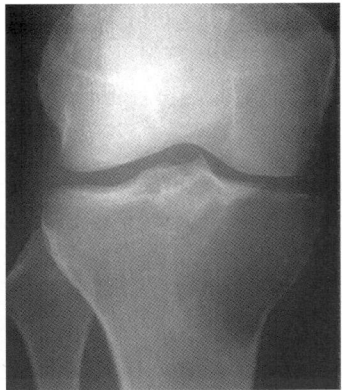

    a. Aneurysmal bone cyst
    b. Giant cell tumor
    c. Simple bone cyst
    d. Osteomyelitis

24. An adult patient was presented with severe low back pain at the level of L5 vertebra with no motor weakness. A CT LS spine was advised. What is the diagnosis and corresponding X-ray sign?

    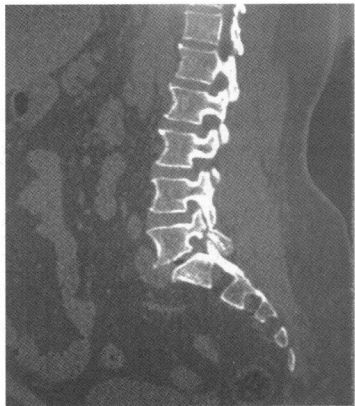

    a. Spondylolisthesis, Scottish dog with collar
    b. Spondylolysis, beheaded Scottish dog
    c. Spondylolisthesis, beheaded Scottish dog
    d. Spondylosis, Scottish dog with collar

25. A child had an episode of seizure and fell unconscious. The child was referred to a neurologist who pre-

scribed for a NCCT head. What is the diagnosis:

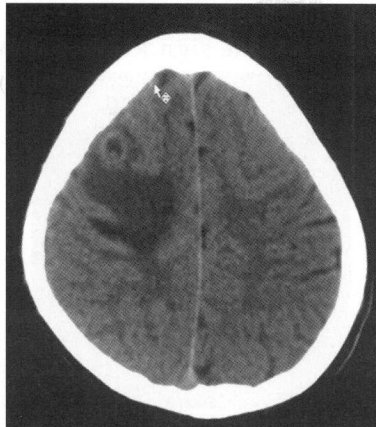

a. Tuberculoma
b. Metastasis
c. Abscess
d. Neurocysticercosis

26. An adult was presented with left scrotal swelling with no constitutional features, having a dull character. An USG was done by a radiologist who diagnosed it a left sided hydrocele. What is the characteristic USG finding in hydrocele.

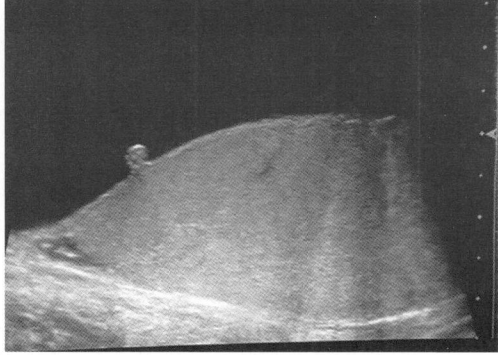

a. Isoechoic collection in scrotal sac
b. Hypoechoic collection in scrotal sac
c. Anechoic collection in scrotal sac
d. Hyperechoic collection in scrotal sac

27. A 36 years old female presented with lump in right breast with no features of nipple discharge, skin puckering or weight loss. USG reveals an oval iso to hypoechoic soft-tissue nodule which shows lateral distal shadow with no surface irregularity. What is the diagnosis.

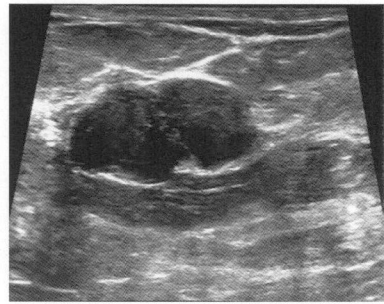

a. Breast abscess
b. Carcinoma breast
c. Fibroadenoma
d. Simple cyst

28. A patient was presented with knee pain and found to have a lytic lesion the X-ray. A NCCT was done for the better evaluation of the lesion and found to be a nonaggressive lesion. All the features are seen on this NCCT except:

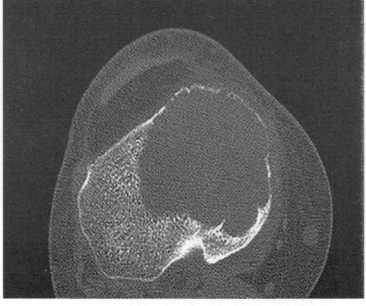

a. Well-defined lytic lesion
b. Narrow zone of transition
c. No surrounding sclerotic rim
d. Associated exophytic soft-tissue component

29. A female patient presented in the ANC OPD for routine checkup. She was found to have twin pregnancy.

USG was done to assess the chorionicity of the placenta. What is the diagnosis and USG sign on given image.

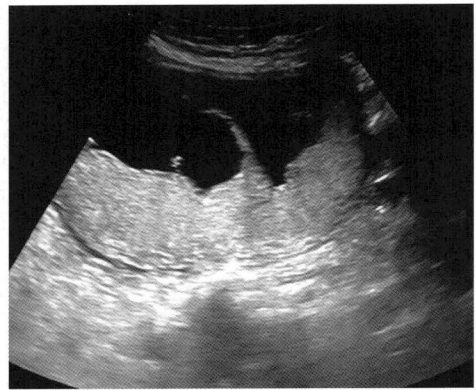

a. Monochorionic diamniotic, twin peak sign
b. Monochorionic diamniotic, T sign
c. Dichorionic diamniotic, twin peak sign
d. Dichorionic diamniotic, T sign

30. What is this USG sign (arrow) known as in the sonography of gallbladder?

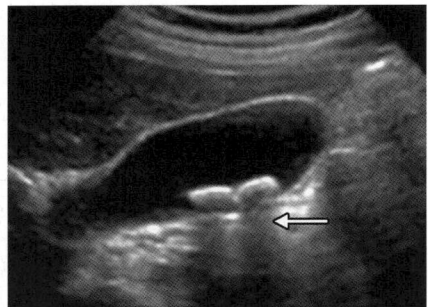

a. Acoustic enhancement
b. Acoustic shadowing
c. Comet-tail artefact
d. Twinkling artefact

31. Where do we see this sign?
a. Gallbladder calculi
b. Kidney calculus
c. Gallbladder cyst
d. Both A and B

32. In a patient with back pain, NCCT spine reveals the following appearance of the vertebra. What is the diagnosis and the sign known on X-ray?

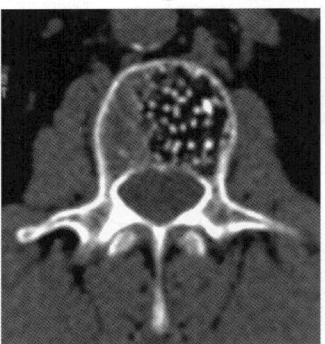

a. Hemangioma, corduroy appearance
b. Hemangioma, polka dot appearance
c. Osteoporosis, H-shape vertebrae
d. Osteoporosis, polka dot appearance

33. A patient presented in the chest clinic for follow-up of pulmonary Kochs post ATT having dyspnea. CT scan was advised which revealed:

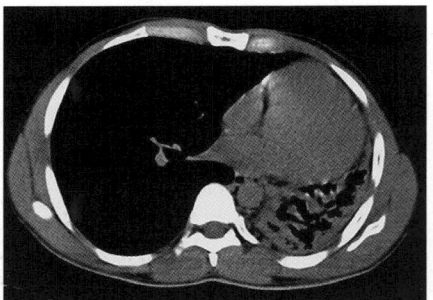

a. Consolidation with airbronchogram with ipsilateral mediastinal shift
b. Collapse with bronchiectatic changes and ipsilateral mediastinal shift
c. Collapse with airbronchogram and ipsilateral mediastinal shift
d. Consolidation with bronchiectatic changes with ipsilateral mediastinal shift

34. A patient presented with acute left lumbar pain of colicky nature. USG KUB was advised which revealed the following finding in left upper ureter (arrow). What is the diagnosis?

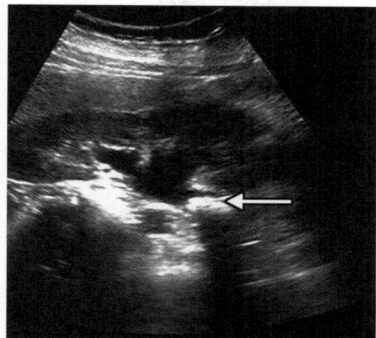

a. Pyelonephritis
b. Renal calculus
c. Abscess formation
d. Cyst with internal hemorrhage

35. A patient presented with dysphagia with pain. A barium swallow was advised. Which revealed multiple alternating constrictions and dilatations giving shish-kebab appearance. What is the diagnosis and gold standard investigation?

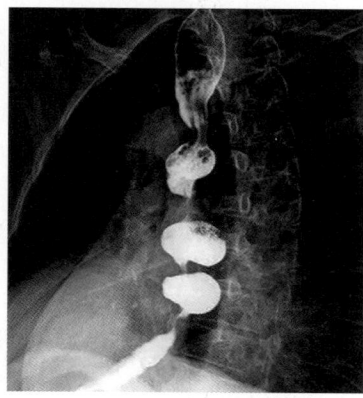

a. Presbyesophagus, barium swallow
b. Diffuse esophageal spasm, barium swallow
c. Diffuse esophageal spasm, manometry
d. Multiple strictures, barium study

36. A follow-up patient of healed pulmonary tuberculosis who had fibro-atelectatic collapse of left lung presented with acute onset respiratory distress, cough and fever. Urgent CECT was advised as the CXR was inconclusive. The CT revealed (arrow) in the right lung. What is the diagnosis?

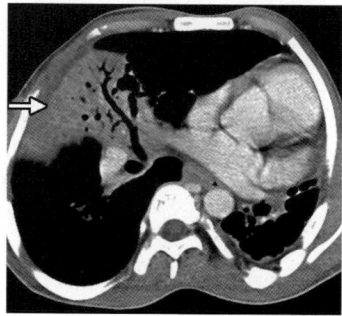

a. Collapse   b. Consolidation
c. Malignancy d. Abscess

37. A patient presented with acute abdomen and came to emergency department. After initial pain management X-ray abdomen was done to rule out acute obstruction. What is the diagnosis and sign known as?

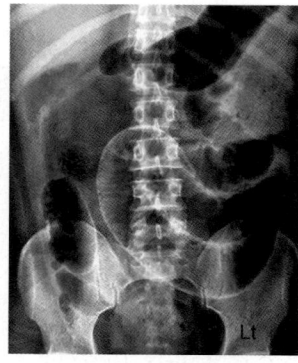

a. Hydropneumoperitoneum, football sign
b. Pneumoperitoneum, string of beads sign
c. Acute small bowel obstruction, string of beads sign
d. Pneumoperitoneum, Rigler's sign

38. An old age patient presented with left lower abdominal pain with bleeding per rectum occasionally. Barium enema was done. What is the diagnosis and sign in the radiograph?

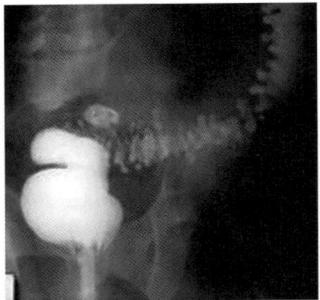

a. Hirschsprung's disease, transition zone
b. Diverticulosis, cork screw appearance
c. Diverticulosis, saw tooth appearance
d. Ulcerative colitis, pseudopolyps

39. An adult female presented with headache which was not responding to conservative treatment. Contrast enhanced MRI was done which shows the following space occupying lesion in the brain. What is the most probable diagnosis.

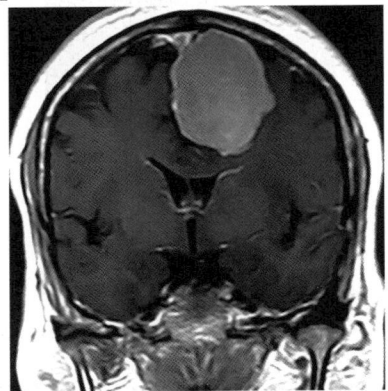

a. Medulloblastoma
b. Abscess
c. Meningioma
d. Ganglioglioma

40. An old aged patient presented with worst headache of his life. NCCT head revealed acute SAH. MR angiography was performed. What is the diagnosis (arrow)?

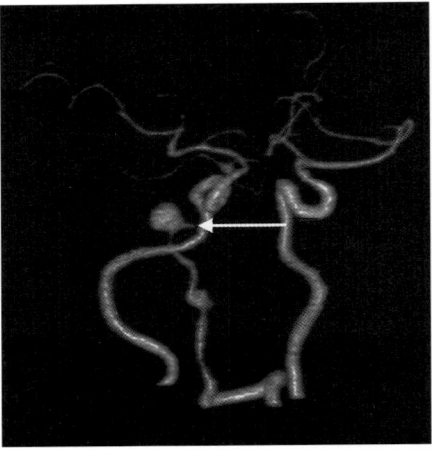

a. Arteriovenous malformation
b. Cavernous hemangioma
c. Fusiform aneurysm
d. Berry aneurysm

41. Identify the investigation done to rule out CBD calculus:

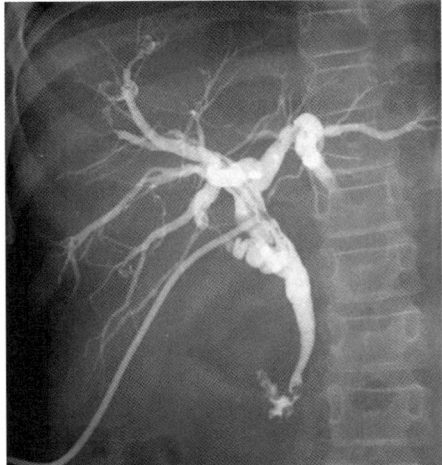

a. T-Tube cholangiogram, invasive
b. MRCP- noninvasive
c. T-Tube cholangiogram, noninvasive
d. ERCP, invasive

42. A diagnosed patient of severe peptic ulcer disease presented in the emergency with severe abdominal pain and abdominal rigidity. An emergency CECT was performed to see the cause of the pain. Which reveals:

    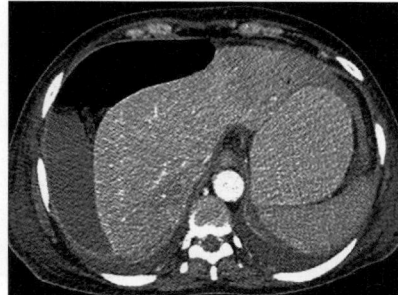

    a. Ascites
    b. Pneumoperitoneum
    c. Hydropneumoperitoneum
    d. Liver abscess

43. A child presented with severe leg pain with fever. On examination, a large soft tissue was noted in the leg. A radiograph was obtained which reveals a soft tissue and periosteal reaction. What is the probable diagnosis and the type of periosteal reaction.

    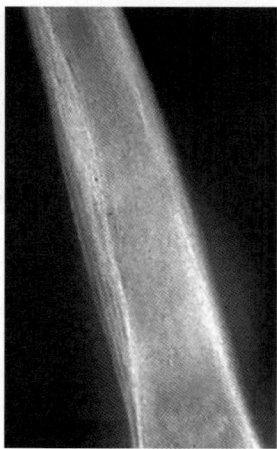

    a. Osteosarcoma, sunburst periosteal reaction
    b. Ewing's sarcoma, sunburst periosteal reaction
    c. Osteosarcoma, onion ring periosteal reaction
    d. Ewing's sarcoma, onion ring periosteal reaction

44. A child presented with pain in right shoulder. X-ray reveals an expansile lytic lesion with the radiographic appearance as shown below. What is the diagnosis?

    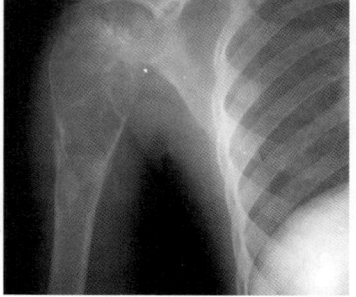

    a. Simple bone cyst
    b. Aneurysmal bone cyst
    c. Giant cell tumor
    d. Osteosarcoma

45. A follow-up case of healed pulmonary tuberculosis presented with hemoptysis. Chest X-ray was undertaken which revealed old fibrotic opacities in bilateral lungs and a focal lesion in the right upper zone (arrow). What is the probable diagnosis.

    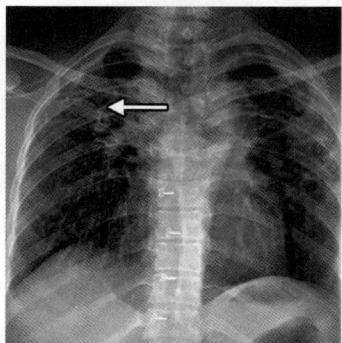

    a. Abscess with cavity formation
    b. Fungal ball with air crescent sign
    c. Hydatid cyst
    d. Consolidation

46. A patient from north east presented with respiratory distress. An NCCT was prescribed which reveals a large cystic lesion with following features. What is the diagnosis?

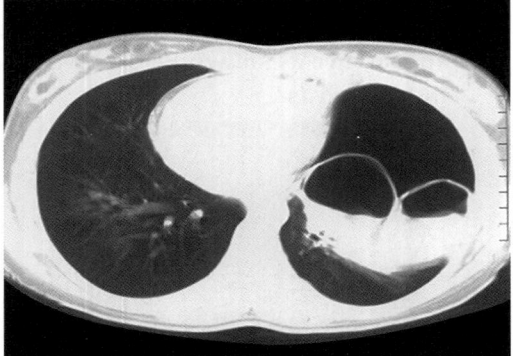

a. Lung abscess
b. Lung cyst (simple)
c. Hydatid cyst
d. Hydropneumothorax

47. What is the diagnosis?

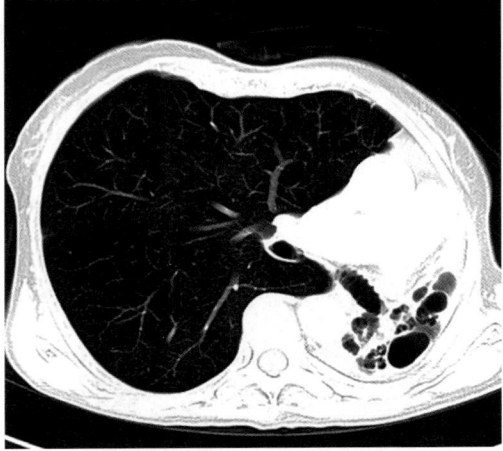

a. Consolidation
b. Collapse with no mediastinal shift
c. Collapse with mediastinal shift
d. Collapse with mediastinal shift with bronchiectasis

48. A child presented with acute respiratory distress. X-ray reveals a life threatening condition. Diagnosis is:

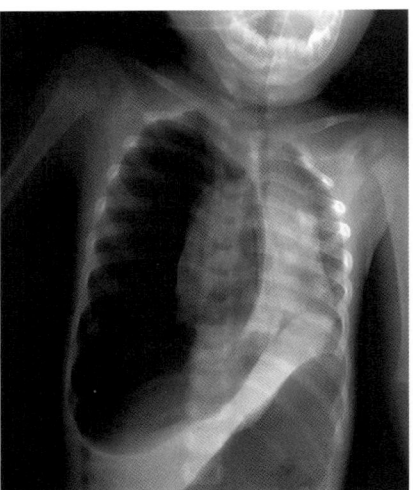

a. Hydropneumothorax
b. Pneumothorax
c. Tension pneumothorax
d. Collapse of lung with hyperinflated contralateral lung

49. A patient of tuberculosis underwent CECT which reveals following findings.

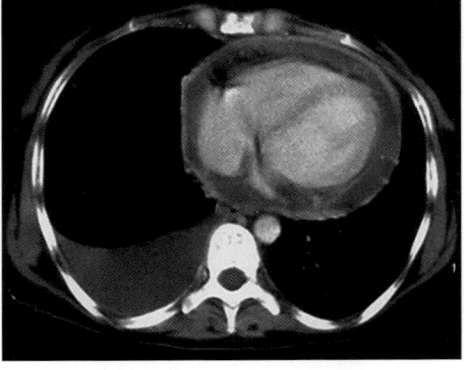

a. Pleural effusion and pericardial effusion
b. Pleural effusion and pericarditis with effusion
c. Empyema and pericarditis with effusion
d. Empyema with pericardial effusion

50. An ICU patient presented with acute respiratory distress and frothy pink sputum. CXR reveals:

52. What is the diagnosis of the X-ray of a patient presented with mono articular pain?

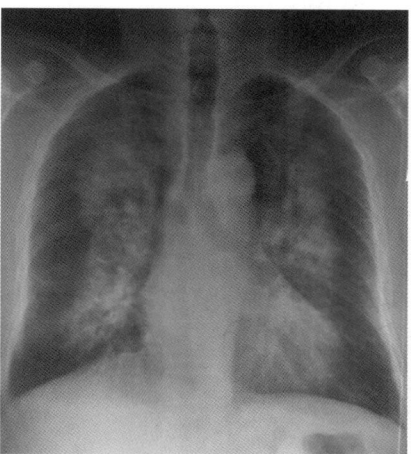

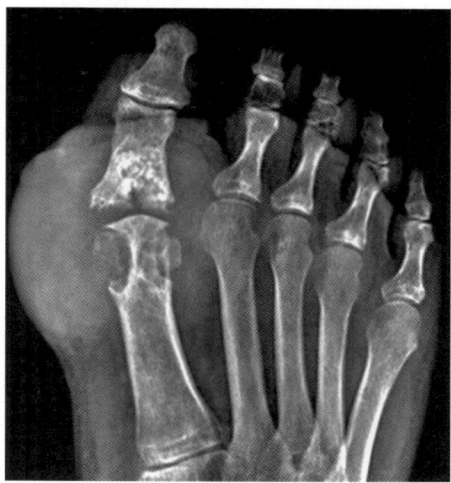

a. Acute pulmonary edema with cephalisation of pulmonary vessels
b. Pulmonary edema with acute interstitial edema and septal thickening
c. Aspiration pneumonia with pleural effusion
d. Frank pulmonary edema with bat wing appearance

a. Psoriatic arthritis
b. Gout
c. Rheumatoid arthritis
d. Osteomyelitis

51. Identify aortic knuckle in the given CXR

53. What is the prominent finding seen in the X-ray of hand?

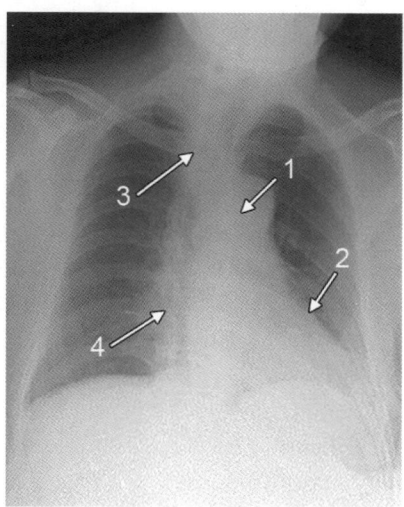

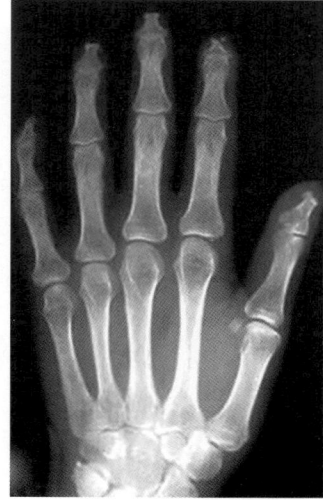

a. 1
b. 2
c. 3
d. 4

a. Sea gull sign
b. Pencil in cup deformity
c. Acro-osteolysis
d. Mouse nibben erosions at articular margins

54. What is the appearance of the CSF in the given MRI image of brain as compared to brain parenchyma?

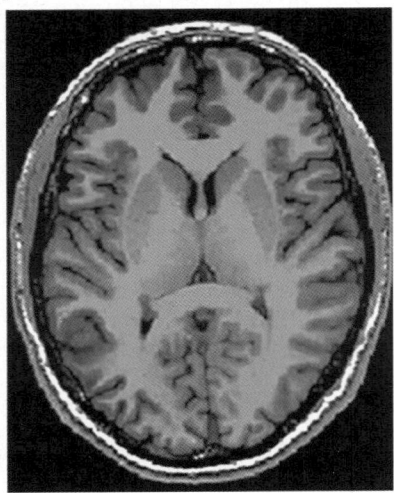

a. Hypointense
b. Hyperintense
c. Isointense
d. Hypodense

55. What is the view of orientation of the given MRI spine image?

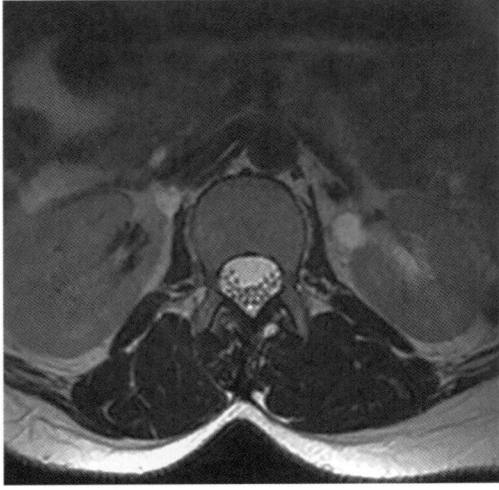

a. Axial
b. Sagittal
c. Coronal
d. Oblique

56. What is pathology seen in the chest X-ray?

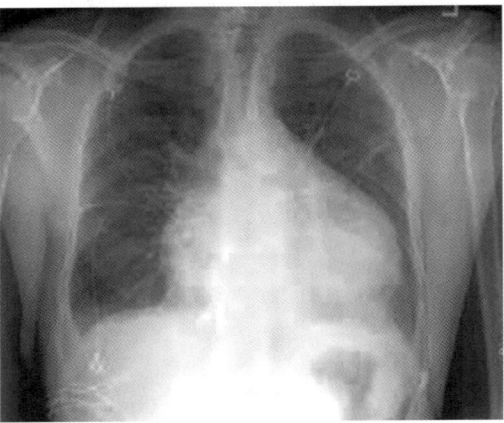

a. Pericardial effusion
b. Pneumopericardium
c. Tetralogy of Fallot
d. Transposition of great arteries

57. What is the most probable diagnosis of the young female presented with shortness of breath with no sputum production?

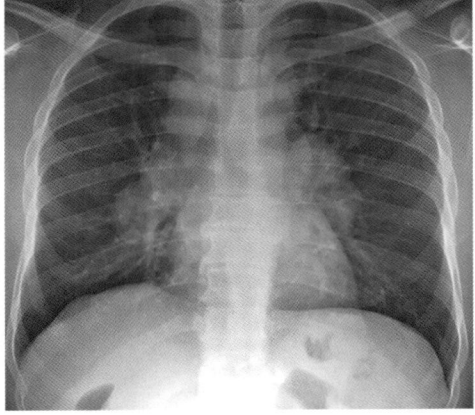

a. Tuberculosis
b. Silicosis
c. Sarcoidosis
d. Pneumonia

58. What are the findings seen in the chest X-ray of a patient of pulmonary tuberculosis?

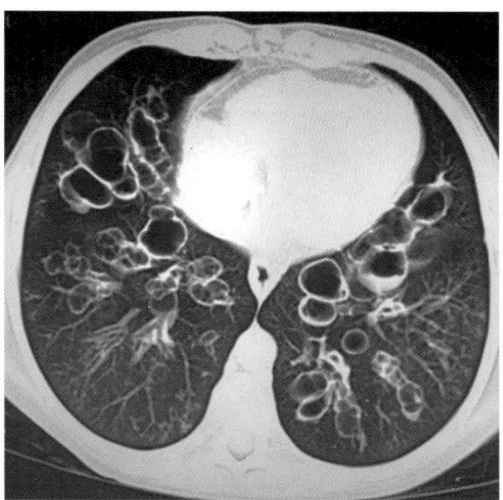

a. Cystic bronchiectasis, tree in bud nodules
b. Cystic bronchiectasis, pneumonic consolidation
c. Cylindrical bronchiectasis, tree in bud
d. Cylindrical bronchiectasis, consolidation

59. Barium swallow of a patient presented with dysphagia reveals following. What is the diagnosis?

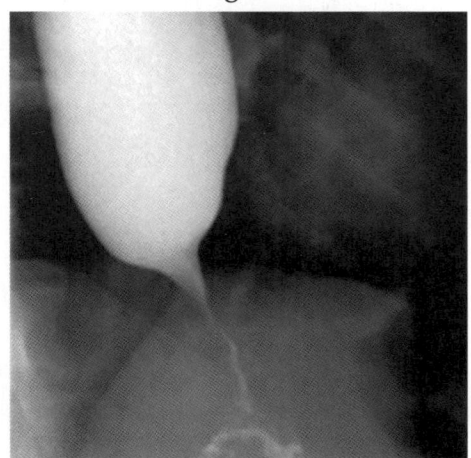

a. Diffuse oesophageal spasm
b. Carcinoma oesophagus
c. Achalasia cardia
d. Schatzki's ring

60. Identify the study?

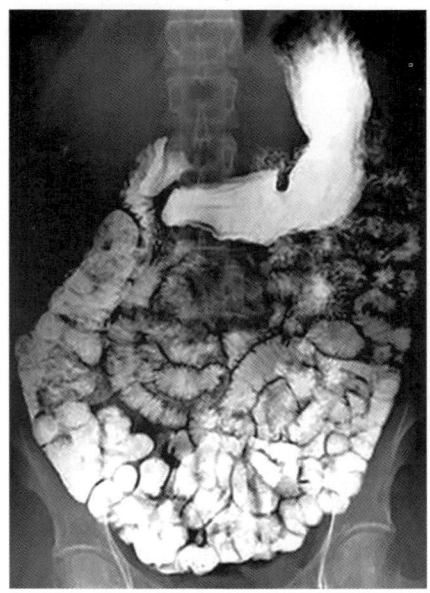

a. Barium swallow
b. Barium meal
c. Barium meal follow through
d. Barium enema

61. Identify the study?

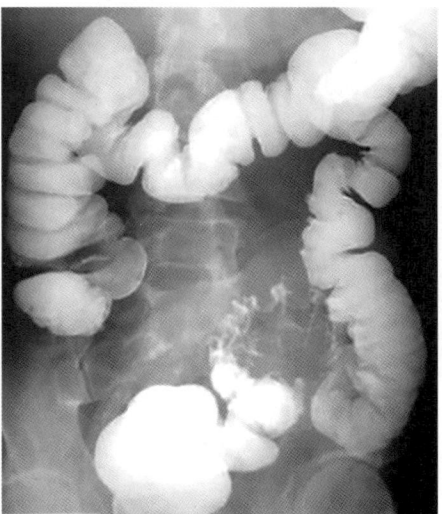

a. Barium swallow
b. Barium meal
c. Barium meal follow through
d. Barium enema

62. What is the diagnosis?

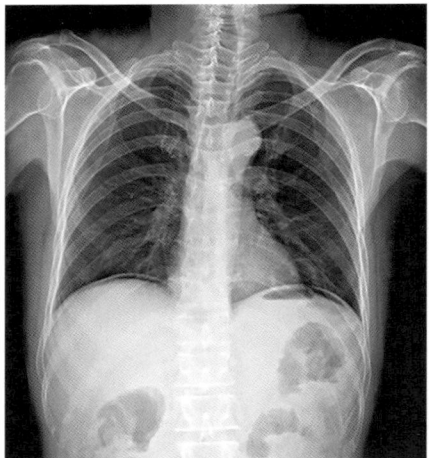

a. Pneumothorax
b. Pneumoperitoneum
c. Pneumomediastinum
d. Chilaiditi syndrome

63. What is the view and diagnosis of X-ray of a patient presented with respiratory distress?

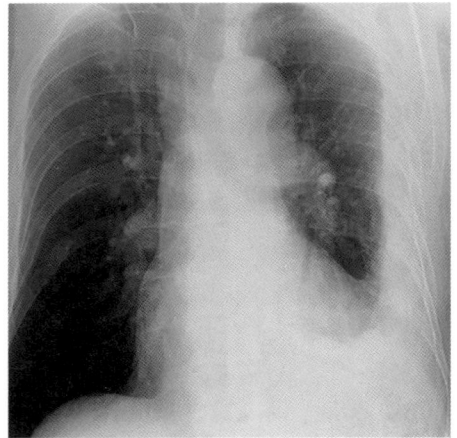

a. Frontal chest X-ray with pleural effusion
b. Lateral chest X-ray with pleural effusion
c. Lateral decubitus chest X-ray with pleural effusion
d. Supine chest X-ray with pleural effusion

64. Identify the caudate nucleus in the axial section of brain at the level of basal ganglia?

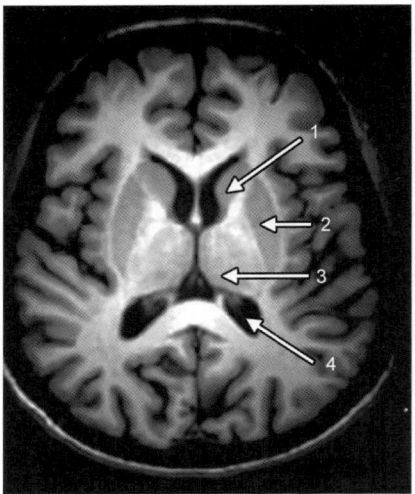

a. 1 b. 2
c. 3 d. 4

65. A patient presents with anosmia for 3 months. He has soft tissue growth from right side of the nose. CT image shows the following. What is your diagnosis?

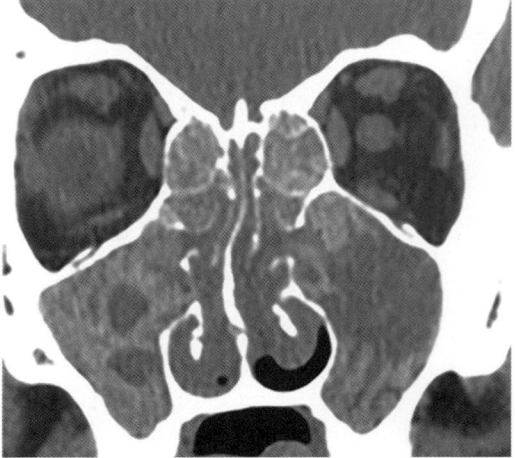

a. Antrochonal polyp
b. Fungal sinusitis
c. Ethmoidal polyp
d. Ethmoidal nasal Ca

RECENTLY ASKED IBQ

66. Identify the investigation done for identifying femoro-popliteal block.

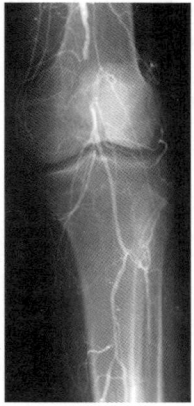

   a. CT angiography
   b. MR angiography
   c. Catheter angiography
   d. Doppler

67. What is pathology seen in the given chest X-ray?

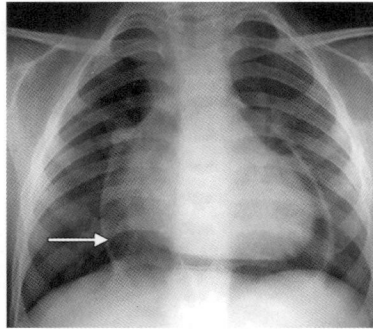

   a. Pericardial effusion
   b. Pneumopericardium
   c. Tetralogy of Fallot
   d. Transposition of great arteries

68. A 33-year-old woman presents to the emergency with diffuse, cramping abdominal pain, nausea and vomiting that began this morning. The abdominal pain is diffuse throughout and the patient also describes her abdomen as looking slightly enlarged. She has a history of chronic pancreatitis, as well as a cholecystectomy and two caesarean sections. The patient states that she has had flatus but no bowel movements since the pain began. On physical examination, there is diffuse abdominal distention and high-pitched bowel sounds without rebound tenderness of guarding present. Given the clinical picture and upright X-ray of the abdomen shown in the image, which of the following is the most likely diagnosis?

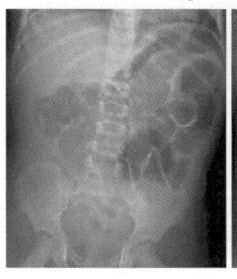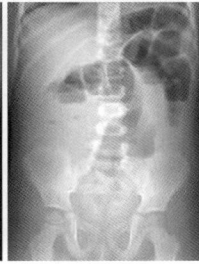

   a. Colon cancer
   b. Mesenteric ischemia
   c. Pancreatitis
   d. Small bowel obstruction

69. What investigation is being shown in the image below?

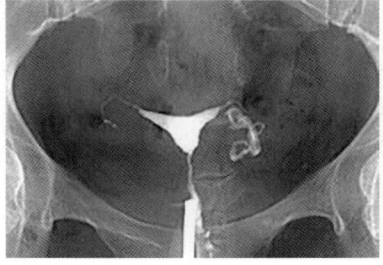

   a. Conventional HSG
   b. CT HSG
   c. MR HSG
   d. USG HSG

70. A 32-year-old man presents with sudden onset pain in the back radiating

to the left leg. A MRI was done and shown below. What is the diagnosis?

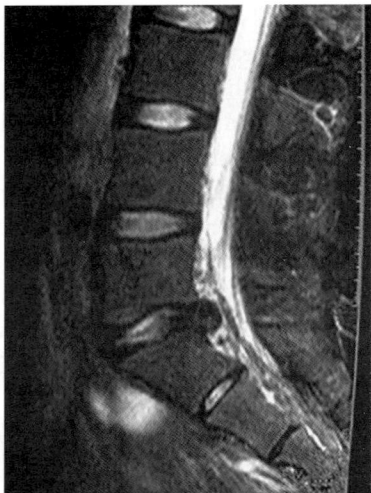

a. L5-S1 prolapsed intervertebral disc
b. Anterolisthesis of L5 over S1
c. Retrolisthesis of L4 over L5
d. Tethered cord

71. A 36-week pregnant female comes for Doppler examination. Doppler of umbilical artery is shown in figure. What is the finding?

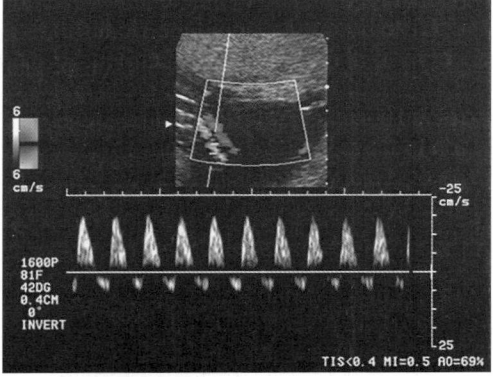

a. Reversal of flow
b. Dampening of forward diastolic flow
c. Presence of diastolic notch
d. Absent diastolic flow

72. A 42-year-old man presents to the doctor with c/o nervousness, sweating, tremulousness and weight loss. A thyroid scan is performed on the patient and image is shown below. The patient's findings are most consistent with which of the following disorders?

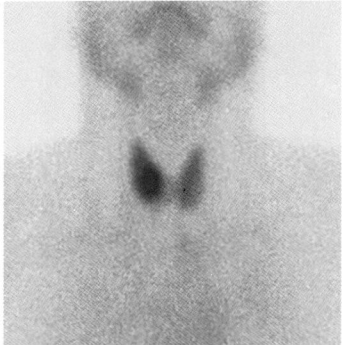

a. Hypersecreting adenoma
b. Grave's disease
c. Lateral aberrant thyroid
d. Papillary carcinoma thyroid

73. A 55-year-old male having bony pains for last two year present with the image as shown below. Most probable diagnosis is:

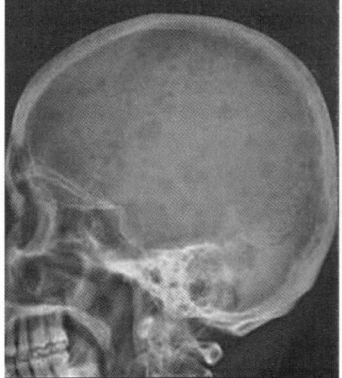

a. Multiple myeloma
b. Paget's disease
c. Hyperparathyroidism
d. Eosinophilic granuloma

74. A 45-year-old female presents with sudden severe onset of headache. There is evidence of neck rigid-

ity but no fever. A CT was done and shown below. An angiography will most likely reveal the aneurysm from which vessel?

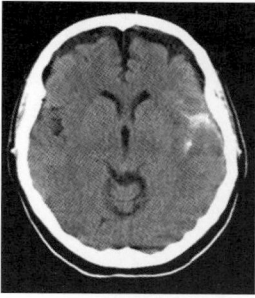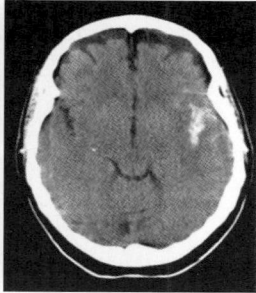

a. Left middle cerebral artery
b. Left posterior communicating artery
c. Left anterior cerebral artery
d. Left posterior cerebral artery

75. A 45-year-old female presented with chest pain and breathless in the causality and below is the representative CT section. What is the most likely cause of her symptom?

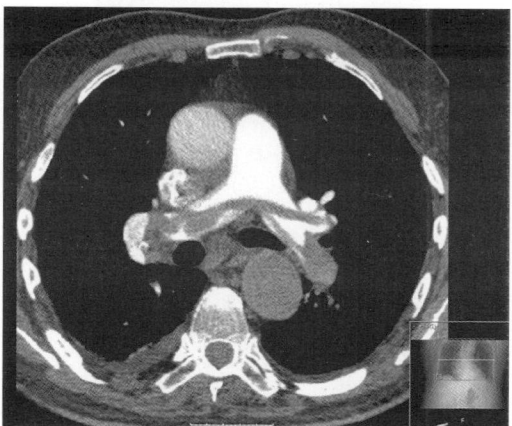

a. Aortic dissection
b. Pulmonary embolism
c. Aortic aneurysm
d. Myocardial infarction

76. A 27-year-old female presents with pain in the right hypochondrium. She is having tenderness at the Murphy's point. A USG is done. What is the diagnosis?

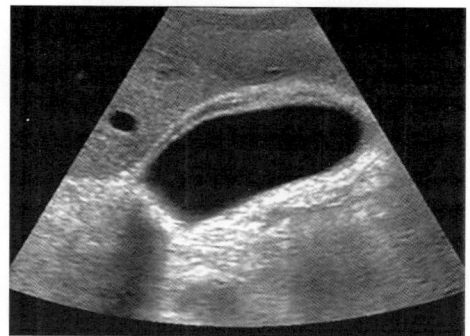

a. Acute calculus cholecystitis
b. Chronic cholecystitis
c. Acute pancreatitis
d. Cholelithiasis

77. A 6-year-old boy has been complaining of ignoring to see the objects on the side of examination. His IQ is normal. His visual acuity is diminished. The radiological image of this patient is shown below. What is the most likely diagnosis?

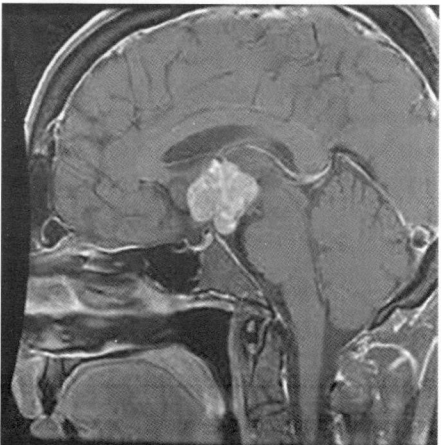

a. Astrocytoma
b. Pituitary adenoma
c. Meningioma
d. Craniopharyngioma

78. Which artery has been shown in the following CT angiographic image?

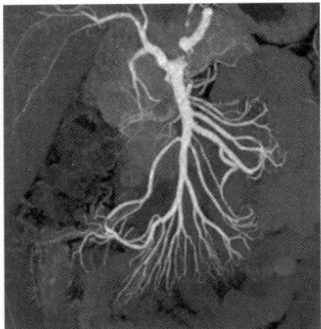

   a. Superior mesenteric artery
   b. Inferior mesenteric artery
   c. Splenic artery
   d. Coeliac artery

79. Identify the structure marked in the given image:

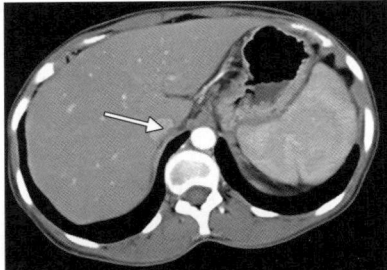

   a. IVC   b. SVC
   c. Thoracic duct
   d. Aorta

80. What is the most likely diagnosis?

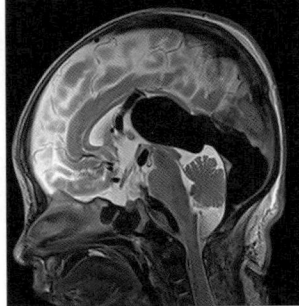

   a. Dandy-Walker malformation
   b. Arnold-Chiari malformation
   c. VHL syndrome
   d. Vein of Galen malformation

81. What is the diagnosis of the image shown below?

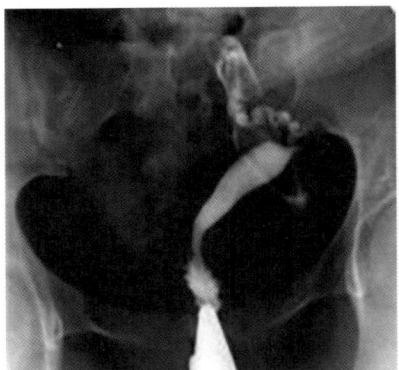

   a. Unicornuate uterus
   b. Uterus didelphys
   c. Bicornuate uterus
   d. Septate uterus

82. A patient has undergone some procedure and after the procedure, following radiograph was obtained. What is the most likely performed procedure?

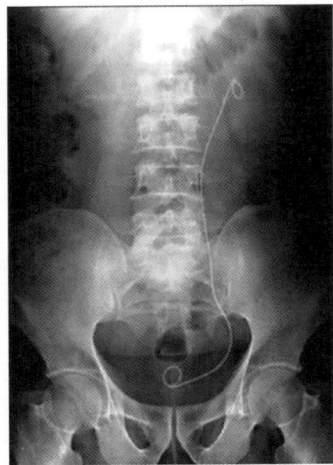

   a. ESWL for renal stone removal
   b. ERCP for biliary stone removal
   c. ESWL for bladder stone removal
   d. Urethral stone removal

83. A patient presented with features of obstructive uropathy. Plain X-ray of the pelvis was obtained and shown below. What is the most likely diagnosis?

Image-Based Questions | 305

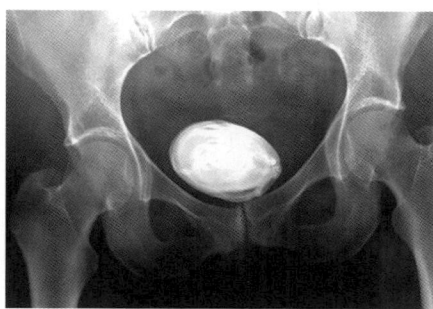

a. Bladder calculus
b. Urethral stricture
c. Benign hypertrophy of prostate
d. Posterior urethral valve

84. A patient presented in the emergency department after head trauma. NCCT was advised. What is the diagnosis?

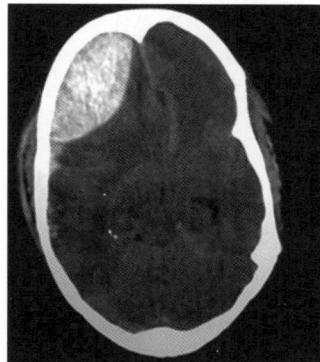

a. Acute EDH
b. Hyperacute EDH
c. Chronic EDH
d. Subacute EDH

85. What is the diagnosis of the image given below?

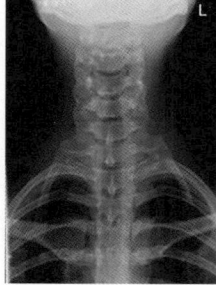

a. Cervical rib
b. Spondylolisthesis C5 over C6
c. Fracture left 2nd rib
d. Costochondritis

86. Which investigation is shown in the given image below?

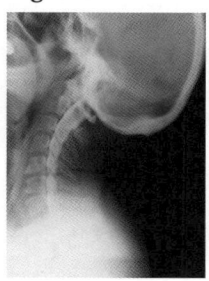

a. Myelography
b. Angiography
c. Neurography
d. Fluoroscopy

87. What is the management of this patient who came to emergency with following CT image?

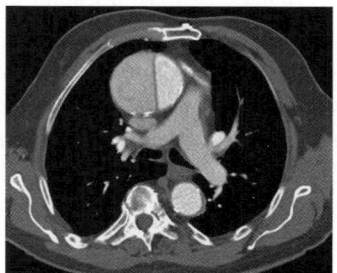

a. TPA
b. Warfarin
c. LMW heparin
d. Immediate surgery

88. Identify the marked structure in figure.

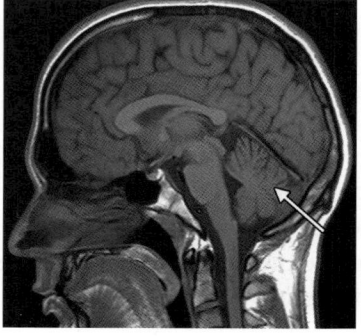

a. Cerebellum
b. Cerebrum
c. Brain stem
d. Corpus callosum

89. Identify the marked structure in figure.

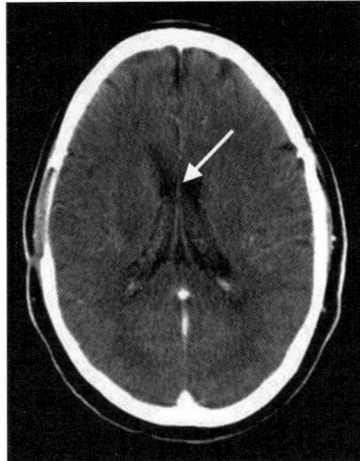

a. Fornix   b. Pineal gland
c. Pituitary   d. Insula

90. A 65-year-old diabetic and hypertensive patient presented with hemiparesis, CT image was shown in figure. What is the diagnosis?

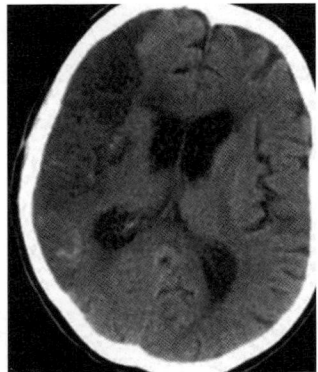

a. Ischemia
b. SAH
c. Intracerebral bleed
d. Glioma

91. NCCT of paranasal sinus was shown in the image. What is the name of the sign shown?

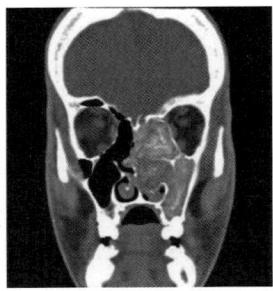

a. Honeycombing
b. Ground glass
c. Onion peel
d. Double density sign

92. Identify the name of the investigation shown in figure?

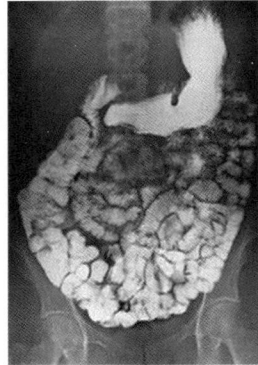

a. BAMFT   b. Ba swallow
c. Loopogram d. Ba enema

93. Chest X-ray of patient with low grade fever is shown in figure.

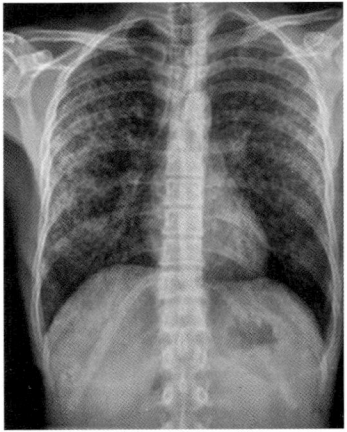

a. Miliary TB
   b. ILD
   c. Bronchopneumonia
   d. Consolidation
94. A patient came to emergency department with some complaints and radiograph shown in figure. What is the definitive treatment of the condition given below?

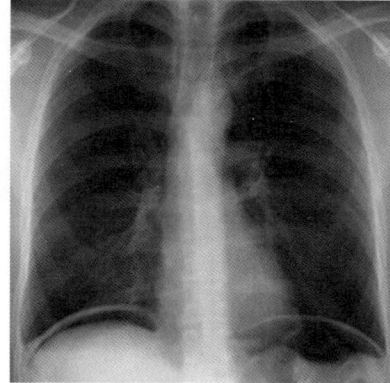

   a. Laparotomy
   b. Intubation
   c. Gastric lavage
   d. Chest tube insertion
95. CT head in figure is showing:

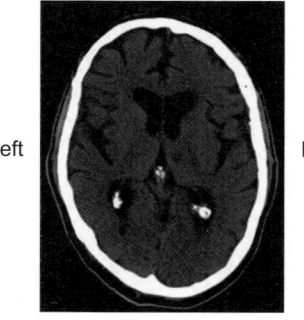

   a. Right lacunar infarct
   b. Left basal ganglia bleed
   c. Normal
   d. Intraventricular bleed
96. A patient who is a known case of acute pancreatitis develops breathlessness, bilateral basal crepitation on day 4 and chest radiograph was shown in figure. Diagnosis?

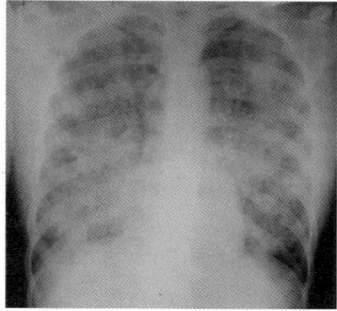

   a. Bilateral pneumonia
   b. ARDS
   c. Carcinogenic PE
   d. Collapse
97. What is the diagnosis of IVP image shown in figure?

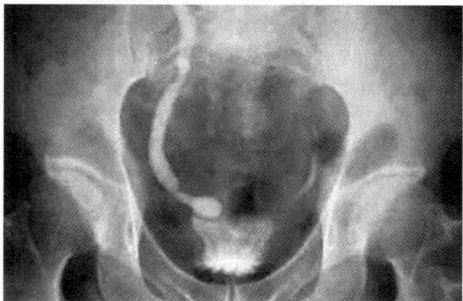

   a. Ureterocele
   b. VUR
   c. TB
   d. Ureteric calculus
98. What is the most likely diagnosis of this 65-year-old lady with backache and following radiograph of the spine shown in figure

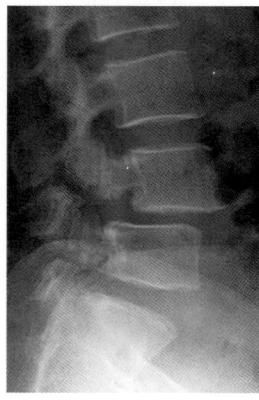

a. Osteoporosis
b. Spondylolisthesis
c. Spondylolysis
d. Discitis

99. Choose the incorrect statement about the following image in figure?

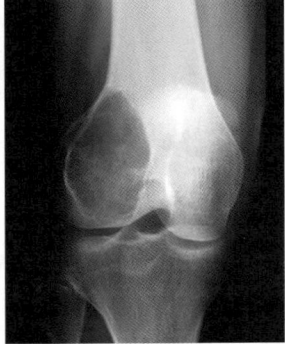

a. Tumour has distinct margins
b. Tumour arise from epiphyseal to metaphyseal region
c. Chemotherapy is the treatment of choice
d. The lesion is eccentric

100. A patient presented with history of diplopia and restricted eye movements. A CT image is given in image.

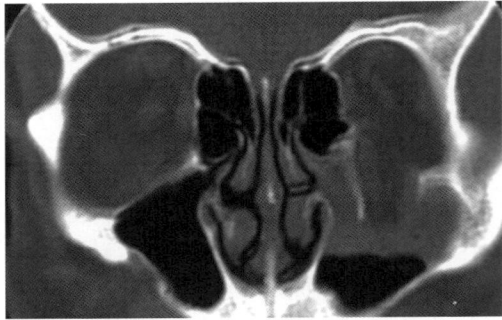

a. Le-Fort fracture
b. Fracture maxilla
c. Fracture zygomatic bone
d. Blow out fracture

ANSWERS

1. a	2. b	3. c	4. c	5. d	6. b	7. b
8. b	9. a	10. b	11. c	12. d	13. b	14. b.
15. c.	16. c.	17. c.	18. c.	19. d.	20. a.	21. d.
22. a.	23. b.	24. c.	25. d.	26. c.	27. c.	28. d.
29. c.	30. b.	31. d.	32. a.	33. b.	34. b.	35. c.
36. b.	37. d.	38. c.	39. c.	40. d.	41. a.	42. c.
43. d.	44. a.	45. b.	46. c.	47. d.	48. c.	49. b.
50. d.	51. a.	52. b.	53. c.	54. a.	55. a.	56. a.
57. c.	58. a.	59. c.	60. c.	61. d.	62. b.	63. c.
64. a.	65. b.					

ANSWERS OF RECENTLY ASKED IBQ

66. c.	67. b.	68. d.	69. a.	70. a.	71. a.	72. a.
73. a.	74. a.	75. b.	76. a.	77. d.	78. a.	79. a.
80. d.	81. a.	82. a.	83. a.	84. a.	85. a.	86. a.
87. d.	88. a.	89. a.	90. a.	91. d.	92. a.	93. a.
94. a.	95. a.	96. b.	97. a.	98. b.	99. c.	100. d.

AIIMS New Pattern Questions

Type 1

Multiple True and False (Each question shall have a stem followed by five alternatives/statements and every alternative/statement will have to be marked as either true or false)

1. The following statements are true/ false regarding a X-ray tube:
   a. Anode is a positively charged end of tube
   b. Speed of moving electrons in X-ray tube is half the speed of light
   c. Focusing cup is a part of anode
   d. Stationary anode is a more efficient type of anode
   e. Target window in mammography is made up of thin glass

2. The following statements are true/false regarding Radiation Units
   a. Conventional unit of exposure dose is Roentgen
   b. One unit of Roentgen= Rem= Rad
   c. Effective dose is related to type of radiation effecting the dose delivered
   d. 1 Gray = 100 Rad
   e. Effect of radiation on human being is damage to DNA by free radicals

3. The following statements are true/ alse regarding investigation of choices in trauma:
   a. NCCT head is IOC in suspected intracranial bleed
   b. MRI is the best modality to pick microhemorrhages after trauma
   c. MRI is the best investigation to detect small pneumothorax
   d. USG is the best way to pick minimal free fluid in abdomen in an attempt to detect suspected solid organ injury after trauma.

4. The following statements are true/false regarding MRI appearance of Meningioma
   a. CSF cleft on T2W images
   b. Areas of signal loss can be seen on Gradient sequences
   c. Hyperintense to grey matter on all pulse sequences
   d. Avascular lesion on contrast studies

5. The following statements are true/false regarding Left atrial enlargement:
   a. Earliest sign is indentation on esophagus
   b. Earliest sign on chest X-ray is elevation of left main bronchus
   c. Straightening of right heart border
   d. Double atrial shadow

6. The following statements are true/false about diagnosis of pneumoperitoneum:
   a. Best investigation is NCCT abdomen
   b. Best abdominal X-ray to detect free air is left lateral decubitus
   c. Erect abdominal X-ray is more sensitive than PA chest X-ray
   d. Rigler's sign on X-ray is pathognomonic of pneumoperitoneum

7. The following statements are true/false about hip tuberculosis:
   a. Wandering acetabulum
   b. Triple deformity
   c. Bird's beak appearance of femur
   d. Mortar and pestle appearance

8. The following statements are true/false about type of radiations:
   a. Beta rays is a type of particulate radiation
   b. Alpha rays are non-ionizing radiation
   c. UV rays are ionizing rays
   d. Microwaves are non-ionizing rays

9. The following statements are true / false regarding MRI signal patterns:
   a. Air is black on T1W images
   b. Fat is bright on both T1 and T2w images
   c. Gadolinium (MRI contrast agent) is bright on T2W images
   d. Ligaments are bright on T2W images

10. The following statements are true / false regarding unilateral translucent hemithorax:
    a. MacLeod's syndrome/ Swayer James syndrome is a neoplastic cause of lucent hemithorax
    b. Most common cause is rotation
    c. Pneumonectomy is a iatrogenic cause of lucent hemithorax
    d. Poland's syndrome is a cause of lucent hemithorax due to absent pectoralis major muscle

Type 2

Match the following type questions (Each question shall have two columns with four items in one column (A) that need to be matched appropriately with the best alternative available in the next column (B))

1. Match the column A with the best possible use in column B

Column A		Column B
1. Filter	a.	Beam restricting device to reduce scatter radiation
2. Grid	b.	Better heat tolerant capacity
3. Collimator	c.	Blocks low energy radiation
4. Rotatory anode	d.	Block high energy radiation
	e.	Blocks scatter radiation to improve image quality

2. Match the column A with the best possible further action plan

Column A		Column B
1. BIRADS- 1	a.	Biopsy
2. BIRADS-3	b.	Continue routine screening
3. BIRADS- 5	c.	Complete/ repeat the study
4. BIRADS-6	d.	Short follow up
	e.	To look for disease in contralateral breast as well as multicentric disease in same breast

3. Match the columns for MRI sequence in column A with their best indications

Column A		Column B
1. FLAIR	a.	Ischemic stroke
2. TOF	b.	To detect fatty lesions in brain
3. Diffusion weighted MRI	c.	Screening for Multiple sclerosis
4. Spectroscopy	d.	Chemical composition of a lesion
	e.	Angiography

4. Match the columns for types of CT with the pathologies in chest:

Column A		Column B
1. NCCT	a.	Interstitial lung disease
2. CECT	b.	Nodal and bone metastasis
3. HRCT	c.	Pneumothorax
4. PET CT	d.	Brachial plexus involvement by cancer
	e.	Lung malignancy

5. Match the columns:

Column A		Column B
1. Tetralogy of Fallot	a.	Box shaped heart
2. Transposition of great arteries	b.	Boot shape heart
3. Ebstein's anomaly	c.	Figure of "8" or Snowman's heart
4. Total anomalous pulmonary venous return	d.	Sitting goose sign
	e.	Egg on side

6. Match the columns:

Column A		Column B
1. Cork screw esophagus	a.	Diverticulosis
2. Claw sign	b.	Posterior urethral valve
3. Drooping Lilly sign	c.	Diffuse esophageal spasm
4. Key hole appearance	d.	Intussusception
	e.	Duplicated excretory system

7. Match the columns:

Column A	Column B
1. Telescoping of bones/fingers	a. Psoriatic deformity
2. Bamboo spine	b. Osteoarthritis
3. Pencil in cup deformity	c. Rheumatoid arthritis
4. Sea gull sign	d. Pseudogout
	e. Ankylosing Spondylitis

8. Match the columns:

Column A	Column B
1. Exposure dose	a. Radiation quality factor × absorbed dose
2. Absorbed dose	b. Radiation necessary to liberate 0.000258C/KG of charge
3. Equivalent dose	c. Equivalent dose × tissue weighing factor
4. Effective dose	d. 100ergs of energy per gram of material
	e. Radioactivity

9. Match the column: Half-life (Column B) of compounds in column A:

Column A	Column B
1. I-123	a. 5.26 years
2. I-131	b. 6 hours
3. Tc-99	c. 13.2 hours
4. Co-60	d. 8 days
	e. 14 days

10. Match the columns:

Column A	Column B
1. Lung hydatid	a. Pneumatocele
2. Resolving staphylococcal pneumonia	b. Golden 'S' Sign
3. Centrally obstructing mass in right upper lobe	c. Water Lilly sign on CT
4. Asbestosis	d. Crazy paving
	e. Round atelectasis

Type 3

Sequential arrangement type (Each question shall have a list of items that need to be arranged sequentially or in order as indicated)

1. Please arrange the following imaging modalities in decreasing order of radiation dose
   a. CT chest   b. Abdomen X-ray
   c. Chest X-ray   d. Bone scan

2. Arrange the following in increasing order of Hounsfield attenuation values
   a. Fat   b. Water
   c. Air   d. Muscles

3. Arrange the following in increasing order of Pathologic stages of Neurocysticercosis
   a. Nodular calcified
   b. Colloid vesicular
   c. Granular nodular
   d. Vesicular stage

4. Arrange the following in spatial order of findings noted on chest x-ray in case of left heart failure: first being the earliest finding seen:
   a. Interstitial thickening with Kerley B lines
   b. Equalization of blood flow in both upper and lower lobes
   c. Frank pulmonary edema
   d. Upper lobe diversion of blood flow with reverse moustache sign

5. Arrange the following antenatal USG visits in sequential order as offered by an obstetrician first being the earliest indication to visit radiology department:
   a. Confirmation of pregnancy
   b. IUGR scan
   c. Nuchal thickness
   d. Anomaly scan

6. Arrange the following bone malignancies in order of increasing prevalence with age:
   a. Giant cell tumor   b. Neuroblastoma
   c. Osteosarcoma   d. Metastasis

7. Arrange the following in increasing order of radiation sensitivity: First being least sensitive, and last being most sensitive:
   a. Gonads
   b. Bone marrow
   c. Cortical bone
   d. Central nervous system

8. Arrange the following in increasing order of radiation quality factor: First being least and last being most ionizing:
   a. Visible rays   b. Alpha rays
   c. X-rays   d. Neutrons

9. Arrange the following barium studies used for various body parts in order of anatomical position of these structures in body proximal to distally: Barium study used for proximal structures being first and barium study used for most distal part should come last:
   a. Barium enema
   b. Barium meal
   c. Barium swallow
   d. Barium meal follow through

10. Arrange the stages of lung sarcoidosis in increasing order with stage 1 being the first and stage 4 the last depending on CT chest findings:
    a. Lymph node and parenchymal changes
    b. Fibrotic parenchymal changes
    c. Only parenchymal changes (peribronchovascular nodules)
    d. Hilar and mediastinal nodes only

Type 4
Multiple Completion

Each question/statement shall have four alternatives/statements of which one or more may be correct and need to be marked using the following key:
1. if a, b and c are correct
2. If a and c are correct
3. If b and d are correct
4. If all four (a, b, c and d) are correct

1. Characteristic features of a mammography X-ray tube includes:
   a. Window is made up of Beryllium
   b. Uses low voltage as compared to Chest X-ray
   c. Requires average four X-ray exposures for a standard screening mammogram
   d. Tungsten is the preferred material used for Target

2. Characteristics of a Dual source CT:
   a. Useful to scan at any heart rates without using beta blockers
   b. Uses two X-ray tubes operating at same potential (Kv)
   c. Can characterize type of kidney stones
   d. Dual source stands for acquisition on two CT scanners separately

3. Causes of ring enhancing lesions on contrast enhanced MRI of brain:
   a. Metastasis
   b. Abscess
   c. High grade glioma
   d. Radiation necrosis

4. Normal hilar shadow on a Chest x-ray comprised of:
   a. Lymph node
   b. Pulmonary arteries
   c. Bronchus
   d. Pulmonary veins

5. About hypertrophic pyloric stenosis:
   a. String sign on barium study is a specific sign
   b. Child presents with vomiting in 3rd week of life
   c. Investigation of choice is USG
   d. It is generally seen in first born female child

6. About periosteal thickenings on X-ray:
   a. Multilamellated/ Onion peel appearance could represent Ewing's sarcoma
   b. Sunburst pattern of calcification is seen in chondrosarcoma
   c. Hair on end pattern could relate to Thalassemia
   d. Osteoid osteoma show discontinuous periosteal reaction

7. About teleradiotherapy:
   a. Commonly used sources for teletherapy are Co-60 and Cs-137
   b. Linear accelerators are probably best source for this technique
   c. X-rays are the most common type of radiation source
   d. Electron beam is used for superficial lesions

8. About effects of radiation
   a. Deterministic effect are dose dependent
   b. Dose threshold exists with stochastic effects
   c. Stochastic effects are responsible for teratogenicity
   d. Disease severity is not dose dependent in deterministic effects

9. About Stroke:
   a. First investigation to be performed in suspected stroke is NCCT head
   b. Investigation of choice for diagnosis of ischemic stroke is MRI
   c. Investigation of choice for diagnosis of hemorrhagic stroke is NCCT head
   d. First investigation in suspected stroke is MRI

10. About pulmonary embolism
    a. Commonest Chest X-ray finding is a normal chest X-ray
    b. Westermark's sign (Focal oligemia) is most specific chest X-ray FInding
    c. Screening investigation of choice is blood D-Dimer level
    d. CT pulmonary angiogram is most useful for diagnosis

Type 5
Reason Assertion

Each question shall have two statements: Assertion (A) and Reason (B) connected by the term "because". The appropriate answer should be marked using the key:

1. Both Assertion and Reason are independently true/correct statements and the Reason is the correct explanation for the Assertion
2. Both Assertion and Reason are independently true/correct statements, but the Reason is not the correct explanation for the Assertion
3. Assertion is independently a false/incorrect statement and the Reason is independently true/ correct statement.
4. Both Assertion and reason are independently a false/incorrect statements

1. a. We increase voltage of X-ray tube to get better contrast in an obese patient
   b. Contrast of an X-ray film is dependent on voltage of X-ray tube
2. a. MRI is safe in patients with IUCD
   b. IUCD is a non-paramagnetic metallic foreign body
3. a. No perilesional edema is seen in vesicular stage of Neurocysticercosis
   b. No inflammatory host reaction (Perilesional edema) seen, when parasite is alive
4. a. CECT is investigation of choice for most of the lung and mediastinal malignancies
   b. Endoscopic ultrasound is investigation of choice for staging of early esophageal cancer
5. a. Miliary pattern of TB on chest X-ray is a result of hematogenous spread of TB
   b. Tree in bud pattern on chest X-ray is a result of endobronchial spread of TB
6. a. Inferior rib notching is seen in coarctation of aorta
   b. Prominent collateral vessels and nerve bundles run along inferior border of rib
7. a Intraoperative radiotherapy is a type of teletherapy used intraoperatively
   b. Intraoperative RT mainly uses electron beam to make margins tumor free
8. a. Power Doppler is most sensitive investigation to diagnose torsion of testis
   b. Power doppler can detect slightest possible blood flow irrespective of angle of insonation
9. a. Previous allergy to iodine is absolute contraindication for I/V contrast studies
   b. Anaphylactic reactions are due to iodine component of CT contrast agents
10. a. Investigation of choice for necrotic acute pancreatitis is CECT abdomen
    b. Investigation of choice for chronic pancreatitis is EUS

Type 6
Extended matching items/Questions (EMI/ EMQ)

Each EMI/ EMQ will broadly have the following components:
- Theme and focus
- Answer option list
- Lead in question
- Scenarios and vignettes

There will be two or more scenario/Vignette related to the overall theme and focus of the question

For each of the following patients as described in the scenarios below, identify the cause from the above answer option list

1. **Theme and focus**
   Non-Ionizing imaging modalities
   a. MRI
   b. Ultrasound
   c. MRCP
   d. Doppler study
   e. Endoscopic ultrasound

   Lead in question
   For each of the following patients as described in the scenarios below, identify the best imaging modality from the above answer option list

   Case 1
   A 10-year-old child came to emergency department with acute pain in right iliac fossa with vomiting. What should be the first investigation to be done from the above list?

   Case 2
   A young athlete comes to sudden onset pain in scrotum with redness and swelling in overlying skin. The doctor in ED is not sure about the diagnosis. What should be the best investigation in the given scenario?

2. **Theme and focus**
   MRI sequences
   a. FLAIR (Fluid attenuated inversion recovery sequence)
   b. DWI (Diffusion weighted sequences)
   c. Spectroscopy
   d. TOF (Time of flight)
   e. SWI: Susceptibility weighted imaging (Gradient imaging)

   Lead in question
   For each of the following patients as described in the scenarios below, identify the best MRI sequence from the above answer option list

   Case 1
   A patient presented with acute onset right hemiplegia and loss of consciousness. The sequence of events are 20 minutes old. Which of the following MRI sequence is investigation of choice for this patient?

   Case 2
   A patient presented with thunderclap headache 3 days ago after a trivial trauma, however, is stable now. Clinician in OPD wants to rule out SAH. Which of the above mentioned MRI sequence is most sensitive in the above scenario?

3. **Theme and focus**
   Pathological calcifications in brain
   a. Periventricular calcification
   b. Sub ependymal calcification
   c. Tram track pattern of gyri calcification
   d. Bracket calcification
   e. Starry sky pattern of calcification

   Lead in question
   For each of the following patients as described in the scenarios below, identify the best calcification pattern appropriate for the case from the above answer option list

   Case 1
   A pregnant lady with TORCH group of infections delivered a baby with microcephaly, who eventually developed seizures. Which of the following calcification pattern is expected in this child's NCCT brain scan?

   Case 2
   A child presented with a pink rash on forehead and seizure. On further investigation by NCCT and MRI a diagnosis of Sturge weber syndrome is made. Which of the following calcification pattern is seen in these patients NCCT scan?

4. **Theme and focus**
   Opaque hemithorax
   a. Massive pleural effusion
   b. Lobar consolidation
   c. Lung collapse
   d. Mesothelioma
   e. Pneumonectomy

   Lead in question
   For each of the following patients as described in the scenarios below, identify the best possible cause for the case from the above answer option list

   Case 1
   An elderly visited medicine OPD for shortness of breath and fever for 1 week. The chest X-ray of the patient revealed left opaque hemithorax, however, there is no associated mediastinal shift. What is the most possible diagnosis from the above list?

   Case 2
   Chest X-ray of a patient revealed right complete opaque hemithorax with contralateral mediastinal shift. What is the most possible diagnosis from the above list?

5. **Theme and focus**
   Urinary tract pathologies
   a. Renal Tuberculosis
   b. Cystic disease of kidney
   c. Horseshoe kidney
   d. Duplicated renal pelvicalyceal system
   e. Ureterocele

   Lead in question
   For each of the following patients as described in the scenarios below, identify the best possible cause for the case from the above answer option list

   Case 1
   An adult presents in the surgery OPD with right renal fossa pain, increase in urinary frequency and low grade fever for 4 weeks. Clinician recommended IVP, which revealed Feathery outline of pelvicalyceal system of right kidney. What is the most probable pathology?

   Case 2
   A patient visited hospital for suspected ureteric colic. IVP was suggested to look for number and positions of calculi and rule out any obstruction. IVP revealed 2 calculi on right and 1 calculus in left kidney with mild hydronephrosis on right side. On excretory phase of IVU the lower pole calyces of both kidneys appear to project medially. What is the most appropriate diagnosis from the above list?

6. **Theme and focus**
   Bone pain
   a. Stress fracture
   b. Osteosarcoma
   c. Osteomyelitis
   d. AVN of hip
   e. Tuberculosis of hip

   Lead in question
   For each of the following patients as described in the scenarios below, identify the best possible cause for the case from the above answer option list

   Case 1
   An old lady presented in orthopedic OPD with diffuse low back pain and pelvic pain slightly worse on right than left. On seeing diffuse marrow edema in sacrum Bone scan was suggested to rule out other areas of bone involvement. However, bone scan revealed only "H" shaped uptake in the sacrum with normal appearance of rest of the bones. What is the most appropriate diagnosis from the above list of pathologies?

   Case 2
   A young athlete has been taking anabolic steroids to increase his sports performance for 6 months. Recently for last 2weeks, he has developed pain in right hip. MRI revealed double line sign on T2W images in head of right femur. What is the most appropriate diagnosis?

7. **Theme and focus**
   Tele radiotherapy agents
   a. X-rays
   b. Beta rays

c. Gamma rays
d. Proton beam
e. Alpha rays

Lead in question
For each of the following patients as described in the scenarios below, identify the best possible radiation beam required for treatment for the case from the above answer option list

Case 1
A patient with known locally advanced rectal cancer and distant metastasis was being discussed in Multidisciplinary team meeting (MDT) for management. It was suggested that long course chemoradiotherapy should be given for palliative care. What should be the most effective way of clearing the tumor burden from the above choices?

Case 2
A surgeon operating on a breast cancer patient after excision of tumor decides to offer her radiotherapy during surgery to improve her chances of having tumor free margins and long term survival. What should be the most appropriate choice of radiation for her?

8. **Theme and focus**
   Ultrasound applications
   a. Elastography
   b. Spectral wave patterns
   c. A mode USG
   d. B mode USG
   e. M mode USG
   f. Blood flow velocity
   g. Direction of flow

Lead in question
For each of the following patients as described in the scenarios below, identify the best possible USG application most suitable for the case from the above answer option list:

Case 1
An alcoholic patient is attending gastroenterology clinics for deranged LFTs with raised ALP and AST. No significant abnormality detected on routine B mode USG, however, clinician is suspecting underlying cirrhosis and does not want to go for any invasive procedures like liver biopsy to start with. Which from the above list would be best non-invasive method to detect liver fibrosis?

Case 2
A patient on annual follow up CECT chest and abdomen post Whipple's for pancreatic cancer found to have a small hypodense non-enhancing lesion in liver. The lesion is equivocal for metastasis with possible differential of benign simple cyst in liver. Which from the above list would be most helpful to decide if the lesion is solid or cystic?

9. **Theme and focus**
   MRI spectroscopy metabolites
   a. Creatine
   b. Choline
   c. Lipid and lactate
   d. Lactate
   e. N-Acetyl aspartate

Lead in question
For each of the following patients as described in the scenarios below, identify the best possible spectroscopy metabolite peak most suitable for the case from the above answer option list:

Case 1
A 4-month-old child is presented with poor motor development with abnormal muscle tone, feeding difficulty and blindness. The child has an abnormally large, poorly controlled head. MRI brain reveals diffuse white matter changes in keeping with Canavan's disease. Which of the following metabolite peak is expected in spectroscopic study of brain of this child?

Case 2
A 67-year-old man presented with headache and left sided weakness for 3 weeks. MRI reveals a large rim enhancing mass in right parietal lobe with perilesional edema. The differentials for lesion are abscess, high grade glioma and tuberculoma. Which of the metabolite peak from the above list would be diagnostic of glioma?

10. **Theme and focus**
    Dysphagia
    a. Achalasia cardia
    b. Peptic stricture
    c. Diffuse esophageal spasm
    d. Esophageal malignancy
    e. Dysphagia lusoria
    f. Systemic sclerosis

    Lead in question
    For each of the following patients as described in the scenarios below, identify the best possible spectroscopy metabolite peak most suitable for the case from the above answer option list:

    Case 1
    A 57-year-old lady with chronic history of acid peptic disorder presented with nonprogressive dysphagia. The dysphagia is more to solids than liquids. Barium study reveals stricture in distal esophagus with irregular mucosal outline. What is the most appropriate diagnosis from the above list for this patient?

    Case 2
    A patient presented with dysphagia and found to have external indentation on upper esophagus on barium studies. CECT chest reveals Aberrant right subclavian artery. What is the diagnosis of this case from the above list?

AIIMS New Pattern Answers

Type 1

Multiple True and False (Each question shall have a stem followed by five alternatives/statements and every alternative/statement will have to be marked as either true or false)

1. **Ans.** T, T, F, F, F
2. **Ans.** T, T, F, T,T
3. **Ans.** T, T, F, T
4. **Ans.** T, T, F, F
5. **Ans.** T, T, F, T
6. **Ans.** T, T, F, T
7. **Ans.** T, F, T, T
8. **Ans.** T, F, F, T
9. **Ans.** T, T, F, F
10. **Ans.** F, T, F, T

Type 2

Match the following type questions (Each question shall have two columns with four items in one column (A) that need to be matched appropriately with the best alternative available in the next column (B))

1. **Ans.** 1-c, 2-e, 3-a, 4-b
2. **Ans.** 1-b, 2-d, 3-a, 4-e
3. **Ans.** 1-c, 2-e, 3-a, 4-d
4. **Ans.** 1-c, 2-e, 3-a, 4-b
5. **Ans.** 1-b, 2-e, 3-a, 4-c
6. **Ans.** 1-c, 2-d, 3-e, 4-b
7. **Ans.** 1-c, 2-e, 3-a, 4-b
8. **Ans.** 1-b, 2-d, 3-a, 4-c
9. **Ans.** 1-c, 2-d, 3-b, 4-a
10. **Ans.** 1-c, 2-a, 3-b, 4-e

Type 3

Sequential arrangement type (Each question shall have a list of items that need to be arranged sequentially or in order as indicated)

1. **Ans.** a>d>b>c
2. **Ans.** c>a>b>d
3. **Ans.** d>b>c>a
4. **Ans.** b>d>a>c
5. **Ans.** a>c>d>b
6. **Ans.** b>c>a>d
7. **Ans.** c>d>a>b
8. **Ans.** a>c>d>b
9. **Ans.** c>b>d>a
10. **Ans.** d>a>c>b

Multiple Completion Type 4

Each question/statement shall have four alternatives/statements of which one or more may be correct and need to be marked using the following key:

1. If a, b and c are correct
2. If a and c are correct
3. If b and d are correct
4. If all four (a, b, c and d) are correct

1. **Ans.** 1
2. **Ans.** 2
3. **Ans.** 4
4. **Ans.** 3
5. **Ans.** 1
6. **Ans.** 2
7. **Ans.** 4
8. **Ans.** 2
9. **Ans.** 1
10. **Ans.** 4

Reason Assertion Type 5

Each question shall have two statements: Assertion(A) and Reason (B) connected by the term "because". The appropriate answer should be marked using the key:

1. Both Assertion and Reason are independently true/correct statements and the Reason is the correct explanation for the Assertion
2. Both Assertion and Reason are independently true/correct statements, but the Reason is not the correct explanation for the Assertion
3. Assertion is independently a false/incorrect statement and the Reason is independently true/ correct statement.
4. Both Assertion and reason are independently a false/incorrect statements

1. Ans. 3
2. Ans. 1
3. Ans. 1
4. Ans. 2
5. Ans. 2
6. Ans. 1
7. Ans. 2
8. Ans. 1
9. Ans. 1
10. Ans. 2

Type 6

Extended matching items/Questions (EMI/EMQ)

Each EMI/ EMQ will broadly have the following components:
- Theme and focus
- Answer option list
- Lead in question
- Scenarios and vignettes

There will be two or more scenario/ Vignette related to the overall theme and focus of the question

For each of the following patients as described in the scenarios below, identify the cause from the above answer option list

1. Ans Case 1. b
   Ans Case 2. d
2. Ans Case 1. b
   Ans Case 2. e
3. Ans Case 1. a
   Ans Case 2. c
4. Ans Case 1. b
   Ans Case 2. a
5. Ans Case 1. a
   Ans Case 2. c
6. Ans Case 1. a
   Ans Case 2. d
7. Ans Case 1. d
   Ans Case 2. b
8. Ans Case 1. a
   Ans Case 2. d
9. Ans Case 1. e
   Ans Case 2. b
10. Ans Case 1. b
    Ans Case 2. e